Cardiac Dilemma: Navigating Your Heart Disease for Positive Results

Marc L. Platt M.D.

www.marcplattauthor.com

The world of your heart is full of wondrous properties that will fascinate your imagination. These properties make the heart the most exciting organ in your body. It takes years to train a cardiologist or an electrophysiologist (specialist in heart rhythms) with the tools and knowledge to care for patients in the hope of curing the multitude of diseases and maladies of the heart. The aim of this book is to teach the workings and treatments of these ailments.

First, we'll delve into the world of insurance and Medicare as an introduction to some of the complexities of medical reimbursement. This will prepare you for the discussion of all the disorders of the heart and what patients, as consumers of medical care, should expect in terms of how to structure their care and what to expect of the doctors and the insurance carrier.

Next, we'll exhaustively review the history of cardiac medicine interspersed with analogies to modern medicine. Armed with this basic knowledge, we'll learn about the cells that comprise the heart, the mechanics of heart function, and the electrical circuits that control all the repetitive functions of the cardiac system. We will further examine the intriguing and complex interactions of the heart with other body organs, including their malfunctions on a cell-to-cell as well as to a larger, whole-body perspective.

The rest of the book will be a detailed review of all the diseases of the heart, their history, and recent developments. Simultaneously, I will cover the complexities of medical reimbursement for your heart care and how to take control of your medical expenses specifically for each of these diseases.

My main goal is to transform you into experts, who can manipulate through the medical mass of knowledge and the options for cardiac interventions and cures. It is my fervent hope that this book will kindle and instill within you the excitement afforded by knowledge and understanding upon finishing it. Ultimately, you'll be able to make effective and informed decisions should you or someone you know be struck by disease.

      The basic premise is to educate people to be proactive in their own care as the patient is the best advocate who can also produce positive results. In the parlance of medicine, this is called positive outcomes where your disease is managed for hopeful cure as well as reimbursement and deductibles which benefit you financially. So, join me as I open the door to the timeless universe that makes up the heart. Let's enter and navigate through the realm and totality of your heart.

Contents

Chapter 1: Navigating The Maze Of Medical Insurance	9
Chapter 2: The Heart In Early History	31
Cro-Magnon	31
Egyptians	32
Chinese	36
Greeks And Romans	41
Modern Era Of The Americans And Europe	52
Renaissance	57
The Beginning Of Modern Medicine	66
Modern Cardiology	70
Historical View Of Cardiac Electophysiology	80
Heart Disease-More On The Arteries And Muscle	103
Cardiac Catheterization	119
Coronary Catheterization Procedure	124
Indications	125
Technique Of Coronary Catheterization	131
Procedure	139
Stent	146
Complete Total Occlusion	148
Hospitalization For Angina Pectoris And Myocardial Infarction	149
Coronary Artery Bypass Surgery (CABG)	153
History Of CABG	157
Electrophysiology	158
Artificial Pacemakers	164

Automatic Impantable Cadiac Defibrillator (AICD Or ICD)	182
Sudden Cardiac Arrest (SCA Or Sudden Cardiac Death)	182
AICD History	185
Newer ICD Technology	190
Contraindications For An Icd Implant; When Not To Implant	198
Invasive Electrophysiological Testing And Syndromes Of SCD	203
Long QT Syndrome (LQTS)	204
Torsades De Pointes	207
Arrythmogenic Right Ventriclar Dysplasia	210
Left Ventricular Hypertrophy; Hypertrophic Cardiomyopathy	213
Brugada And Early Repolarization Syndromes	216
Catecholiminergic Ventricular Tachycardia	220
Sick Sinus Syndrome, Tachycardia-Bradycardia Syndrome, Paroxysmal Supraventricular Tachycardia (PSVT), And Atrial Fibrillation.	220
Paroxysmal Supraventricular Tachycardia (PSVT):	225
Radiofrequency Ablation	235
Indications For Radiofrequency Ablation	237
Complications Of Ablation	240
Atrial Fibrillation Ablation.	242
Ablation For Atrial Flutter	249
Ablation For Ventricular Tachycardia (VT)	250
Ablation Of Non Scar Related Ventricular Tachcardias	255
Ablation For Polymorphic VT And Ventricular Tachycardia	255
Insurance Coverage	256
Cardiac Catheterization, Heart Attacks, And Bypass Surgery	259

Coronary Artery Bypass Surgery	264
Peripheral Vascular Disease And Vascular Bypass Surgery	271
Congestive Heart Failure And Cardiomyopathy	283
Cardiomyopathy	295
Valvular Heart Disease	298
Pericarditis And Pericardial Effusion	307
Syncope	311
The Heart And The Mind	323
Conclusion And Summation	332

Chapter 1: Navigating the Maze of Medical Insurance

Before we venture into a discussion of the heart, I feel that it's critical to establish a dialogue regarding medical reimbursement issues for common cardiac procedures and hospital admissions. We start with this section principally because of how important having the exact knowledge of the cardiac procedure or the hospital diagnosis is to you. And ultimately, you need to know how much money will be your responsibility versus reimbursement by Medicare or a private insurer.

Let's face it. Only a firm understanding of your cardiac disease will give you some control over the amount you have to spend on your medical care as well as contributing to better and safer hospital admissions. Armed with this invaluable knowledge, I hope that you can circumvent what I feel is the intentional result by private insurance coverage and under Medicare, which is now under the Affordable Care Act as of 2014 (Obamacare), to specifically create an environment where a much larger proportion of the medical bill both for the hospital and to the doctor comes out of a patient's pocket.

In general, as of 2014 under Obamacare, the amount of money paid by the insurer or Medicare decreased proportionally while the patients' co-payments increased. The private insurance companies are compelled by law to embrace the edict of covering six to seven million newly uninsured people. It's at the expense of canceling (double the number uninsured people) the employed individuals' policies for more expensive and higher deductible policies.

Isn't it exciting to know that if you are a working woman at the age of 60, you're paying for comprehensive insurance that covers pregnancy care? The uninsured are often subsidized to be only given insurance with deductibles up to 20% of their income, which most can't afford to pay. As a result, hospitals are short changed and patients end up in debt. Although it covers for pre-existing conditions, at the same time it only markedly increases the insurance expense and deductibles.

To make matters worse, most patients are totally ignorant of what their procedure or hospitalization entails or what they cost.

Furthermore, the patient is completely unaware if there are extra procedures ordered by the physician that are actually unnecessary, can be done in the less expensive outpatient setting, or can be done in the doctor's office rather than the acute care hospital. Lastly, it's crucial to become empowered, so the patient knows the hospital admission status in terms of being an "inpatient" versus an "outpatient" or "observation" service. This designation has critical implications because you could be saddled with an incredibly large and unexpected medical bill, which you assumed would be covered by your insurance.

Before I proceed with more detailed explanations, I want to briefly clarify the words inpatient admission, outpatient, and observation services. This classification is essentially determined on your presentation to the hospital by your physician. It's even more disturbing that the hospital has no obligation to reveal your admission status unless you absolutely insist or threaten to sue. I feel that this is a direct affront to patient's rights.

This is just one of the insidious ways the system is designed to basically keep the patient uninformed and ignorant of the reality of what is being done during their hospitalization. In this circumstance, it's essential for the patient or the family to simply demand to know if the status is inpatient, outpatient, or observation. It's up to the doctor to spell out to the patient clearly the admission status and the reason for the classification in no uncertain terms or ambiguity.

The patient must insist that the doctor relays this information even if the doctor might be offended. It's truly imperative that after reading about the various forms of cardiac disease, you're properly categorized in the appropriate classification of hospital services.

Now, you're probably wondering what the heck I'm talking about. Well, as I've said before and will continue to repeat in this book, it's a historic change like this that is a deceptive way of sticking a significantly higher proportion of the medical bill to the unsuspecting and ill-informed patient who has no clue of what was being done during their hospitalization. This includes the cost of things being done to you in the hospital whether it was necessary or not.

This is called transparency of care and is the new catchword for the insurance companies. I might add that there are a multitude of new websites to give the consumer (patient) some reasonable insights about their proposed hospitalization or the cost and what the responsibility of the patient would be. Unfortunately, these websites give no clue whatsoever regarding the types of admission: inpatient, outpatient, or observation.

Also, they absolutely don't even attempt to delve into the very contentious issue of what happens if Medicare refuses to pay for the hospital time at all! However, at this time, most of these websites are basically worthless and charge for regurgitating information that is free to a privately covered patient, Medicare enrollee with or without a coinsurance, and patients under every large insurance carrier.

First, let us revisit the concept of inpatient versus outpatient or observation services (status). This is based on what's called the Acute Care Hospital Inpatient Prospective Payment system (IPPS) in which the hospital contracts with Medicare to furnish acute hospital inpatient care and agrees to accept Medicare as payment in full based on the diagnosis or the DRG (diagnosis-related groups). This is the principal diagnosis and possible complications that are assigned for your complete admission. Also, Medicare has the option to review this DRG and make the decision that some or all parts of the DRG are arbitrary and not related to the principal diagnosis. Then they simply don't pay for the service and you may be responsible for the payment.

Now, if you're admitted as an inpatient by the doctor, Medicare Part A pays for the inpatient hospital stay and Medicare Part B pays for the doctor's services during hospitalization. I know it sounds complicated, but it isn't. Most patients have Medicare part A that pays for inpatient hospital services, and some have Medicare part B (or private insurance via your employer) that pays 80% for outpatient and/ or the doctor's charges for rendered hospital services.

The problem arises when the doctor assigns you the wrong status such as observation instead of inpatient. There's absolutely no way the doctor can change that status once you're discharged, and this has a substantial effect on how the hospital is paid. This impacts the amount the patient is obligated to pay. In general, the amount out of your pocket is substantially more if you're observation or outpatient and may not show for up to a year after your discharge as Medicare reviews the merits of the services rendered. This is called an audit, which is a review of the charges and the services under an inappropriately assigned inpatient verses observation or outpatient service.

As of October 2013, it's been made infinitely more complicated by what is called the "two midnight rule". This was implemented to save Medicare a substantial amount of money. Frankly, although this rule seems arbitrary, it's actually revealing the amazing abuses by the physician and some hospitals' incorrect use of admission status. The decision for inpatient hospital admission is a complex medical decision by your doctor's judgment as to the complexity and the anticipated services to be rendered as part of the medically necessary hospital care.

Furthermore, as of October 2013 and now 2015, the doctor must certify or discuss in his chart at the time of or during your inpatient admission that you're expected to need two or more midnights of medically necessary hospital care (benchmark). This requires the doctor's signature and the hospital's formal implementation. This two-midnight certification or documentation is a very complex decision for the doctor, and if the doctor doesn't document correctly or simply sign (even write) the order in the first place, then the admission upon discharge review will be assigned as an observation. Even worse is payment as outpatient status when you were in the ICU with a life threatening condition!

Obviously, this is a catastrophic loss to the hospital in terms of payment as well as the patient now being Medicare Part B outpatient or observation status. So, the patient has the potential of having to pay for a major part of the hospitalization! This situation may seem unacceptable, but unfortunately, this is simply the reality as of 2015. This is further compounded by the fact that many, if not most of the doctors in the United States, have the attitude that all this is beneath them.

They feel that they don't have the time for such bureaucratic nonsense. The problem is that there are incredibly negative consequences for the patient and the hospital. As of October 2015, this problem may be partially alleviated by Medicare rule 541, which was previously opposed by almost every doctor and lobby group in the United States.

Previously, the hospital wasn't paid for the inpatient versus observation or outpatient service, but the doctor was paid. However, with 541, the doctor risks not getting paid for all of his services, and that loss of income might finally compel the physician to take the responsibility to properly classify, document, and sign the inpatient two-midnight order. As far as I am concerned, this rule 541 is the best thing that Medicare has done in the past 20 years for the ultimate benefit of the patient. The real question is that it's questionable whether or not Medicare will enforce what is already on the books.

I'm sure you've noticed that I've been talking mostly about Medicare and not the private insurers or Medicaid. This was on purpose because they've not yet adopted the same limitations and rules. However, if precedent is applied, they will all abide with such rules and follow the lead of Medicare in the near future. For me, the rather revolutionary two-midnight rule and rule 541 are testaments to Medicare because they benefit the patient in the long run as the doctor conforms to the rules. This represents Medicare actually confronting organized medicine when it had the doctor's interests held above that of the patient in the past. This is in contradistinction to the age old adage since antiquity of "do no harm to the patient."

We'll discuss some examples in a moment. There are some websites run by Medicare represented by CMS (Centers for Medicare and Medicaid Services) that deal with all of these issues (cms.gov). However, you have to be a combination of Harry Houdini and Albert Einstein to make heads or tails of the contents as they're not meant to be user friendly. I feel that CMS pays individuals to sit around all day to make the language as incoherent and ambiguous as possible. The rules, which is often part of new law, are purposefully ambiguous so that they can simply conform to the legislature and fit the agenda of whoever is interpreting the law.

Additionally, if you call Medicare for guidance and lucky enough to get someone on the phone, they can be of great help. However, unless you record the call and think about it at your leisure, the information is so complex and abundant that it is hard to digest quickly. The whole purpose of this book is to guide the patient through the maze of the cardiac medical care from a disease state and the payment for its treatment.

As of now, it's certainly not inconceivable that if one is hospitalized when it should've been inpatient service that this is a result of the doctor or the hospital not filling out the appropriate documents for inpatient intensity of care or didn't sign the inpatient two-midnight certification for inpatient treatment. This omission can create dire consequences to the patient.

After a year or more, if Medicare denies the inpatient service claim, it's possible that the patient could get a bill for tens of thousands of dollars for the hospital and doctor to make up for their lost payment! This is not ludicrous. With the knowledge learned from this book, you'll have the power to see through what is being done and hopefully reject such notions. For now, this unfortunately may require taking legal action to set a precedent for such irresponsible behavior.

There's belief and faith in our medical providers that they have our best interest at heart. This may have been our wish and trust since posterity, but unfortunately, it's now becoming just a naive fantasy. In other words, you have to know the right questions to ask as a well-informed patient because you're at the mercy of a medical system that no longer works in your best interest. Think. You'd never buy a car without first knowing its price. In addition, it's in the salesman's best interest to sell you pricey accessories, but a smart consumer won't be talked into buying unnecessary accessories and upgrades.

Thus, the knowledge of the heart and heart procedures will empower the patients to make informed decisions regarding their care. One might say that this book is the "Kelly Blue Book" for the heart. Like purchasing a car, your healthcare is simply no longer off limits to free discussion. It's open season for exchange with your doctor about what various procedures and the relative costs of these procedures. The thought that discussing costs and implications about your health care are somehow going to offend the doctor is simply an antiquated fear. Openness regarding healthcare is no longer a sacrosanct topic and should be the same for hospital admissions and protocol and can be as easy as ordering meals from the hospital menu. Transparency is the catchword for 2015.

Next on the agenda is a brief overview of how Medicare and private Insurance reimburse for various illustrative scenarios and cardiac procedures. This may include procedures such as a cardiac catheterization, ablation of a cardiac arrhythmia, a heart attack or congestive heart failure, and procedures done in a doctor's office or outpatient facility such as a treadmill or even an electrocardiogram. Although this seems an overwhelming task, I think that for this book, only the salient points are appropriate. In this respect, I'll explain how these apply to both Medicare A and B and how the doctor and the hospital can affect the ultimate monetary and clinical outcomes.

First, we must initially take a look at Medicare because most of cardiac diseases become an issue in the patient's life as one moves onto Medicare coverage at the age of 65. I fervently hope that it is ingrained in your minds. As of October 2014, as well as beginning with the implementation of Obamacare, the Medicare reimbursement game has radically changed to the significant detriment of the patient. With the dramatic increase in patients' payment and less cost to Medicare, the odds have shifted to favor the cost savings for the government.

In my opinion, this is a disgrace to the elderly, who can barely afford these severe and cruel rule changes—especially when there was no communication to the patient regarding these radical rule changes. The main revolution that we will discuss is what is referred to as the "Two-Midnight" rule. Simply put, it used to be that a procedure or hospitalization could be considered an "inpatient" admission after you were in the hospital for only one midnight. Thus, if you had a condition that warranted by its severity or complexity inpatient status, you only needed to be in the hospital one midnight to qualify for inpatient services and almost complete payment by Medicare A for hospital services.

This may seem trivial, but you'll see its enormous ramifications in the cost of your care. As of October 1, 2014, this changed to require the need for an expected or actual two midnight hospitalization in order to qualify for inpatient versus outpatient status. Note that it's two midnights, and not two days. This is intentional and is the specific criteria utilized by Medicare as outlined by CMS (Centers for Medicare and Medicaid services).

CMS is the principal government agency responsible for implementing the Affordable Care Act (Obamacare) and Medicare rules. I will delve into details in a moment, but suffice it to say that Medicare Type B pays for outpatient and Medicare Type A pays for inpatient status. For a complex procedure such as a cardiac catheterization, this could be the difference of an inpatient procedure with a minimal amount of money you pay versus an outpatient procedure that costs possibly two to three thousand dollars. And this cost is not fully paid by Medicare part B, which means you or your coinsurance must pay after deductible!

It's time that you take notice and become vigilant to what is a truly profound fact. This rule is now the subject of multiple civil suits by hospitals and consumer groups that contend the two-midnight rule as "arbitrary and capricious." However, as I've stated, I think the two-midnight rule is a double-edged sword. The doctor must properly apply the rule under the right circumstance. If you're having a complex inpatient procedure that's qualified and could potentially require a two-midnight stay, the rule may actually be of significant benefit in protecting your pocketbook.

The real problem is that the doctors, in many if not most cases, don't document properly. I feel it has to take some patient and family input to right the situation as an example of demanding transparency of one's care. The doctors' proper certification has been improving, but as of Jan 2015, the doctor only has to document in the medical record. I have no doubt documentation will become an even more daunting problem for the doctor and hospital with increased enforcement of the requirements of CMS. Only heaven knows why CMS changed this rule as of 2015 other than to get more hospitals to classify patients as outpatients when they should be inpatient. Due to the increased demands of the rules placed on doctors and hospitals, this misclassification ends up costing Medicare less and more for the patient because it costs Medicare less to pay for an outpatient procedure that would've been paid for the properly billed Inpatient hospitalization.

I would like to go into some examples. It's important to make a mental note of these cases because the rest of this book will be about explaining these diseases and their complexity. My goal is to give you a better understanding of whether, if faced with this situation, you should be an inpatient or outpatient. Although there are remarkable private companies in the United States that facilitates the correct status of your admission, a proactive approach by the patient and family specifically aimed at the care and status given by the physician will significantly affect the patient's financial responsibility and remarkably lead, in many instances, to a more positive medical outcome. You must remember that it's only possible when you "know what you're talking about."

So, let's start with the first scenario. Let's say you go to an emergency room with chest pain, which is one of the most frequent reasons for emergency room visits and subsequent hospitalization. Your knowledge of diseases of the heart will start off saving you money right from the get go. Let me tell you as a Cardiologist that I, along with probably every human being in the world, have had some episode of chest pain.

Even as a doctor, I often wonder if I should seek medical attention, so I understand how hard it is for others to make such a decision. A majority of chest pain complaints admitted to a hospital turns out to be a false but a very expensive alarm. In most cases, if properly managed, a visit to the family physician for recurrent pains would be safe and far less expensive. Additionally, an appropriate referral to a cardiologist's office would ultimately lead to far better medical care. So let us take the following examples:

1. You are in the emergency room (ER) with chest pain. The ER doctor does an EKG on you and orders various blood tests to see if you did have a heart attack. Hopefully, he checks the character of the pain such as pressure or sharp and if you have a history or family history of documented heart disease such as a previous cardiac stent, heart attack, or coronary bypass surgery. At this point in the ER, you're considered an outpatient and Medicare B is paying the doctor and all your tests. The doctors then see you and ascertains that you have had or are at high risk for having a heart attack. He plans to do a cardiac catheterization in the morning or even that night as an emergency procedure that was not previously scheduled or planned. Please note that this will be an emergent procedure in contradistinction to a scheduled, elective cardiac catheterization.

Due to the complexity of the situation and the fact that the doctor plans a complex emergency procedure, it's absolutely appropriate that you're qualified to be admitted as an inpatient at this point. It's categorically critical that at this point the doctor "certifies or documents" as a part of declaring the status as inpatient and that your condition is consistent with the need for a two-midnight stay. Now, if Medicare agrees with this determination and the doctor properly certifies and signs, then you're paid for by both Medicare A for the hospital services and the cardiac catheterization while Medicare B pays for the doctor's services.

The true catastrophe arises if the doctor writes for outpatient (observation) status and *never* changes this order before your discharge an even if you're in the hospital for two midnights. In that case, the whole hospitalization is deemed outpatient and Medicare B pays the doctor's services and some of the hospital costs such as for the cardiac catheterization. But that's it! The rest of the bill is absorbed by the hospital, and a big portion of the bill may be your responsibility.

2. You come to the ER with chest pain, and initially, the doctor needs to hospitalize you for further tests, and he feels you have a low probability of a heart attack or coronary heart disease. Let's say that all the tests are negative, and you have a normal EKG (we'll go into detail about the EKG later). You're kept in the hospital overnight, and the doctor doesn't admit you as an inpatient and sends you home the next morning. In this scenario, you're considered an outpatient or observation. Therefore, Medicare B pays for the doctor's services and hospital outpatient services such as lab tests, intravenous medicines, and many others of the services considered outpatient.

Your deductible is rather large, but it is manageable. The disaster arises when the doctor improperly orders inpatient and certifies two midnights. The problem is that your situation realistically doesn't qualify, so upon Medicare review, they now have the power to deny the whole hospitalization, or after they have paid Part A, demand repayment from the hospital. Subsequently, the patient receives a far larger second bill for the hospitalization possibly even a year or more after being discharged!

3. Here is an example of one of the biggest problems to be faced by the patient that is remarkably common in American medicine, which places the patient at sizable, financial jeopardy. You're placed in the hospital and immediately have an emergency cardiac catheterization. And all the inpatient orders and certification are appropriate for Medicare Part A payment. You're about to be discharged, and the doctor tells you that you have something of concern on your chest x ray. You're completely without symptoms or medical need for immediate evaluation.

For many reasons, the least of which is to the patient's benefit, the doctor's desire for sheer convenience is to evaluate this with tests that can easily be done at another time as an outpatient or in the office. However, for many other reasons that we'll discuss later in the book, it is my opinion that this is done for the fear of a lawsuit. This arises out of your or the doctor's desire to immediately and quickly resolve the issue with various outpatient tests ordered while you're still an inpatient in the acute care hospital.

Upon Medicare review and if the hospital bills for these non-emergent tests, it's conceivable that Medicare will pay the *whole* hospitalization as outpatient or Medicare Part B but not pay the doctor. This all depends on whether or not the hospital bills for what is obviously excessive and unnecessary outpatient tests done out of convenience. Some hospitals wisely don't bill and just absorb the cost with the distinct possibility that they could try to bill the patient for the lost income! This problem is probably one of the most prevalent problems with medical care as it is delivered under the American system. I will provide another similar example.

4. You're hospitalized for an outpatient test such as a cardiac catheterization, which is not as an emergency, so it's scheduled ahead of time as an "elective" procedure. You're experiencing chest pain that the doctor suspects is due to coronary artery disease, but you're stable. And there's no other reason to suspect that you're about to have a heart attack. The cardiac catheterization is done, and the doctor says that you need a coronary bypass surgery.

99% of the time, you can be discharged as an outpatient to have the coronary bypass surgery scheduled at a relatively early date because there's no medical reason for an emergency surgery. But in reality, you're kept in the hospital for no conceivable medical justification for a surgery that may be done in three or four days for the convenience of the doctor or the hospital. Again, this occurs countless times every day in this country.

In this case, if the hospital tries to bill for these "custodial" care days and if you are now an inpatient for the coronary bypass surgery, then Medicare actually has the capacity to deny payment or reimburse as outpatient Medicare B until the hospital rebills properly. And that's if the hospital is not "sanctioned" by Medicare. Nevertheless, there's a tremendous capacity for the patient to be held responsible for a much higher percent of the bill especially if the whole hospital stay that could be one or two weeks is billed as Medicare B rather than properly as Medicare Part A.

5. Here's an even more egregious practice. Let's say you're scheduled for an elective cardiac catheterization for angina, but the doctor ascertains that you don't need surgery but rather a coronary stent. In the overwhelming circumstances, there's definitely no medical justification for the doctor not doing the stent at the same time and subsequently sending

you home the next day. However, let us say that the doctor who does the heart catheterization is not trained to do a stent but must call in an "invasive" cardiologist to do the intervention on your coronary arteries. Often, the intervention is done as a second procedure the next day, which will result in a two midnight stay and inappropriate consideration as in inpatient rather than simple outpatient procedure.

An even more absurd practice is that the first procedure is done at a doctor's office or a free standing clinic outside the hospital that is not equipped to do the intervention. In this case, you're transferred to the hospital for the subsequent intervention probably the next day. This is simply a very contentious situation and places the patient not only clinically in added danger, but the billing consequences are monumental and can only lead to basic noncompliance with Medicare guidelines. In these two circumstances, the procedure can be considered an inpatient "emergent" procedure or spans two midnights and billed as potentially inpatient. Both of these possibilities are simply inappropriate for a basically outpatient procedure. Again, Medicare denial and sanctions for improper billing, which in can be sheer fraud at times, can lead to very negative billing consequences.

6. Next is a situation that's unfortunately increasing in our country. Your doctor writes an order and certification for inpatient services. But upon review, either by their own in-house reviewers or an outside contracted service, it's changing your hospital status to outpatient or observation. Your doctor must agree, and the hospital must tell you in writing before you're discharged that your status has changed. If the doctor does not agree, some hospitals have procedures in place to deal with such ridiculous, and what I consider perilous and unacceptable, doctor's behavior. It's interesting to note that some hospitals don't choose to sanction these physicians for their ludicrous behavior because the doctors bring business to the hospital. Needless

to say, this behavior is detrimental to the patient rather than the hospital.

7. You're brought in for a test called an electrophysiological study for a heart rhythm abnormality or passing out that tests for a possible electrical abnormality of the heart. The doctor ascertains that you need a pacemaker or a surgery called a radiofrequency ablation as a solution to the problem. Both of these procedures can be done on the same day, but they're done the next day for non-medical reason. If the doctor certifies for inpatient status, the hospital may inappropriately bill for inpatient services because of the two-day stay and thus opens the door for a Medicare audit.

The real problem occurs again like in the previous examples. Let's say the service is qualified only for outpatient services, but Medicare deems the two midnight stay unnecessary. The potential inpatient Medicare A services will be downgraded on discharge to an outpatient Part B service where the patient is responsible for a much greater proportion of the bill. And in some circumstances, it means denial for the whole hospital service.

These are but just a few of the examples, and I will strive to communicate those practices and possible solutions that will be facilitated by the "power" of knowledge.

However, as of January 1, 2015, this two-midnight rule has been somewhat modified. As far as I'm concerned, this is the most treacherous and underhanded move that I have seen CMS try to accomplish. The new rules are guised in hundreds of pages to hide the true intent of the rule change. After reading through reams of simply hokum, there are two basic changers that are rationalized to actually make is simpler for the hospital to assure that the patient requires a two midnight stay.

1. "Documentation" is substituted for the word "certification." A two midnight stay is need for hospitalization in the medical record and not necessarily in the signed doctor order. And now, Medicare in its audits can search the medical record or even the doctor's office notes to justify

for the complexity of the procedure or care with the need for inpatient hospitalization.

2. The basic change is that Medicare will now have access to the doctor's office records for additional documentation that will justify the inpatient service. It's a move that actually makes it easier for Medicare to prove fraud on the doctor's part as it may conflict with his hospital documentation and rationalization for the inpatient status. In other words, if the office notes documents that the physician discussed a relatively "simple" procedure in the office but in the hospital chart records a "complex" procedure and inpatient status, this would trigger a Medicare audit and possible punitive damages against the hospital and the doctor.

It does not get rid of the "benchmark" of a two midnight stay or perceived need, but it substitutes the word "documentation" for certification. This simple word change is rationalized by CMS to make it easier for documentation and classification. However, it's no different than a smoke and mirrors illusion. The smoke is the change from certification to documentation under the pretense of appeasing those that disagreed with certification. All they got was something more ominous, and the mirrors are that it was substituted by something with a multitude of interpretations at the whim of the reviewer, which will ultimately be in the favor of Medicare.

In the present situation, the reviewer is paid 25% of the recovered Medicare over reimbursement and is no different than a "bounty hunter." The fabrication that it's represented as more efficient and precise is simply a lie. As we have seen with much of Obamacare and CMS rules, the deceptions are hidden in such indiscernible language that it's nearly impossible to understand. Luckily, I'm a trained doctor in the field of medical necessity review, so the true intent and treacherous nature of these changes was obvious to me.

In actuality, it gives some false "legal" means for Big Brother CMS to access to your private doctor records. It's most likely through the electronic medical records that Obamacare had legislated the need for a doctor to have operational in 2015. In many ways, the requirement of an electronic medical record is just an underhanded means to breach your privacy through your computerized records. As we shall see, the electronic medical record may have some advantages. But like any computer record, if a false diagnosis is entered into the silicon system, it simply perpetuates forever in your record as in any computer, "junk in and junk out".

Second the law justifies itself with the rational that it will make it easier to ascertain the real need for inpatient status. That is a bunch of hogwash that it truly defies sensible reality. Now that hospitals have mastered the act of certification of inpatient need in the orders, CMS just wants to make it difficult to justify inpatient status, Medicare A payment, and facilitate the downgrade default to outpatient Medicare B services. They have substituted a subjective system that can be interpreted in a capricious manner from an objective arrangement that was easily verifiable and could be in the patient's best interest.

It's crucial for the proactive and knowledgeable patient to know that your financial responsibility is multiple with Medicare B service as Medicare pays less. With Medicare part B, the bill is primarily paid minus your deductible by approximately 80% of the bill; thus, it's far cheaper for Medicare to bill and admit you as outpatient than as inpatient. This is all some great lie. As we've seen with most of Obamacare and CMS rules, it's a simple ploy to make the patient bear more payment and shifts the responsibility to assure the patient's proper care and admission status to the patient. By reading this book, you'll hopefully become an expert to fight the forces that are legislating medical care to your detriment.

Before we leave the subject of medical insurance, I'd like to proceed with a short note about Obamacare and your insurance. This comment is based upon recent revelations that this legislation was the result of the voting public being too "stupid" (Jonathan Gruber 2014) to understand the implications of the legislation. I prefer the word "uneducated" about the implications of the legislation. There is no doubt that the bill lacks "transparency." That is a word I will use repeatedly to refer to the rules that are too complex and unobvious that they don't even lend themselves to an understanding.

It must be understood that Obamacare basically created a system where every uninsured person suddenly feels empowered to have medical insurance, not realizing that the insurance may have a $10,000 dollar deductible. Most of these individuals, who could barely afford the insurance in the first place, can't possibly pay that amount. Nevertheless, this give the facade of being "insured," and the hospital loses money in the long run as the public is left to pay the bills.

Almost seven million uninsured received these absurd deductible insurance plans. At the same time, up to 15 million of the previously insured lost their insurance or had it changed. It cost the same or more money for one of these ridiculously high deductible, and honestly, useless plans. Therefore, Obamacare is just a complex "bait and switch plan" that is detrimental to the working class individual, and it changes the whole face of medicine to an "entitlement" system that will lessen the quality and effectiveness of reasonable medical care. In the end, Obamacare is a useless and dangerous piece of medical legislation.

Here's an additional example of the capricious nature of Medicare. If you were admitted for an atrial fibrillation ablation and the doctor certified an expectation of a two midnight stay, Medicare was appropriately obligated to accept inpatient services. As we shall discuss later in the book under atrial fibrillation, this procedure is complex enough that you should be considered for inpatient admission status. Under this new system, the need for two midnights must be justified by Medicare's purposefully nebulous guidelines and somehow be documented to be complex and dangerous enough in the medical record or the doctor's office. Because it's totally subjective, Medicare can accept or deny the doctor's argument at its whim and to its monetary advantage at the totally inappropriate expense to the patient.

I know a black man, aged 68, who works as a guard and greeter at the place where I work. He's a hard-working individual who is trying to live in semi-retirement from being a truck driver. He is apparently sick and could've gone on disability. But this man is too proud and lives by the principle that as long he can work, he will earn his money. He asked me how the changes in Medicare under Obamacare is suddenly costing him more money, and now, he can barely afford his medication.

What could I say to a man of morals who is suffering under this new oppressive system? In the case of hospitalization, there are ways of having your insurance pay the bills, but in the case of this guard, I had no answers, which made me feel very sad. That's why it is imperative that all of you heed my warnings and gains the knowledge to navigate the maze of the system for your benefit and the benefit of your loved ones.

Lastly, before we leave the complexities of Medicare and insurance reimbursement, I want to cover one last topic of importance. It's the Medicare Beneficiary Notice Initiatives (BNI). This is a fairly unknown aspect of Medicare but is very important for the patient to understand or have some knowledge of its presence. In actuality, these initiatives are primarily for the benefit of the provider whether it's the hospital or the doctor. Unfortunately, as with almost everything with Medicare, these guidelines have nothing to do with protecting the patient and thus leave little options for the proactive consumer of medical care.

In general, Medicare rules and initiatives just leaves the patient out to dry. I can assure you that under most circumstances, the hospital will not inform you of its existence as it can have a large effect on their profit. Most hospital and doctors have no real clue as to its effects, and it's partially to have the public ignorant of the consequences of this act. Honestly, I doubt if there is any doctor who has any knowledge of its actual existence. I asked every doctor I know and none of them any idea of the existence or consequences of the BNI initiative.

In addition, when an average person visits the CMS website and reads about BNI, it looks like nonsensical gibberish. When I read the rules, it took me days to completely understand. Also, when I called the Medicare provider service with multiple consultants, it was obvious to me that very few of them have any reasonable knowledge of the consequences or workings of the BNI. My best friend, who is a doctor, likes to say that Medicare rules and guidelines are "intentionally made obscure" as is most legislation that comes out of our government. I look at it a different way; these rules and regulations have nothing to do with protecting the patient and are not written for the average person to understand. One needs a PhD in linguistics just to make sense of the language or its meaning. However, with the changes in Medicine, it's necessary for the patient to be proactive and understand some of its complexities.

Basically, BNI has two major components: The Advanced Beneficiary Notice (ABN) and the fee for service Hospital-Issued Notices of Non-coverage (FSS or just HINN). Primarily, hospitals are obligated to issue a HINN prior to admission, at admission, or any point during an inpatient stay where the hospital determines that the care the beneficiary (patient) is receiving or about to receive, is not covered by Medicare because it is:

1. Medically unnecessary.

2. Not delivered in the most appropriate setting (inpatient when it should be done in an outpatient setting).

3. Is custodial in nature (waiting for a test that's not being done in an expedient manner due to scheduling conflict or overbooked hospital).

The key to these provisions is that the hospital in 99% of the cases doesn't properly issue a HINN when it knows that Medicare won't pay for service. They should not bill for the service, and the patient won't be liable for paying the hospital for the service not covered by Medicare. The problem with this scenario is that if the hospital bills for the service knowing Medicare won't pay but feign ignorance, then Medicare could audit. And there lies the possibility of patient financial responsibility.

The catch 22 in all this is that if Medicare doesn't review the hospitalization, and the hospital is in no jeopardy if they don't issue a HINN or an ABN, Medicare will reimburse the whole service and the hospital and the patient will not be financially liable. However, if the hospital is aware of the fact that Medicare won't pay for like sitting around for a procedure that was canceled and then Medicare audits the case, the hospital will be subject a censure, and the money will be requested to be returned by the hospital. But this doesn't protect the patient from eventually receiving a new bill for that uncovered hospital day. This is the point not to be forgotten!

The ABN can be issued (but isn't required) if the hospital knows Medicare won't reimburse for what it doesn't cover but can still bill even with the prospect of a future denial in a Medicare audit and the subsequent financial responsibility to the patient.

There's only one actual recourse for the patient to deal with this dilemma. The patient must know that the hospital doesn't issue you a valid HINN on the day that the test was canceled. They cannot bill you, so you must remember and demand that the hospital issues a HINN after the event has occurred. If the hospital allows you to wait without issuing an ABN or HINN, you cannot be billed even though Medicare will not pay in case of an audit.

Conversely, if you demand the ABN or HINN after the fact, the hospital is free to bill you even though they know that it's not an item or service that Medicare will cover. There's no doubt that if your procedure is canceled, they should know to send you home to return at a later date. Once the hospital issues the HINN, you'll still be billed for the day. If Medicare doesn't audit the case, Medicare will automatically pay. However, the moment you receive your Medicare bill, you must go to the Medicare website and obtain the phone number for recipient inquiries and billing questions.

Once you get a service agent on the phone, inform them that you've received a HINN for a service when the doctor didn't properly discharge you from the hospital. There is no alternative and it's rather painstaking. I think it was purposively designed to dissuade you from such appeals. Nevertheless, once the inquiry is launched and Medicare is aware of your HINN and the billing for a custodial day, you financial responsibility will be exonerated. So, you and Medicare will not pay for the service, they will ask the hospital for a return of their money, and to return money to you if they collected any deductible for the unnecessary service. As I said, it's certainly a roundabout way to be proactive, but Medicare is unquestionably designed for the hospital's benefit, not yours.

I know this sounds convoluted and complex—and it is. The hospitals have no obligation to make the patient aware of the process of issuing an ABN or a HINN, and obviously, it's in their best interest to refuse transparency and forthrightness to the patient in this procedure. In addition, it definitely isn't in the best interest of the doctor because if he proceeds—as in the example of the heart catheterization—without sending you home on the canceled day and properly readmitting you to the hospital for a later time, he has the possibility of Medicare denying his payment for the whole procedure and hospitalization. This obviously places the patient and the doctor at immense financial liability.

This same situation applies when the doctor does a heart catheterization and deems it necessary to do a further "elective" and not emergent procedure such as a second stent or even a cardiac bypass surgery. If you're just sitting around with custodial care, which is not covered by Medicare, the hospital isn't required to issue a HINN to bill Medicare and risk a future audit; however, you can demand a HINN, so the hospital can bill Medicare and further promote your discharge. The real problem lies when the physician doesn't agree to discharge you or document the reason for your stay in the hospital. Then you'll ultimately pay unless you demand the HINN and appeal at a later date. Undoubtedly, 99% of the time, the doctor doesn't do the appropriate discharge when indicated and has no idea or care to know about HINN and ABN.

Before leaving this section, I want to capsulize this incredibly convoluted concept of the ABN and the HINN again. It's critical to understand this concept and to reread this section until you have a firm understanding. First, the last thing the hospital wants to admit is that they're aware that a part of your care is just custodial management and does not require acute hospital care. However, by issuing a HINN, that is exactly what they're admitting to knowing the care is inappropriate, yet they're still billing after informing you of this transgression. On the one hand, Medicare is saying it's legal to bill even though it's inappropriate.

CMS is talking out of their mouths and their rear end at the same time to their advantage. The sheer lunacy of such a rule is beyond me. As far as Medicare is concerned, the patient is supposed to get up and leave the hospital. This is sheer madness and cannot be reasonably accomplished, especially if the doctor disagrees that it's custodial and unnecessary care. So, these rules place both the patient and the hospital in jeopardy and leave little for the patient to rectify the solution other than to stay in the hospital, demand a HINN letter, and submit the letter to Medicare immediately after leaving the hospital and receiving the bill.

Well, now that you've had an earful, it's time to proceed to the meat of the matter: the history of the heart, the specifics of disease states, and how to deal with your treatment and hospitalization.

Chapter 2: The Heart in Early History

Cro-Magnon

I guess the place to start is at the earliest recorded beginning. The heart symbol as an icon of the heart that we all know was first depicted before the last Ice Age. In cave pictograms, Cro-Magnon man (or woman) depicted the heart we envision as a simple valentine depiction (Fig.1). It's hard to know how early humans could've conceived of this image but is certainly intriguing that we use the same schematic to this day. Some of the opinions calls this a drawing of a leaf, but I still like to think that a power beyond human somehow garnished our early ancestors with primal knowledge.

There's another possibility that is certainly less spiritual. It's that the hunter became aware after one of them was splayed open by a saber tooth tiger or a mastodon tusk that there is something other than air inside their bodies. They saw that there was the dead person with this big thing in the middle of the chest, which is the heart that looks very much like in the cave pictograms.

It's known that even in this early social structure, there was a shaman or healer of probable high intelligence and spirituality that added cohesiveness as the one who was trusted with care of the sick. The present doctors shouldn't forsake this essential function that places them in high regard based upon the ageless trust in doing what is best for the patient. I fear though, as we'll uncover as we read on, this function has been inexorably and relentlessly eroded over the past six years by the ill-conceived and often ignorant bureaucratic intervention. Inevitably, the ageless one-to-one intimacy between the patient and his or her cardiologist is slowly being replaced by the surrogate physicians who are guided by a microchip brain with steel hands and no conscience or soul. In the coming chapters, we'll see how this affects a patient's care and how to defend against this authoritarian delivery of your medical upkeep. Now that we compared the beginning and the present, let's learn more about the past and how each step might affect the future.

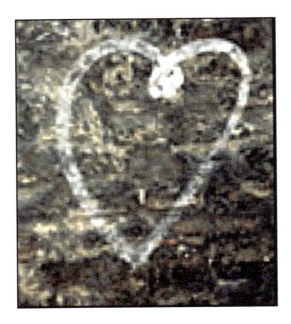

(Fig.1) (Pbs.org-Paul Silverzweig) Cave art with the depiction of the heart by Cro-Magnon man.

Egyptians

Between 2,500 to 1,000 B.C.E. the Egyptians believed that the heart, or iab, was the center of all consciousness—the center of all life and mortality itself. When someone died, it was said that their "heart has departed." It was the only organ left in the body during the mummification process. According to the Book of The Dead, after death, one's heart was taken to the hall of Maat to be weighed and either sent to Osiris in the afterlife or to the demon of Ammut to be eaten, which resulted your soul vanishing from existence.

One can certainly envision that the Egyptians witnessed the beating heart in the open chest of the injured during warfare. Thus, we have the symbolic depiction of the heart as the center of the soul. One cannot help but be amazed at the beautiful spiritualism and symbolism centered on the heart. It has been said that the symphony of the mind is a reflection of the beauty and order of nature.

Therefore, the heart was regarded in Ancient Egypt as the organic motor of the body, the seat of intelligence, and a principal religious and spiritual symbol. It was considered as one of the eight parts of the human body. Unlike other organs, it remains carefully intact in the mummy to ensure its eternal life. In Ancient Egypt, the concept of heart included three components: heart-haty, heart-ib, and the spiritual seat of intelligence, emotion, and memory. The hieroglyphs representing the heart early in the first dynasty were drawn with eight vessels attached to it (Fig.2).

Although it is written that that the heart was the only organ not removed from the mummy, some mummies were discovered without the heart. It is probable that although most mummies are of the wealthy or influential, these families didn't think the person earned a valued place in the afterlife by thus removing the heart after death (post mortem). Unequivocally, Egyptian doctors elaborated on the original conception of cardiovascular physiology and the principal importance of the heart, which have endured since the beginning of mankind.

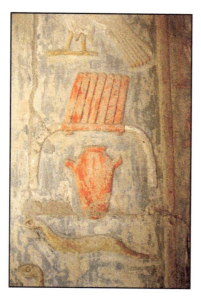

(Fig.2) (belovedegypt.com by Ruth Shilling) This picture is an Ancient Egyptian hieroglyph representing the heart and one of the eight vessels attached to the heart. Each vessel represents an emotion such as joy, sadness, or remorse that expresses all the feelings that were understood to reside in the heart. In these wall writings, it's said that when the soul felt an overwhelming emotion, the heart would "...feel like it could burst." It's interesting to think that this might this be the early description of the rapid and strong heartbeat called sinus tachycardia that's often accompanied by emotional upheaval or excitement such as making love.

The clay jars that have symbolic meaning as the hearts were usually left in the corpse. Interestingly, one of the vessels would often be drawn broken, so the other world would look upon the soul with a broken heart as a tragedy of their worldly lives such as a person who lost a child. In this depiction of the heart vessel, there is the picture of a necklace flowing upward to the heavens, representing the emotions ascending to the afterlife. This is a beautiful example of the Egyptian spiritualism and the primary significance they placed in the heart.

As a side note, after studies on the heart of mummies in the 3,500 years old jars, it's been reported by researchers that the Pharaoh Merenptah had severe atherosclerosis-coronary artery or hardening of the arteries and had a premature death. Upon investigation in the tomb, many others in the Pharaoh's entourage were found to have had a similar affliction.

The interesting solution to this revelation relates to modern times epidemiology—a branch of medicine dealing with the cause of disease—which finds that the high status Egyptians led them to eat fatty meats from fowl and livestock. These foods were high in cholesterol and fatty acids that we now know is related to the development of atherosclerosis in the coronary arteries as well as hardening of the arteries in the legs—leg pain or claudication. (Fig.3) This may be the most remarkable illustration in this book.

It's a computerized tomography, CT scan, of an ancient mummy. Basically a CT scan is a very precise X-ray that looks at a slice of the mummy and is a virtual picture of the various body parts. In this CT scan, the white we are looking at is at the level of the coronary arteries and the aorta with the large iliac arteries leading into the legs. If you remember, atherosclerosis is the depositing of cholesterol and fats into the lining of the arteries. This is also called hardening of the arteries because of the cholesterol which causes deposition or collection of calcium, which is the same substance that makes up bones; thus, the artery becomes brittle and less flexible.

In this fascinating CT scan on the left, we see the calcification of the right coronary artery (RCA) and the left coronary artery (LCA). Don't worry if you don't understand the anatomy as we'll go over this down the line. It's clear that these coronary arteries are severely calcified, which suggests advanced coronary artery disease (CAD). Additionally, one can see significant calcification of the aorta and the iliac artery or what is called peripheral vascular disease (PVD). Thus, this ancient Egyptian most likely suffered chest pains or angina pectoris and leg pains, or claudication. Let's wrap this up by noting that now a patient may undergo a CT scan of the heart to visualize coronary calcification with a "calcium score" to determine if it's minimal or severe CAD.

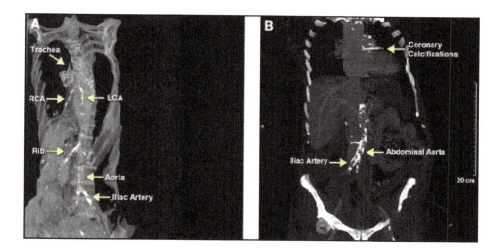

(Fig. 3) (Journal of the American College of Cardiology; Cardiovascular Imaging, April 2011 Volume 4:4 pp. 315-327) In this remarkable CT scan of a mummy, the presence of coronary and vascular disease is depicted in white that represents the calcium deposits in these arteries. It's obvious that the arteries are highly calcified, and the person probably had severe chest pains and severe leg pains.

I sincerely hope that this historical review of cardiology isn't putting you to sleep because I strongly believe that the understanding these historical milestones will aid in your understanding of modern cardiology as it relates to the anatomy and physiology of the cardiovascular system. Soon, we'll delve into the enlightened age of the Renaissance and modern times, which I think you will find more palatable.

Chinese

The ancient Chinese physicians (5,000 B.C.E.), in their incredible wisdom, were impressed by the importance of an irregular heartbeat. As a side note, it's important to understand that Egyptian medicine evolved independently over the same time as Chinese medicine. The resultant Chinese "pulse theory" can be said to have laid the foundation for cardiac electrophysiology as the study of heart rhythms as a unique and integral part of cardiology. They described the pulse as being irregular to the point of being unpredictable. What's amazing is that this "irregularly irregular" heartbeat is still observed during a physical examination and is used to describe atrial fibrillation.

Another early description of atrial fibrillation is from The Yellow Emperor's Classic of Internal Meda Medicine (Huang Ti aching Su Wen). This emperor, whose line ruled between 1,696 and 2,598 B.C.E., had physicians who recognized the poor prognosis and shortened lifespan that was associated with a chaotic irregularity of the pulse. These physicians were known to have used herbal preparations to be ingested or used as a balm for treatment of this irregular heartbeat. Although not described in Chinese writings, we know that digitalis derived from the plant foxglove can help control the fast heartbeat associated with this arrhythmia (abnormal beat of the heart). Thus, it's intriguing to contemplate whether these doctors from antiquity deducted from clinical experience an observation that wouldn't be recognized until over 4,000 years later.

As long as the heart was in motion, the Chinese recognized that blood circulated through the vessels and the patient was alive and could bleed. In reality, the heart is an elaboration of blood vessels that first manifests as a one chamber heart that is seen in the lower animals and fish. However, in Humans, a child can survive with effectively only a one chamber heart called Hypoplastic heart syndrome. Interestingly, the Chinese were the first to observe the embryonic development of the heart. They correctly observed that the blood vessels first appear followed by the appearance of the heart and the apparent modification of the blood vessels. It was recognized that the vessels developed and supplied nourishment to the liver, spleen, and intestines with blood.

It was recorded that when the heart pumped normally with blood flowing through the circulation, the face and the tongue would have a rosy complexion. If the blood became sluggish or obstructed, the face and tongue would become gray. And this condition would ultimately result in death. As a principal theme of this book, the physician's keen observation of a patient and change over time is of great importance in the diagnosis of heart disease. This gray complexion is now referred to as cyanosis and perioral (around the mouth) cyanosis. They knew that this cyanosis was a harbinger of severe illness and premature death.

For example, in the CT scan (Fig.3) of the mummy with hardening of the arteries leading to the legs, this peripheral vascular disease would lead to cyanosis first to the feet and progressing up the leg. In its last stages, the feet would develop non-healing ulcerations or simple wounds of the feet, resulting in infection that leads to sepsis and death. In modern day, most smokers are unable to fully oxygenate their blood in their diseased lungs and develop perioral cyanosis. Again, as in the majority of smokers, this is a sign of premature death due to the myriad of fatal disease that develops in the smoker.

In addition, the pericardium, which is the sack containing the heart, seemed to have an important role as documented in Chinese manuscripts. They seemed to believe that the pericardium was a separate organ and that blood must pass through to enter the heart. Obviously, that's incorrect, but certain aspects of their observations have a stunning correlation to modern medicine. Blood stasis to the Chinese was when the blood became sluggish in the vessels and became "dead," referring to blood clots or thrombosis. Referring to the CT scan of the mummy (Fig.3), if the hardening of the coronary arteries or the leg arteries becomes severe, the blood will initially slow and give inadequate blood to the heart muscle or leg tissue.

The Chinese described the stasis of blood in the heart as the cause of the chest pain and the development of pain in the legs. They attributed this to the heart and occurring within the pericardium. This is true as the coronary arteries run over the surface of the heart muscle that is covered by the pericardium. Ancient text further describe a heart attack as being caused by the clotting of the blood within the pericardium or coronaries: sudden chest pain, loss of voice, lips and face turning blue, and the hands and feet becoming cyanotic and cold. In this regard, they considered this a result of "polluted blood is attacking the heart" and causing thrombosis of the coronary vasculature.

Interestingly, they made the correlation of having a heart attack with the preceding chronic findings of palpitations, dizziness, pale face, and fine, weak, and often rapid pulse. To the Chinese, treatment of the heart ailments took on a rather logical approach. If the pulse was slow or weak, and there was the danger of heart thrombosis, they turned to herbal remedies that would "invigorate" the heart and pulse with the dispersal of the "shen" or disease focus.

On the other hand, if the pulse was too quick and irregular, the herbal remedies were used to settle the heart and prevent chest pain. In that case, they often formulated Tang-kuei, which was four combinations (Siwu Tang) of herbs as the treatment of these heart disorders. It's interesting to note the frequency of the use of ginseng (reshen) and Ophiopogon (opiates) in treatment of palpitations and shortness of breath with chest pain that is aggravated by physical activity (exertional angina pectoris).

What I've mentioned before, and a recurrent theme in this book, is that the power of observation was well recognized by these early physicians. These ancient physicians didn't have the machines we have today or the distractions of the Internet or computer games. The basis of their practice was the observation and interactions with the patient. Unquestionably, these healers utilized all of their senses in making a diagnosis and plan of action. It's been said that one can peer into the soul of the body through the eyes. The hands feel the essence of the patient by the beat of the heart and the temperature of parts of the body. The nose inhales the fragrance of disease like the smell of infection and the odors of impeding death. To realize what these Chinese physicians deemed from senses and observations is truly amazing. This is a lesson that is being lost rapidly to the ages.

Before we continue, I would like to reflect on some contemporary issues as we're amazed at the wisdom of the Chinese physicians and the depth of their physician-patient interactions. If it isn't obvious to you by now, the only way these physicians were able to ascertain things, such as when an irregular pulse was an ominous sign, were through documenting these findings. They would discover these correlations as they followed up with the patient through the years.

The modern physician knew this to be true until recently when this fine balance of patient and physician exchange has been impacted by a multitude of external factors. The greatest change may be the limited time of patient-physician interaction. It's without question that 90% of the deduction in ascertaining disruption in a patient's body begins with the handshake. It may take only 15 minutes of face-to-face exchange between doctor and patient rather than a surrogate or computer hologram of the patient. As they say in computer lingo, "junk in junk out."

The young resident and intern are on eight-hour shifts where they pass on the patient to another shift doctor and no longer have the luxury of taking care of the patient in a continuous fashion. It leaves them simply unprepared for the rigors of acute medicine. In my career, I have been in surgery for 13 straight hours. If an emergency arose, I often would respond reflexively like I could do it in my sleep. When human life is at stake, I'm thankful that I was trained to do it even when I had not slept for 48 hours.

It's no different than what Navy Seals go through during their training. They train until they're near physical and mental breakdown. Mistakes made during training translate into survival in the battlefield. Additionally, it weeds out those who cannot make it or possibly need more training. We forsake the old because we think we now know more than Huang So, who was in ancient China. That is such a ridiculous notion.

Those in power legislate what they think is good for us as if they have some intellectual superiority. Knowing what we've learned, we know that appointing an "accountant" rather than an MD to head Medicare is beyond absurd. Such an appointment for the largest medical bureaucracy simply defies the imagination and is a reflection of the idiots who lead (I use this word lead very loosely) this country.

After reading this book, it's my hope that we'll rise up to vote for men and woman, who have intelligence with vision and will let our voices be heard. Creativity is squashed out of our doctors with rules, quotas, limited skills, and less guided practice with the multitude of procedures. Medicine will be rationed and patients will die waiting for a heart bypass or coronary angiogram. Your loved one who dies waiting will be a cost savings factored into the bottom line by bean counters and lauded by the leaders as an effective reduction in the bottom line. Dehumanization of medicine and forsaking ancient knowledge are now becoming a stark reality.

To finish, the critical question for the Chinese was in their quest for understanding the heart. When is death? Is it when the heart stops, or when the soul ascends to heaven? "When the pulse is irregular and tremulous and the beats occur at intervals, then the impulse of life fades; when the pulse is slender "smaller than feeble, but still perceptible, thin like a silk thread", then the impulse of life is small; when the pulse stops, the soul leaves the body." This was actually written in ancient Chinese medical literature (Fig.4).

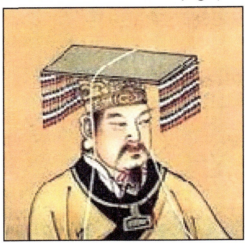

Huang Ti Nei Ching Su Wen (Fig.4), ancient Chinese physician and philosopher, was also a budding poet.

Wow, what a beautiful and profound description of the heart rhythm reflecting the symmetry of existence and the intimate connection to our environment and essence of being.

Greeks and Romans

Well, enough of the Chinese. We now see that observational knowledge about the heart flourished during the time of the Ancient Greeks (400-200 B.C.E.). In general, most of the physicians and philosophers were "cardio-centrist" in that they believed the heart to be the center of the soul and reason. In part, this was because when the person was knocked out the body continued to function and the essence was not lost. They held the heart to be the center of the man and the source of heat within the body.

They most certainly deduced this from the fact that the body rapidly cools down when the heart stopped beating. The earliest description of the circulatory system was developed in 500 B.C.E. by the mathematician, Alcmeon, who wrote that the "breath, or the spirit, was sent around the body by the blood vessels." Within the same time frame, we come to Hippocrates of Cos or in Greek Hippocrates of Kos (460-360 B.C.E.), who was an Ancient Greek physician of the Age of Pericles and is considered one of the most outstanding figures in the history of medicine.

Referred to as the father of western medicine, he was the first physician recognized as the founder of modern, scientifically-based, observational medicine (Fig.5) and as the spiritual rector of the Hippocratic manuscript collection. He gained paramount importance for establishing the medical profession's tradition of education. For that matter, he was considered the descendent of Asclepius, the legendary god of medical science in Greek mythology.

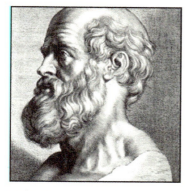

(Fig.5) (www.pbs.com) Hippocrates, who is considered the father of western medicine.

It is important to understand that much of the knowledge of human anatomy flourished during the time of the Greeks and Romans because these societies allowed the practice of "vivisection." It means the dissection of the human body on the living, which was generally prisoners sentenced to death. In this way, in a systematic manner, the physician was able to deduce certain relationships—when the heart pumps, the blood is moved and gushed out especially when certain vessels were breached. When the body died, they noted, the heart seemed to be the last thing that stopped. And when it did, the blood stopped flowing, and there was no pulse. The heart was described as "the knot of veins and the fountain of blood."

It's hard to imagine the agony of these condemned individuals. Although the practice seemed barbaric for such an advanced society, the logic was very efficient in that it advanced society and knowledge. There was some redeeming usefulness of the wrongdoer, cleansing the society of those who threatened their social and moral structure. I suppose their reasoning is debatable and could be a reminder to modern day society that grapples with the question of the death sentence and whether these bodies should be put to use as organ transplants.

To continue back to the ancients and to advance this science of observational medicine, Hippocrates stated in his Aphorisms: "Those who are subject to frequent and severe fainting attacks without obvious cause die suddenly." This might be the first description of Sudden Cardiac Death that we now know is caused by ventricular tachycardia (VT) and ventricular fibrillation (VF). These observations could be linked to electrical diseases of the heart such as the Long-QT syndrome, Brugata's syndrome, Dilated cardiomyopathy, and Idiopathic Ventricular Tachycardia.

Furthermore, Hippocrates and his students made the observation that sharp pains irradiating toward the breast bone and the back were ultimately fatal. It was the first description of what we now know to be angina pectoris or cardiac ischemia related to coronary atherosclerosis or "hardening" of the arteries. In this respect, they made the further observation that with this chest pain, one should rest immediately to relieve the pain (modern day exertional angina). Those with this pain at rest were more likely to die, and that the obese were more likely to die from this affliction.

Additionally, another Greek author described various ways to treat this chest pain while it was occurring. These included drinking wine (to relax), the bleeding of the patient (to lower blood pressure), and the encouragement of the physician. Lastly, although dissection of the body was relatively prohibited during the late ancient Romans and through the Medieval Era in Europe, Arataeus of Alexandria was able to deduce that the measured pulse rate of the circulation was the reflection of the beating of the heart, an observation substantiated in due time. Aratacus also noted that the heart was responsible for the peripheral pulse measured at the wrist and groin (femoral artery). Interestingly, the Greeks also noted that the pulse would increase in young woman with the discussion of their lovers!

According to the Hippocrates treatise, the heart is a deep crimson color shaped like a pyramid and contained in a membranous sac filled with a small amount of fluid, which we now know as the pericardial sac. He also made the observation that, sometimes, this fluid can accumulate and interfere with the heart function, a condition we recognize as pericardial tamponade. Once the blood is in the heart, it leads to the lungs where it draws air. He described the heart as a very strong muscle with the left chamber much thicker and with more abundant muscle compared to the right side. He further observed correctly that the inner surface of the heart is rough compared to the smooth outside and that the inner left side is rougher than the right. We know this to be true with the "roughness" due to the inner trabeculae of the heart muscle.

It was described in the treatise that when the top of the heart is removed, it exposed the various orifices of the heart. Most remarkably, Hippocrates correctly identified that the vessel leading out of the right heart led to the lungs, and although this was blue blood, he called this conduit the pulmonary artery. It's also for the first time that Hippocrates recognizes that there were valves of different functions within the heart.

He didn't know precisely how the valves functioned except that they allowed the uni-directional flow of the blood, and sometimes, there was backward flow through the valves if corrupted. We now call this valvular regurgitation. He described the valves as a "masterpiece of nature's craftsmanship." It's truly amazing the accuracy of these observations as it applies to modern day anatomy and physiology.

The Hippocratic Oath is recited by every new physician as he or she graduates medical school and enters into this noble and ageless profession. It has perpetuated through the ages and reflects the balance of trust that is endowed upon the patient-physician relationship.

Next, in the fourth century B.C.E., the important Greek philosopher, Aristotle (Fig.6), noted that the heart was the first to form in chick embryos and felt it was the most important organ of the body. It was the center of "intelligence, motion, and sensation." He added, the heart is a three-chambered organ (we now know it to be four chambers) that is the center of the body's vitality, and the other organs existed to primarily cool the heart. It's interesting that it's both correct and incorrect.. The heart pumps the warm blood and maintains the body's heat. It could've been from observing moving things like a wheel of a chariot that generate heat due to friction. Thus Aristotle deduced that the heart was always moving as it beat, so it would simply heat up!

According to Aristotle, the heart had three chambers without mentioning the valves with two significant vessels connected to it: the vena cava and the aorta. The right chamber was described as having the hottest and most abundant blood, the left chamber had the cooler blood and least abundant, and the middle chamber had the thinnest and purest blood. Aristotle incorrectly believed the heart to be the starting point of the veins when it's actually the starting point for the arteries.

A part of the observations came about as Aristotle strangled an animal to prepare it for dissection. It resulted in the right side of the heart being engorged with blue deoxygenated blood while the left side of the heart was drained of red or oxygenated blood. In his drawings, he doesn't recognize the heart valves, but he does recognize the difference between arteries and veins. Also, he correctly described the heart as two primary chambers with their own set of blood: blue and red.

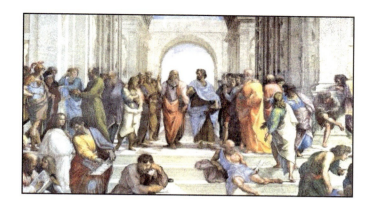

(Fig.5) (frankdevita.wordpress.com) Aristotle with his students during a heated conversation as the medical students congregate around the great teacher as is done so frequently with an influential medical school teacher. When I was a student, I'd walk across the snowy streets of Chicago across two hospitals in heated discussion with my popular, infectious disease professor. We totally ignored the 20 degree temperature in our short, white coats as we learned important "pearls" of information that we valued like gold.

Continuing on with the discussion, the second century physician Galen of Pergamon reaffirmed in his treatise, On the Usefulness of the Parts of the Body, that the heart was the source of the body's heat and the center of the soul (Fig.7). It's important that we learn more about this amazing man. He may not be as well known as Hippocrates or Aristotle, but Galen has earned the reputation as one on the greatest of all ancient physicians. I think his history speaks for itself.

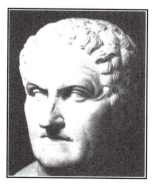

(Fig.7) (www.general-anesthesia.com) Galen of Pergamon.

First of all, he came from a very wealthy family. Then and now, the cost of medical education can be very expensive even with the help of some wonderful scholarships. But I don't think there were scholarships in ancient Greece. Galen's father was an architect and died when Galen was 19 years old, leaving his fortune to his son. This money allowed him to follow the Hippocratic teachings, ultimately traveling to and attending the great medical school of Alexandria where he studied medicine until he was 28 years old (8 years).

Now, here's the interesting part. He returned home as head physician to the gladiators of the High Priest of Asia, who was the wealthiest man of the times. It certainly seems like a contradiction that a priest would be super wealthy and owns a hoard of gladiator slaves. Nevertheless, it's said that Galen earned this position by eviscerating (cutting open the stomach and exposing the bowel) an animal in front of the priest and successfully repairing the damage with surgery and saving the animal.

Although Galen was said to have learned much of his knowledge and technique from dissection of apes and pigs, his work shows that there may have been some surreptitious dissection of the human body. At that time in Alexandria, dissection of humans was no longer allowed. His remarkable knowledge of human anatomy and surgical technique resulted from his attending to the gruesome trauma cases of the wounded gladiators. Like modern trauma surgeons whose craft is honed on real life experience, Galen's proficiency made him, without question, the expert of his times.

Unlike Aristotle, Galen regarded the heart second to the brain as he realized that both brain and heart injury in the fighting arena was always a mortal and fatal wound. When he'd put pressure on the inner brain exposed by a wound, the person rendered first "immediately without sensation or movement" followed by death. He also made the observation that wounds that pierced the heart didn't lend themselves to experimentation because the patient died immediately. Because this seemed unique to this organ, the heart came to be understood the primary importance in sustaining of life.

Galen became the most prolific writers of medicine during his times. Observing wounded warriors, he became aware of the difference in mortality and the color of the blood. It's venous with low oxygen having delivered the oxygen through the capillaries to the cells and bluish in color under low pressure on its way back to the lungs where it is deoxygenated and then to the heart. He recognized that it was reversed when the blood was red while blood was gushing through the wounds and was being pumped from the heart with a fresh supply of oxygen back to the capillaries.

He didn't call them veins and arteries but did describe that they were like the "intricate threads of a fisherman's net which not the hands of man could compete with the delicacy of their composition or the complexity of network." One of his greatest observations is that one of the largest and most important parts of this network was the large artery (carotid), which takes off from a larger artery (ascending aorta) that starts at the heart and goes to the brain (Fig.8).

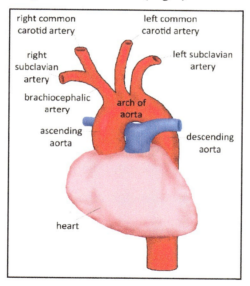

(Fig.8) (Wikipedia) This is a very important picture. The heart is depicted as the pump that supplies and circulates the blood through the body. All the blood leaves the heart through the ascending aorta as depicted. All subsequent arteries like pipes that supply water to your household initially emanate from the aorta. In this picture, you can see the carotid arteries to the brain coming off the aortic arch as the aorta makes a 180-degree turn to supply the lower body.

Also, Galen made some wonderful observations that are important in terms of what we're going to review later, which are depicted in (Fig.9), which is from the works of Galen and his pupils. Like the previous image, this anatomic figure from the works of Galen reveals some astounding relationships. First and foremost, look at the lungs and the right ventricle on the left side of the picture (remember that the right ventricle is the right side of the heart from the bodies perspective). Note that blue blood enters the right ventricle and is pumped into the lungs through the "Vena Arterialis."

This is key. It's the first time that attention is brought on this pathway, which is the pulmonary artery and the only artery in the body that carries blue or deoxygenated blood. Obviously, Galen was ambivalent and covered his bases by calling it both an artery and a vein, while something that can cause confusion is the fact the this vessel is a blue blood artery. In similar fashion, he labels "Arteria Venialis," the vessel that leads out of the lungs with oxygenated red blood into the left ventricle that is then pumped into the aorta.

Again, Galen covers his bases and is ambivalent about the name of this structure, which we now know as the pulmonary vein, the only vein in the body that carries red blood. The pulmonary vein has some very important implication, and later, we'll discuss atrial fibrillation and its cure with what is called "Pulmonary Vein Ablation and Isolation." Please remember for now that these relationships are the key importance.

Note that the right and left ventricle is separated by the septum. If you refer to (Fig.9), you'll see nicely that the septum is a muscle that is between the right and left ventricle. This septum is important to understand as some people are born with a ventricular septal defect, a varying size hole in the septum that allows blood to flow between the ventricles in both ways—red to blue blood or blue to red blood bypassing the lungs.

Additionally, there's a condition that runs in families called idiopathic hypertrophic obstructive cardiomyopathy. This disease is where the muscle of the interventricular septum becomes very thick (hypertrophied) and blocks the blood as it leaves the ventricle through the aortic valve into the aorta. So, this leads to inappropriate hypertrophy of the left ventricular muscle and can have ominous implications in terms of sudden cardiac death. Again, we'll cover all these conditions later, but I hope that you just note the names and how these diseases relate to these anatomic drawings.

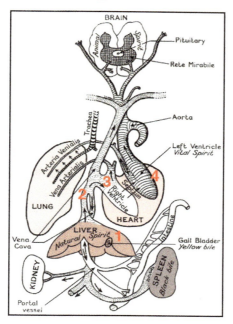

(Fig.9) (jap.physiology.org) This is a remarkable picture from Galen that should be studied and understood in detail.

It's exciting to realize that Galen was the father of modern vascular surgery, cardiac surgery, and neurosurgery. He laid the framework for the specialty of cardiology in the domain of internal medicine. He wrote "The heart is, as it were, the hearthstone and source of the innate heat by which the animal is governed." Most importantly, he observed that the heart was made up of "fibers" that were hard and not easily injured. He correctly envisioned that the heart enlarges then "collapsing" and expelling its contents to perform nature's job in ridding the body of its "residues." However, he incorrectly argued, in contradiction to Aristotle, that the heart was in secondary importance compared to other organs such as the liver that produced "healing humors." His ideas predominated medicine until up to the seventeenth century when it was realized that immediate death followed when the heart stopped.

Lastly, Galen may have made his most important contribution to modern cardiology by being the first physician to describe the heart as consisting of two major chambers: the right and left ventricles. He deduced that these were the chambers responsible for pumping the blood, but there is no evidence that he understood or recognized the other two chambers of the heart: the right and left atrium. Interestingly, he described the valves in the heart that separated the upper and lower chambers although he didn't know their important function.

I think it's time to advance to the next level in understanding the anatomy of the heart. We will build upon what was learned from (Fig.9), tracing it step by step like Galen. Thus, in (Fig.10), we see the four chambers of the heart: the right atrium, right ventricle, left atrium, and the left ventricle. In (Fig.8), we saw the aorta as it came off the heart, which was depicted as a rather basic single chamber "pump." Now, however, we can see that the aorta emanates from the left ventricle. I know that it's difficult to translate a 2D picture into a 3D object, but it's essential that you study this depiction of the heart to construct in your mind the spatial relationships of these chambers and see in your mind the aorta as it comes out of the left ventricle.

Of equal importance in the anatomy of these chambers, we have to go one giant leap further. There's a very specific translation of the heart's structure into its functionality; there's an almost mystical way the physical makeup of the heart. I know this sounds rather esoteric, so I'll make it simple. If you know the structure of the heart, then how and why it functions will make all the sense in the world.

So, let's take a look at the blue and red colors in (Fig.10). On the right side of the heart is the blue blood. As we discussed before, the blue represents flowing blood that is low on oxygen as it has dropped off its oxygen load to the body. The blood then comes back to the right side of the heart to be given a "boost" in its speed and force as the right side of the heart pumps blood into the lungs to receive a new load of oxygen. Thus, the blue blood first arrives at the right atrium then pumped by the right ventricle directly into the pulmonary artery into lungs.

At this point, you may wonder why the need for two chambers rather than just the right ventricle. For now, you just need to understand the road the blood takes and the exact need and function. The right atrium working with the right ventricle will be discussed later. The depiction of the blood low on oxygen as blue is simply a reflection of this blood being darker and somewhat bluish with a depleted and low oxygen content as compared to the reddish blood that exits the lungs filled with life sustaining oxygen. Once the blood picks ups oxygen from the lungs, it flows into the left atrium and empties into the left ventricle where it pumps the high octane oxygenated blood into the aorta and to the body.

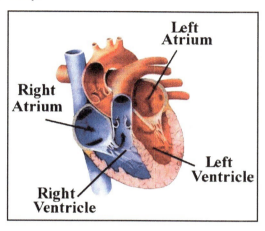

(Fig.10) (www.topnews.in) Again, a very important figure of the heart and the path of oxygenated and deoxygenated blood.

Next, it's the ancient Romans from 43 B.C.E. to 200 C.E. They understood the life-sustaining importance of the heart as evidenced by a quote from Ovid: "Although Aesculapius himself, who is the Greek deity of medicine, applies the herbs, by no means can he cure the wounds of the heart." In this same era, the most important classical physician of the time was Claudius Galenus, who was the personal physician to the Roman emperor, Marcus Aurelius. He makes several important points concerning the heart that apply today including the description of the heart valves and two ventricles with a further distinction between veins and arteries.

MODERN ERA OF THE AMERICANS AND EUROPE

We now enter the modern era of early Americans (100 C.E.-900 C.E.) that recognized the importance of the heart. The ancient Teotihuacan culture in Mexico believed the Teyolia, the spiritual force associated with the heart, must remain within the body at all times, or the person will die. One can only assume that they must've made this empirical observation during ritual human sacrifice!

A great deal of cosmological thought and spirituality seems to have underlain each of the Aztec sacrificial rites. The most common form of human sacrifice was heart extraction. The Aztec believed that the heart (tona) was both the seat of the individual and a fragment of the Sun's heat (istli). To this day, the Nahua considers the Sun to be a heart-soul (tona-tiuh). In the Aztec view, humanity's "divine sun fragments" were considered "entrapped" by the body and its desires. And the round pulsating heart gave heat and life to the body. Human sacrifice was documented in the "Codex Nagliabechiano" seen in (fig.11) that vividly illustrates the central theme these cultures placed in the pulsating heart. It's amazing that the depiction of the heart is similar to the cave pictograms of early man in (Fig.1).

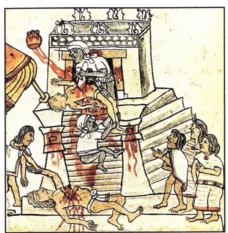

(Fig.11) Human sacrifice before the temple and the priest with cutting out the heart. Heart extraction was viewed as a means of liberating the istli and reuniting it with the sun, wherein a victim's transformed heart flies Sunward on a trail of blood.

Next, we enter an age of relative enlightenment (1000 - 1400). During this time, the Church contributed much to the knowledge of the physical world as it related to theology. Importantly, images of the Sacred Heart became "of paramount importance as emitting ethereal light and suffering wounds which is seen equating to Jesus Crist and his love."(Fig.12).

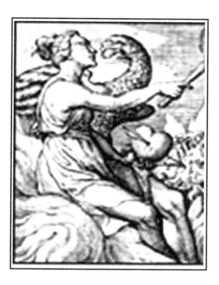

Fig.12 (photobucket.com) The depiction of the holy heart and his wounded heart as he gave his life depicted as an arrow in the heart with the serpent of worldly sins."....Only the Heart of Christ who knows the depths of his Father's love could reveal to us the abyss of his mercy in so simple and beautiful a way" from the Catechism. P:1439.

Next, we see the central place of the heart as depicted in the images of Christ (Fig.13) and the Immaculate Mary (Fig.14) and how much of a central theme was placed on the heart as to the soul of Jesus Christ and Mary. During the middle Ages, devotion to the Sacred Heart is constantly seen in prayers and doctrine, which remains today.

During this time period, the teachings of Galen and Hippocrates are followed. But there are no new medical advances regarding the heart. Middle age physicians relied mainly upon observation, palpation of the pulse, and examination of the urine. Referring back to the teachings of Galen, they recognized that an irregular pulse was often associated with weakness, shortness of breath, and premature death. Like their predecessors, they relied on herbal remedies but did perform some basic surgery such as amputation in case of gangrene of the feet. They also recognized syncope (fainting or the loss of consciousness) as a malady of the heart and was often associated with extreme heat or occurring in the Church. We now know this as a syndrome called "Church Syncope" caused by long periods of sitting still or kneeling in prolonged prayer then suddenly standing often with mild dehydration and heighted emotions in the praise of Christ.

Christian physicians were strictly forbidden to dissect the human body. Thus, little of our knowledge regarding the heart was advanced during this time. In medieval Europe, there was an emphasis on human suffering as experienced by Jesus and this severely limited study of the heart and the practice of medicine as a healer of the suffering. This was done by the church. The biggest event in the popularization of the heart symbol was when it began to be included on playing cards during the 15th century. Painters and sculptors started using the symbol more frequently without the previous association with Christ. Hearts were now everywhere from coats of arms to gravestones. The meaning of the heart took on love, fidelity, and bravery.

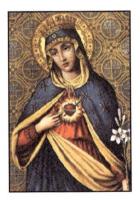 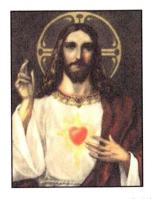

(Fig.13) Immaculate Mary   (Fig.14) The heart of Christ

Thus, the research into the heart was severely limited in Medieval Europe. However during this time, there was an Arab physician, Avicenna, who made significant strides in his astute study of the heart. Most importantly, he challenged previously accepted doctrine regarding the process of oxygenation of the blood. First, he felt that there were no pores within the muscular interventricular septum that allowed blue blood and red blood to mix. This was the way previous scholar hypothesized that blood became oxygenated.

Avicenna was the first to correctly assert that the blood was mixed with air in the lungs, and obstruction with this process would cause severe shortness of breath. Although not specifically described, he was probably referring to chronic obstructive pulmonary disease (COPD), which severely restrict the exchange of air into the blood within the lungs. He knew of no specific cause of this disease but did recognize the association of this syndrome as well as others such as chronic abscess or infection—also a long-term association with death from heart disease.

Interestingly, this association of chronic infection and heart disease has only recently been understood in that the festering long term infection is related to inflammation of the coronary arteries and lead to premature collection of fat and hardening of the arteries. Equally compelling is the reason Avicenna was able to describe these diseases, which was that contrary to Medieval Europe, smoking of the hookah or water pipe with "shisha" or tobacco was ingrained in the social structure of Arabic and Persian society.

This method of inhaling vaporized tobacco was associated with large concentrations of nicotine, tar, and cyanide, which is a primary cause of heart attacks and vasculopathies. This was the result of diffuse atherosclerosis of the body's arteries including: carotids and strokes (arteries of the arms and loss of digits.), arteries leading into the kidney with resultant hypertension and kidney failure with dialysis, arteries of the leg with claudication or pain in the legs with non-healing sores and gangrene with loss of limb, and premature vascular dementia (hardening of the brain arteries with resultant loss of mental function and dementia with multiple strokes.)

Now, there's a 50-70% increase in these diseases in smokers over nonsmokers, which is an astounding statistic. It's interesting to hypothesize whether these Arabic doctors made the association to the multitude of other syndromes and diseases associated with smoking including premature aging, ulcers and bleeding, early facial wrinkles, cancers and growths in the breasts, GI tract masses, and skin disease with obvious inflammation. As a cardiologist, it never ceased to amaze me that within 20 seconds of observing a patient, I was able to determine if a patient was a chronic smoker 99% of the time.

These smokers were frail beyond their years, thin limbed with atrophied muscles, pale or even cyanotic with a bluish complexion, short of breath with distended chests and abdomens, wrinkled skinned, chronically ill with a multitude of complaints, and often prematurely, even at a young age, intellectually challenged. Avicenna noted these chronically ill patients from suffering difficulty in oxygen exchange in the lungs, but there is no indication he made the association of these conditions directly to smoking.

It truly seems amazing to me as a cardiologist that these early observations seem to fall on modern day deaf ears in all levels of society and government with billions of dollars in unnecessary medical cost and loss of life and limb simply due to smoking with any form of tobacco as the vaporized nicotine have essentially the same toxins. As usual, the quest for money simply overshadows rational and reasonable prohibitions for those who simply are addicted and know no better do invariably become a medical burden on society and their families.

As a closing piece of literary license, it's my strong belief that an aspect of the vicious cycle of ghetto life and poverty is directly related to smoking. The number of heart and vascular disease in the black poverty level far exceeds the national average. Thus, it's not surprising to see that the greatest number of smokers in the United States is within the poor, black population. Subsequently, this sociological group remains also the greatest medically uninsured. When heart or vascular disease strikes this group, they can't afford the massive expense. There's increase probability for early death of a child's parent and the psychological trauma of a one parent childhood.

Furthermore, the highest exposure to second hand smoke occurs in the homes and the cars, and the children are exposed to smoke, which can lead to stunting of their intellectual development. It only perpetuate the cycle of poverty as they underachieve at school and end up with menial jobs. The scourge of drugs and smoking simply doom this population to remain forever "chained to the slave ship" of poverty and illiteracy while our leaders do absolutely nothing to recognize the problem. And the tobacco companies simply enslave the ghetto and make fortunes off people's misery and despair.

RENAISSANCE

Well, enough talking about smoking and the ancient physicians. Let's cover the most exciting time of the Renaissance, which I consider truly the beginning of many new developments that shaped modern cardiology and our anatomic knowledge of the heart. This will be an extensive review of the principal anatomists of the time. As you may have noticed, I referred to them as anatomists, not doctors because medicine and surgery was practiced primarily by "Barbers." Some were trained in the medical schools of the time, but most were individuals with practical knowledge of medicine and surgery passed down through the generations and who just put out their shingles.

There was an exponential explosion of intellect, observation, and knowledge with the renewed practice of dissection and analysis of disease that could've been due to the decline in the power of the Church to govern everyday life and stifle creativity. The Renaissance revival of anatomy facilitated the physicians to redefine and resolve much of the ambiguity regarding the structures of the heart. The development of cardiology as an off branch of medicine began. The relationship of the structures of the heart became evident, and the function of the heart was found to be a primary organ that's essential for life.

Here's an interesting story in the late Renaissance. A son of an aristocrat survived a devastating accident that left him with a gaping hole in his chest. With his heart exposed, it could be seen and touched while it was beating. With this, the coronary arteries running on the surface of the heart could be seen as well as the pounding of the heart, which corresponded to the pulse in the wrist and was correlated with the blood circulating through the body. Thus, the anatomist could compare what he saw in dissection to the basic functions and anatomy seen in a real beating heart. This allowed them for the first time to bridge the anatomic knowledge with the real time functioning of the heart (Fig.15).

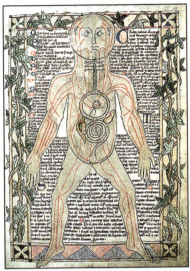

(Fig.15) With this Renaissance rendering of the circulation, this drawing shows that the physicians were aware that red blood emanated from the heart in the center of the chest and supplied the blood to the brain, organs, and the extremities.

Next, we'll cover Flemish anatomist and physician, Andreas Vesalius (1514-1564), who published the book "De Humani Corporus Fabrica (On the structure of the Human Body)" in Greek, Latin, Arabic, and Hebrew, and is considered the father of modern anatomy. He performed dissections with a collection of students in an amphitheater, making a detailed investigation into the circulatory system. With printing available during this time, distributing highly detailed and reproducible pictures of the anatomy was possible. Also, he attended various medical schools, but at last, he graduated Magna Cum Laude with a Doctor of Medicine after passing two days of rigorous tests. He was versed in many languages. His work was disseminated throughout the civilized world, which led to a significant expansion in medicine in many countries.

In terms of the heart, Vesalius confirmed that the beating of the heart corresponded directly to the timing of the pulse. However, he went one step further and described that when the heart beats irregularly, the pulse also beats irregularly, and the power of the pulse seemed to vary from beat to beat. Therefore, this corresponds to what we now know as atrial fibrillation in that the magnitude of the blood ejection from beat to beat changes and affects the power of the pulse. It's a very distinct observation in atrial fibrillation on physical examination and is the cause of many symptoms such as palpitations.

In addition, because of his interest in the brain, he was the first to describe the branches of the arteries that came off the aortic arch (the part of the aorta as it leaves the left ventricle and turns to the left). It included the carotid arteries that lead to the brain, and the major arteries that supply the upper extremities. Through his study of traumatic injuries, he was able to deduce that injury to these arteries led to malfunction such as paralysis or stroke in the areas that they supplied.

In (Fig.16), we see the rendering of the heart by Vesalius. The importance of this picture is that he was the first to describe the valves of the heart. In this representation, R stands for the left ventricle. Blood leaves the right ventricle and passes through the aortic valve labeled in this picture as A, B, and C. This valve has the three parts to it (leaflets) and acts as a one way "spigot" that in health prevents blood going backward called aortic regurgitation, which is a disease state we'll discuss later. The valves are no different from a valve in a water pipe that prevents water from flowing the wrong way.

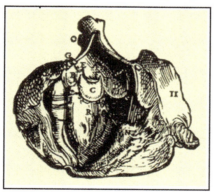

(Fig 16). (faculty.humanities.uci.edu) As discussed above, in this rendering of the heart by Vesalius, A, B, and C represent the three leaflets of the aortic valve as pouch-like structures that separate the left ventricle (R) from the aorta (O). Also, the structure labeled II is the left atrium with the little extension like a tail at the bottom of the left atrium appropriately called the left atrial appendage,

In these next two pictures (Fig.17) and (Fig.18), we see the modern day picture of the four heart valves. If you notice the aortic and pulmonic valve are shaped like a pouch. These two valves have three leaflets shaped like the crescent of the moon, so they're also referred to as the semilunar valves. In his brilliant study of hydrodynamics, we'll soon discuss Leonardo Da Vinci who drew and deduced that these pouch like structures (Fig.19) would balloon back and keep the valves closed after the blood is ejected. And the forward and the backward pressure closes the valves and prevents the blood from going back (regurgitating) into the left and right ventricle.

We now know that this pathological condition creates an audible "murmur" in the heart called aortic regurgitation of the aortic valve and pulmonic regurgitation of the pulmonic valve. Remember, these two valves are very strong, are exposed to high pressure, and are supposed to function properly your whole life. Just try to imagine a car valve lasting that long! One cannot help but be taken aback at the very beauty in nature of such structures.

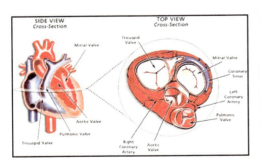 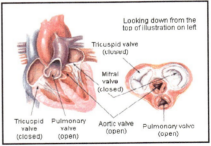

(Fig.17) (www.wwk.in)

(Fig.18) (Wikipedia) In these two figures (17 & 18), one sees modern day drawings of the heart. And it's four valves: the aortic, pulmonic, mitral, and tricuspid. First, the aortic and pulmonic valves are thick and pouch-like. With the aortic valve between the left ventricle and the aorta leading to the systemic circulation, the pulmonic valve between the right ventricle and the pulmonary artery leading to the lungs. Similarly, the tricuspid and mitral valves are thinner and tethered to the heart muscle by chordae. The tricuspid valve separates the right atrium from the right ventricle, and the mitral valve is between the left atrium where the oxygenated blood comes from the lungs and flows into the left ventricle.

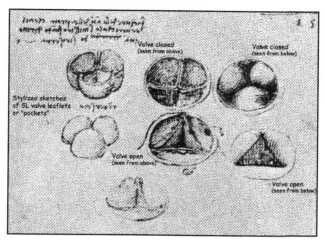

(Fig.19) (www.bbc.co.uk) In this drawing by Da Vinci, the aortic valve or the semilunar valve (SL) is depicted correctly. This pouch-like architecture allows the valves to balloon back and close after the blood is ejected from the left ventricle into the aorta and systemic circulation. The thick and robust nature of the aortic valve allows it to perform under the very high pressures generated during left ventricular systole. If this valve is abnormal at birth or becomes diseased with age, the valve doesn't close completely after systole and the blood can leak back into the left ventricle, which is called aortic regurgitation. If the aortic valve becomes partially closed and won't open completely with systole, this condition is called aortic stenosis.

I introduce the last picture (Fig.19) to you so that you are aware of two more valves of the heart: the mitral and tricuspid valves. If you look, the mitral valve controls the flow of blood from the left atrium into the left ventricle while the tricuspid valve separates the right atrium from the right ventricle. Thus, the heart is a four-chamber structure in contradistinction to previous belief of the heart being a two-chamber organ. At the time of the Renaissance, the atrium was seen but its function was unknown. We'll soon discuss the atrium and their valves, which are subjected to lower pressures than the semilunar valves and have somewhat different structure.

Leonardo da Vinci was an inventor, anatomist, artist, and had a very keen interest in hemodynamics or the study of the flow of liquids. Though he wasn't a physician, his anatomic drawings and analysis were accurate and truly brilliant. First, he correctly established that the heart had two major chambers—the left and the right ventricle separated by a septum that had no mixing of blood through "pores" in the septum. However, he was more accurate in making the observation that the heart had two other chambers with relatively thin muscle that is separated from the ventricles by valves.

The function of these minor chambers was not known then, but we now know the right and left atrium are separated from the right ventricle by the tricuspid valve and separated from the left ventricle by the mitral valve. With his knowledge of the flow of liquids, he correctly deduced that with the blood separated by the valves could not flow in opposite directions. Although this seems intuitive, it was when the separate function of the atrium and the ventricles was realized.

He felt that the right ventricle contracts and expels blood while the atrium dilates to accept blood to feed into the ventricle. Although this concept seems logical, I think it's important that the readers of this book ends up with a firm understanding of these relationships. In the same light, he also drew the function of the aortic valve, which separated the left ventricle from the aorta and how blood is ejected into the body. These atrium and atrial-valves are essential to the function of the heart and the maintenance of the heart beat specifically when we delve into the electrical mechanisms of the heart. The doctor of this specialty is called an Electrophysiologist who specialize Electrophysiology.

Initially, Da Vinci's knowledge came from the dissection of bovine and pig's hearts. We know this because his initial study of the heart contained moderator bands which are much larger in the bovine heart than in the human heart. These are interesting structures whose function was unknown until recently. These thick ridges of muscle prevent the heart from dilating (enlarging) when the heart is under critical stress such as while one is engaged in heavy exercise. These bands can enlarge (hypertrophy) pathologically (causing disease) in professionally trained athletes. In this case, they can obstruct the outflow of blood from the ventricles, lead to congestive heart failure, and pathological dilation at rest in the ventricles.

More importantly, these bands contain electrical fibers (conduction system), and these can actually become the source of fatal irregularities of the heart and "sudden cardiac death," which is becoming more common in the trained athletes. Da Vinci's astute observations have a great implication for modern medicine. It's astounding to me what a keen mind and observation can achieve it the advancement of science.

It's also said that Da Vinci was one of the first to establish the result of aging on the coronary circulation of the heart. He dissected the body of a 100 year old man shortly after he died and described the coronary arteries as thickened and tortuous, and totally occluded often at places where the vessel was most tortuous. He noticed, due to his interest in hemodynamics, that the most sand and deposits are accumulated at the bends in a river. So, he compared these same processes to the coronary circulation, which is due to the accumulation of fat or "atheroma." In the drawing of the heart by Da Vinci (Fig.20), it's clear that he accurately noted the coronary arteries as they traveled across the outside or the epicardium of the heart.

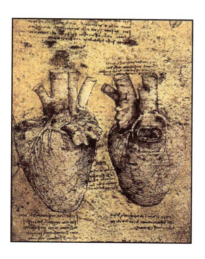

(Fig.20). (www2.warwick.ac.uk) In the left drawing, the small arteries that run along the surface or epicardium of the heart are the coronary arteries. Generally, there are three major arteries: the left main (LM) artery that divides into the left anterior descending artery (LAD), the circumflex (CX), and the right coronary artery (RCA). They seem to emanate from the aorta, which is true but they actually start at the pouches of the aortic valve at the coronary ostium (origin). With this examination, Da Vinci became aware that the coronary arteries of an old person is hard and full of buildup, which we now know are collections of fat and calcium called atheroma that leads to heart attacks.

These examinations of the older heart were followed by the dissection of a two year old child. In this, he observed that the arteries were without thickening, and were straight, without folds or tortuosity. He made the distinction between an old river with bends and a young stream that is straight and without sandbars collecting at the bends of the river. Da Vinci was keen on making observations that the body mimics what's found in physical nature that was mirrored in inventions such as his flying machines that mimicked a bird's wings.

By the middle of the sixteenth century and following the teaching of Da Vinci, many physicians started to accept the fact that the arterial and venous blood were truly separate, and in health, there was no mixing of the blood from the right to the left ventricle through the septum. Yet it wasn't until English physician, William Harvey, in his visionary book, On the Circulation of the Heart (1628), established these concepts and modern ideas of circulation.

Harvey made another key observation in his book. He wrote that the heart is actively working when the ventricles are small and expel the blood into the lungs and the body (systole). When dilated and relaxed (diastole), the ventricles are receiving blood to be subsequently pumped. 100 years later, these ideas were generally accepted, but they're the basis for how the heart functions as a pumping organ. Harvey was the first to advance the concept that the circulation is a closed system that continuously pumps the blood in a circle from the left ventricle to the aorta, the vena cava, right ventricle, the lungs, and back to the left ventricle. However, he wasn't aware of the function of the lungs, which didn't occur until the nineteenth century.

Various calculations that Harvey made challenged the notion of Galen by deducing that that blood is continuously being generated heart beat to heart beat rather than at times lying stagnant. He based this on the following calculations.

1. The weight of blood in the body was 2 ounces. Thus if the heart beat 70/minute the heart would pump: 70 X 2 oz. = 9 pounds of blood per minute.

2. In an hour, the heart would pump 540 lbs. of blood: 60 min X 9 lbs. = 540 lbs.

3. In 24 hours, the heart would pump 6.4 tons of blood: 24 hrs. X 540 lbs. = 6.4 tons.

Now, if you're not amazed by 6.4 tons of blood pumped by the heart per day, I certainly am. What is humbling is that this goes on every day for a lifetime. Certainly, no man made pump can even come close to this in terms of longevity and sheer volume it produces. So, Da Vinci concluded that the heart kept the blood flowing through the body in a never ending continuous circle throughout one's lifetime.

I'd like to point something out at this point, which may be intuitively obvious. Of course, there's continuous regeneration and maintenance of all the cells of the heart. Some organs such as the brain have none or limited function to replicate and repair damaged cells. However, heart has a constant replacement of the cells, which are simply worn out. Thus, the organs of the body can maintain themselves in health for a lifetime. When a part of the heart is damaged in a heart attack, that part is irreversible damaged. A heart attack occurs when the closed artery deprives blood to the part of the heart—myocardial infarction—where the section of the heart muscle is dead. In this circumstance, the heart muscle cannot regenerate because there is no effective blood supply.

However, over time, arteries of the heart can actually grow and supply blood from another artery to the damaged section. These are called collaterals. Some of the cells are in limbo (stunned) yet not dead. They cannot operate normally because the blood supply is marginal and most of the muscle is dead. Recently, some investigators have actually been injecting stem cells into the damaged arteries, and miraculously, actual growth of new cells around the architecture of the heart structure replaced the dead cells. Obviously, this is truly an amazing discovery and certainly brightens the outlook for patients who have suffered a myocardial infarction with resultant death of some heart muscle and severe failure of their hearts (cardiomyopathy and congestive heart failure).

At this time, there was no conjecture of how and what made the heart beat in this regular and synchronized fashion on the average 70 times per minute. We now know it's the function of the conduction system of the heart, which is the realm of study called Electrophysiology. It's the complex yet organized interplay of the mechanics and electrical conduction system of the heart, which keeps healthy heart beating regularly (normal sinus rhythm) for our lifetime. It's only diseased heart that beats irregularly, which disrupts the pumping of the heart (arrhythmias). Common examples are atrial fibrillation (AF), paroxysmal supraventricular tachycardia (PSVT), and ventricular tachycardia (VT) with premature ventricular contractions (PVCs).

THE BEGINNING OF MODERN MEDICINE

The eighteenth and nineteenth centuries saw an explosion of knowledge regarding the heart as well as the modern medicine for the treatment of certain heart ailments.

Extremely important in this endeavor was the British physician and botanist, William Withering (1741-1799). He was called upon to evaluate a folk remedy that seemed to be effective for a condition that was called dropsy, which was the accumulation of the fluid in the body. We now know that it's congestive heart failure in which one of its manifestations is edema of the body (Fig.21). In his analysis, the concoction consisting of twenty herbs and with trial and error in his patients, he found that the herb foxglove was the active ingredient. I can't stress enough the discovery of foxglove as it's the active ingredient in the medicine digitalis or digoxin that are used extensively in contemporary medicine to strengthen the heart and to aid in the control of the rapid and irregular heart rate principally in atrial fibrillation, atrial flutter, and atrial tachycardia.

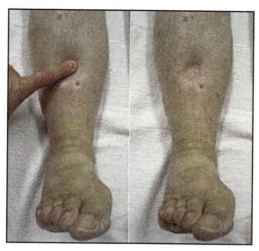

(Fig.21) (en.wikipedia.org) In this photograph, we see the physical finding of edema of the leg due to increased fluid in the body because of congestive heart failure. Placement of pressure on the leg causes the physical finding of pitting edema were the excess fluid is temporarily expelled from the pressure point on the leg. Undoubtedly, Doctor Withering in his treatment of congestive heart failure with foxglove observed that much of this swelling would resolve after treatment with the drug. In patients with congestive heart failure, this edema of the legs is often the initial complaint of patients with fluid retention due to weakening of the heart.

This active ingredient, foxglove, is part of a group of drugs call cardiac glycosides. Not only did Withering document the efficacy of foxglove in the treatment of dropsy, but he and his contemporary physicians published an article for the College of Physicians in London that described the successful use of foxglove in treating dropsy and what was called cardiac consumption. Cardiac consumption is now known as pulmonary edema where there is excess fluid accumulation in the lungs or edema in the body seen with dropsy or congestive heart failure.

They made the observation on its effect to rid the body of excessive edema of the legs. In more advanced case of dropsy, the excess edema affected the whole body, which is called anasarca. They also realized that the drug cleared these conditions by apparently increasing the urine output, or in modern terms, act a diuretic. In actuality, the drug is not a direct diuretic on the kidney, but foxglove acts to augment the heart muscle strength and makes it more effective in clearing the fluid "backed up" in lungs or pulmonary edema (Fig.22).

In addition, Withering described the action of foxglove in slowing the often rapid and irregular heart rate or pulse associated with dropsy. The cardiac glycosides block the electrical connection from the atrium to the ventricles, which basically make it slow the heart rate especially in atrial fibrillation, the heart rhythm often seen in patients with congestive heart failure (Fig.23).

Now, we know this to be the effect of digitalis to effect the sodium-potassium (Na-K) pumps that are seen in both the heart muscle and the fibers of electrical connections in the heart and to augment the inotropic effect (strengthening of the heart muscle pump) that is the main action of digitalis. Simply put, this observation led to the development of other cardiac glycosides and similar drugs that greatly enhanced the efficacy of digitalis in these conditions.

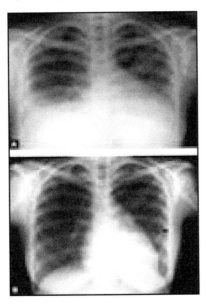

(Fig.22) At this point, I want to introduce a picture of a chest x-ray that illustrates the finding of pulmonary edema or the build of fluid within the lungs due to congestive heart failure. On the bottom, you see a chest x-ray with the white heart in the middle and the lungs around it in black, indicating that they're just air with no opacities that tells pathology within the lungs. In contrast, in the upper chest x-ray, one can see the heart borders are not as well defined and much of the bottom part of the lung is replaced by white. That is the x-ray manifestation of fluid buildup in the lung or pulmonary edema. Obviously, chest x-rays were developed a long time after Withering, but without question, he was able to hear the patient wheezing and see severe shortness of breath, and again, there is resolution of much of these findings and symptoms after the administration of foxglove along with limiting the patient's salt intake.

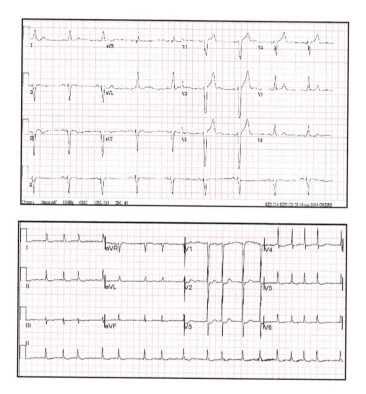

(Fig.23) I introduce these electrocardiograms (EKG) at this time to explain the rhythm of atrial fibrillation in which digitalis is utilized to treat. The EKG machine was not invented until the 20th century, but it's familiar to most people because they get hooked up to a bunch of electrodes to record the EKG at the doctor's office.

Basically, the EKG is a recording of the electrical activity of the heart. In the top tracing, we see an EKG with normal sinus rhythm (NSR). The large deflections are called the QRS and represent one heartbeat. It's important to notice that these deflections are regular in nature with the intervals between the QRS's evenly spaced meaning that the heart beat is regular in nature as in should be in health. Thus, Withering would've noted a regular and slow pulse in the normal patient. However, the second EKG represents the abnormal rhythm of atrial fibrillation.

Note that the intervals or spacing between the QRS complexes are now irregular and of different durations. Also, the spacing is less than the EKG of NSR, meaning that the pulse rate is both faster and irregular. This is how Withering would've diagnosed atrial fibrillation, which he treated with foxglove and salt restriction. With the slowing or reversion of the heart to a regular rhythm, he would've regarded this as success. Today, this method of finding the right treatment out of repeated successful outcomes is called "evidence based medicine."

Lastly, Withering also described the side effects of ingesting too much foxglove. In cases of accidental or purposeful ingestion of the drug, the patient would present with profound nausea and vomiting with actual increase in the amount of fluid in the body. This was simultaneously associated with a marked slowing of the heartbeat, which could lead to loss of consciousness or fainting (syncope). Basically, too much digitalis causes an overwhelming of these Na-K pumps in the heart and makes them malfunction. This leads to a block in the conduction of electricity in the heart and makes the muscle weak in its pumping action, both resulting in death.

MODERN CARDIOLOGY

Well, now we come to the exciting period of an explosion in medical knowledge regarding the heart that heralded modern medicine. Our main focus will be on the heart and cardiology, but we'll also make a special effort to review the advances in electrophysiology, the study of the heart rhythms. We've reviewed atrial fibrillation and the electrical system of the heart. This time period was highlighted by a multitude of small advances that added up to how medicine and cardiology are practiced today. So, let's delve into this exciting period of time from 1800-1950.

Many of the medical milestones have been discussed, but I'll often digress and discuss the effect to the practice and the process of diagnosis and treatment of cardiological diseases. These discussions will become more frequent as we approach the multitude of cardiac diseases, so take note if you want to be enabled to navigate the remarkable complexities of modern medical care. Unfortunately, most of patients have the expectation that somehow modern medicine will take care of them and lead to a cure. This is simply not true anymore, and there has been a dramatic loss of this trust as it has been since antiquity and at the beginning of modern medicine.

The day of the private practitioner making house calls and practicing medicine to the benefit of the patient are long gone. As we learned, your best interests aren't the top priority when it comes to insurance reimbursement and Medicare. If the purpose of this book is to empower the patients to optimize their care, the discussions of contemporary medicine becomes increasingly important to navigate through the increasingly complex and expensive modern cardiological care. With Obamacare, bureaucratic and "corporate" medical care don't operate for the betterment of the patient but rather to increase patient turnover. Ultimately, it's to increase profits and delivery of optimal medical care for patient's unique needs isn't part of the equation.

One of the principal tools of the physician is the physical examination. A weaknesses in contemporary practice is that the physician does a cursory examination of the patient, forgetting about, or not having learned, the importance of a timely physical examination. This is mainly due to the time restraints placed upon the physician. More often than not, medical schools rely more on computers to teach rather than hands on examination of the patient, so the modern day physician is simply not equipped to utilize these appropriate tools of physical diagnosis.

Equally, with the advent of "corporate" owned medicine, the physician is often on a quota system and just doesn't have the time for an adequate physical examination. Under these circumstances, the doctor's skills are not measured in his ability to make a successful diagnosis but the profit he makes for the business. Thus, as the patient, one must be aware of these realities. During the physical examination, demand this level of care or approach the results of limited attention with caution as you take the next step of your cardiological care.

As we go on in the rest of this book, I will point out the pitfalls of such care, and teach the patient to realize optimal medical outcomes (cured) and in a cost-effective manner.

For instance, Austrian physician Joseph Leopold Auenbrugger (1722-1809) found that one could detect forms of heart disease by laying a hand on the chest and tapping the finger over the hand to sense the noise made by this tapping motion. This maneuver is called percussion that is mainly utilized to detect areas of the lungs that contain too much fluid. The dullness in the sound signifies fluid buildup in contrast to a crisp hollow sound of clean air in the lungs.

In actuality, it's a very effective technique, especially in skilled hands, in evaluating the cause of shortness of breath and detecting pulmonary edema without the benefit of the chest x-ray, which would be developed years later. There's similarity in utilizing evidence-based medicine such as the employment of foxglove that led to a cure, the normalization of percussion of the lung, and advanced the use of digitalis for the treatment of dropsy. These techniques are rarely utilized today as they've been replaced by the chest x-rays and CAT scans.

Although these newer modalities are certainly effective tools, they're also far more expensive especially in the case of the CAT scan. And in most cases, percussion would've been sufficient. Truthfully, all that's needed in 99% of the case is percussion in conjunction with a chest x-ray. Often, unnecessary CAT scans of the chest are done, adding more medical expense to the patient and significant profit to those who own the CAT scan machine. These organizations and hospitals need to justify the purchase of incredibly exorbitant machines without any overall benefit to your medical care or clinical outcome and simply add to your costs.

Before moving on to the next subject, I want to add an important component that you as the patient should understand. It relates to the example of the modern day diagnosis and treatment of congestive heart failure. As I've said, the technique of percussion is very accurate in detecting fluid on the lung, and with the chest x-ray, the diagnosis of congestive heart failure can be made 99% of the time. But the use of the CAT scan for the chest doesn't add anything to the diagnosis, except in 1% of the difficult cases. Unfortunately, new physicians and cardiologists have lost good physical examination as a tool and rely on unnecessary scans just because they exist as a modality.

For that matter, many doctors orders CT scans over the phone before they ever see the patient. This certainly increases the profit for the entity who owns the machine, but it increase the patient's bill by $4,000-$5,000 for an unnecessary test. The stark fact is they depend on profits generated by costly but unnecessary, excessive diagnostic and interventional procedures that have a high medical reimbursement to justify their existence. The long term solution would be physician-driven utilization management where every doctor's goal is cost-effective and quality health care system that operates in the best interest of the patient.

An important factor in this equation is the "WIIGS" syndrome (What-if-I-get-sued-syndrome). We'll discuss this more in the last chapter along with the cure for the dysfunctional American medical system. This is where the doctor practices defensive medicine, with the only aim in defending against a possible lawsuit. An effective health system should replace the fee-driven, adversarial malpractice system. In the American litigious arrangements, there are tremendous returns on malicious and unfounded medical lawsuits, yielding ridiculous awards. A system that relies on unbiased arbitration based on the standard of medical practice would alleviate the common legal concerns of physicians, who has to order unnecessary and expensive diagnostic tests just to "protect their butts."

Since our legislative system seems incapable and unwilling to change, it becomes the educated patient's duty to protect themselves, monitoring and questioning what they see as unnecessary and excessively expensive tests for their cardiological care. Now, medical insurance companies properly require preapproval for many tests to prevent abuse of the ordering of elective procedures or surgeries, but the patients should be vigilant as well.

Unfortunately, the "WIIGS" syndrome is present in the majority of our physicians in American medicine. The basis of this situation is beyond the scope of this book, but the fact is that the tort system of medical malpractice is totally abused and distorted. The fear of a lawsuit accounts for up to 90% of useless tests being ordered just because the tests exist and their omission could be used in a malpractice suit. In the case of congestive heart failure, there is a lack of knowledge or skill in percussion, so the physician has little trust in the defense of his diagnosis and must utilize these newer modalities. Also, lawyers, with no clue and no personal gain to learn the proper practice of medicine, can convince a jury, who have no medical knowledge, that these newer tests are necessary.

Because our legislators and Obamacare refuse to rectify this appalling situation, the uneducated patient will simply see his medical bill skyrocket if he cannot defend his own care. In the example of a CAT scan, you can simply tell the doctor that it's unnecessary or have him explain why he feels the need for your case. If he's aware that you know what you're talking about, he won't feel so compelled to do so and maybe even feel fearful of retribution in its abuse.

The problem is a small proportion of patient can suffer from allergic reactions including death, renal failure and dialysis, or shock because of the unnecessary CT scan. This is an example of how defensive medicine can actually be not only expensive but deadly. So, you, as the patient, must direct your care for the correct and cost-efficient diagnosis when it comes to the multitude of heart diseases. Although the physician may resent the "uppity" behavior of the patient, his fear of the consequence of abuse may ultimately result in your proper care.

Another significant advancement, which permanently changed medicine especially in cardiology, was the development of the stethoscope by Rene-Theophile-Hyacinthe Laennee (1782-1826) (Fig.23). Before this invention, Harvey listened to the sounds of the heart by simply putting his ears to the chest. Laennee utilized an amplifying head or diaphragm made out of a paper cylinder and set upon wooden earpieces to amplify the sound of the heart to make it easier to evaluate their abnormalities. The stethoscope greatly expanded the cardiologists' knowledge of various heart murmurs and sounds, which are noises created when blood moves through diseased heart valves. This process is called auscultation of the heart and lungs.

The stethoscope allowed the physician to diagnose disease much earlier thereby improving the chances for survival. For instance in dropsy or pulmonary edema, the stethoscope identified the noise made by fluid in the lung called rales and rhonchi, which corresponded to the fluid buildup seen in the chest x-rays. This finding is aided by percussion of the chest. Additionally, the cardiologist could further define pulmonary edema by identifying certain heart murmurs that could be associated with the heart failure such as aortic valve narrowing or stenosis.

Although the CXR added to the certainty of the diagnosis, in reality, the chest x-ray simply confirms the diagnosis already made by the physician utilizing percussion and auscultation. The consumer of medicine must be very skeptical of further technology, which doesn't necessarily improve your care but only serves to exponentially increase the cost of medical care. The old adage "if it is there utilize it" only adds superfluous tests for your care.

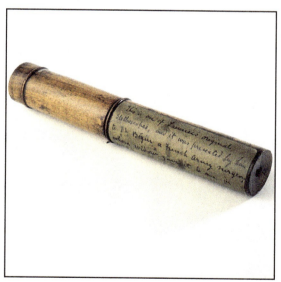

(Fig.23) (www.sciencemuseaum.org.uk) This is a photograph of the first stethoscope utilized by Laennee to listen and record the sounds of the heart and the lungs. It's monaural in nature and is intended to use just one ear, which is placed over the wooden end on the left. The black piece at the other end with a small hole is called the diaphragm that amplifies and defines the sounds of the heartbeat. This piece is placed on the chest at various places over the heart to hear specific pathological heart sounds coming from the ventricles or the atrium.

In the best case scenario, the exam takes a minimum of at least 2-5 minutes, not just a few seconds as is so often done now. Again, it's an art and takes many hours of trial and error practice to get the full benefit and proper information to aid in the diagnosis of cardiac pathology. As a patient, it wouldn't be inappropriate to ask the cardiologist to do a thorough examination in auscultating the heart and to tell you what he heard—now that you're armed with all the information from this book.

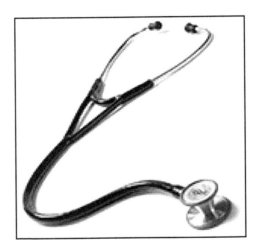

(Fig.24) This is a photograph of a modern day cardiological stethoscope. As I have said, you "know a man (or a woman) by their tools," and it's no different for a physician. This instrument is binaural in that it's intended to be used by both ears. There are two earpieces attached to the metal tubes appropriately called the binaural. These in turn attach to the black, extra thick tubing that's in this stethoscope and has a triangular construction at its origin. This triangular arrangement amplifies and refines the sound from the heart and lungs, making this a very precise stethoscope. Lastly, the tubing attaches to the bell and diaphragm. It's placed on the chest for low and high pitches sounds such as heart murmurs, sounds of disease S3 and S4, opening and closing of heart valves, and lungs rales and wheezes that can be the sign of fluid in the lungs or COPD (chronic obstructive lung disease) and asthma.

When fluid collects around the lungs or the heart, the tissues create a rubbing sound called a friction rub, which is useful in the diagnosing an emergency heart condition called pericarditis. It can mimic the pain of a heart attack and is similar to pleurisy, which is an inflammation of the lining of the lungs. Believe me. You'd gain an instant respect of the doctor if he says that you may have pericarditis, and you ask him if he heard a friction rub!

When I was in medical school, the students spent countless hours in the teaching hospitals listening (auscultating) patient's hearts and lungs of those with specific pathology. We became experts at detecting rales and rhonchi in pulmonary edema. Also, we were able to identify specific heart sounds as murmurs and to what valves these murmurs identified pathologically. We had records that played on old record players that had recordings of all these pathological heart and lung sounds, so we were able to hone our skills further.

It was at this time I realized that I wanted to be a cardiologist and tried to become as perfect as I could be in utilizing my stethoscope. This type of exam takes a very quiet environment and sufficient time. Most of the new cardiologists in the ER take a brief cursory listen to the heart and lungs and probably learn nothing. The ER is too noisy and frenetic to make an accurate assessment with the stethoscope. Since Leannee's development of the stethoscope, its design has been refined over time.

Now, there's a sophisticated kind just for cardiology that is far more sensitive than the simple stethoscope, which is still utilized today and called a nursing stethoscope. This is not to demean the nurses, whom I consider angels of the earth. But the nurse's stethoscopes are usually very basic and unable to detect the fine points of cardiac diagnosis. So, I find it a shame that many doctors, including cardiologist, use or borrow them to listen to the heart. This is why more advanced and expensive testing is used over the right stethoscope to make what could've been an equally accurate diagnosis and could've instantly guided the physician to the proper path of care.

When a patient comes to the ER with pulmonary edema and fluid in their lungs interfering with oxygenation of the blood, expeditious diagnosis with the stethoscope can lead to instant treatment and a much better outcome for the patient without sophisticated, time-consuming tests. It's the basic teaching of medicine that the physicians "do no harm." This is basic to the tenets of the Hippocratic Oath. However, in many emergent cardiac conditions, this is exactly what happens as doctors aren't able to or weren't trained to make a timely diagnosis with observation, palpation, auscultation, and a basic history.

Actually, the CXR and certainly the CT of the chest are just a confirmatory test in many cases, not the primary tool in the making of an immediate and possibly life-saving diagnosis. For example, the problem can be compounded if the patient has a mild headache too, and the doctor orders a simultaneous CT of the head. Such absurd practices by, frankly, ignorant physicians only place the patient's life in jeopardy.

Another unfortunate development in medicine is the utilization of the "Hospitalist" for the initial care of the patient often times directly from the ER. Hospital corporations hire these physicians to direct the care of the patient as simple employees with no real long-term involvement or investment in the patient. When their eight-hour shift is done, they turn over the patient to the next hospitalist. To make matters worse, sometimes, the family, a consulting physician, and even the nurse are unable to identify which hospitalist is taking care of the patient.

Importantly, these hospitalists are most often fresh out of medical school usually with no specialized training or practical experience in the care of the cardiological patient. The blunt reality is that many of them work cheap because they have a hard time finding jobs as recent graduates. The barrage of newly uninsured patients as a result of Obamacare is entering the system, and there's the simultaneous need for the veterans administration to hire government M.D. employees to care for the onslaught of ill veterans. This practice of Hospitalists and the consequences will spread like a malignant cancer. They further ask for specialist consults who come within few days, forestalling the correct diagnosis and treatment and prolonging the hospitalization.

To me, this is very dangerous development in medicine and is only being perpetuated by Obamacare to shift the initial diagnosis and care to the hospitalist, the physician assistant, or nurse practitioner. In the past, morning rounds were done solely by the physician responsible for the continuity of patient care, but now, we have "interdisciplinary rounds," which means rounds with the doctor, nurses, case managers, dieticians, physical therapists, and whoever wants to be involved with patient care.

These interdisciplinary rounds are done daily by physicians who are so busy with impossible patient loads that they dilute the care and responsibility for patient treatment. Now, we have nurse practitioners and physician assistants (which might not be a bad thing as most are honestly better than doctors) writing orders and substituting for the doctor who is too busy to adequately diagnose and properly treat the complex cardiological patient that he has no clue of.

I once had a patient who came to the ER at 2 am with acute pulmonary edema and congestive heart failure. The patient was seen by the ER doctor on his shift and a hospitalist was called in to take over her care. I was on-call for my cardiology group and also got a call at 2 am. Frankly, I did not want to come in at that time of the night to see the patient. However, at about 2:15, I got a call from the patient's daughter who was a physician and a professor at a local university. She demanded that I go to the patient and asked me how old I was.

Then she told me that she wanted me because she felt my older age meant I'd have the skills to diagnose her mother. Also, she was aware of the fact that I was taught in a period of time when the doctor was trained to work late at night under adverse conditions. Now, due to the totally misguided belief by the legislature, the M.D. trainee is to work only 8-12 hour shifts because this would supposedly prevent errors.

For example, navy seal trainees are trained under extremely adverse conditions to learn to keep their heads down because they'd get them blown off in real combat. While coddling the M.D. trainee, they forget about the future doctor errors that will occur due to the lack of similar training once they're out of supervised care. It's frightening to realize that much of this medical legislation is guided by a bunch of lawyer politicians, who have limited intelligence when it comes to medical reality. In fact, they're just dopes.

Let's go back to the case we were discussing. So, I ended up going to the hospital and saw the patient. During the examination, I heard a rub in her heart and the signs of pericarditis. Within minutes, she went into cardiac arrest. Although dead tired, I acted out of trained reflex. We drained the fluid from her heart in the ER after a cursory echocardiogram administered by me and successfully resuscitated the patient. If I didn't diagnose the constricting fluid around her heart but rather had sent her for a time consuming CT scan, most likely, the patient would've died.

If the case had been presented to the hospital for morbidity and mortality review if a CAT scan had been ordered and the patient died, all the peer physicians in the hospital probably would've agreed because they didn't know better. And the avoidable death would've been left to rest with no punitive action against the doctor. This is just one of a multitude of examples where my training saved the patient. If she had died, it would've just gone down as a statistic with no validation that the delay for a more sophisticated test was actually the ultimate cause of the patient's death.

Well, now we come to the British physician, James Hope, who in 1839 used curare for anesthesia and did open heart surgery on live dogs. This was a major advance that, as in least in dogs, it demonstrated a successful surgery on a beating heart. In his extensive observations, he was the first to describe two widely seen disorders of the mitral valve. The first was mitral stenosis where the valve is calcified with resultant constriction, impeded the flow of blood from the left atrium into the left ventricle, and produced a characteristic mitral stenosis murmur.

Additionally, he described mitral regurgitation where the valve does not adequately close when the left ventricle pumps blood, creating a backflow of part of the blood into the left atrium and producing the characteristic murmur of mitral regurgitation or mitral incompetency.

HISTORICAL VIEW OF CARDIAC ELECTOPHYSIOLOGY

Let's jump from the historical perspectives of general cardiology into the electrophysiological milestones that are critical to understanding at least half of the diseases that affect the cardiac system. After this exhaustive review, we'll finish with a discussion of the chronology of general cardiology from the 1800s to the present. This rest of the the bulk of this book will review the cardiological and electrophysiological diseases of the heart and how to deal with each one if faced with hospitalization for these maladies. This will include the cardiac catheterization, angina or heart attack, and end with the complex issues of cardiac transplantation and stem cell therapy.

First, an extremely important finding about the heart occurred in 1838 when the Italian physicist, Carlo Matteucci, discovered that the heart muscle generated electricity. This was a remarkable discovery, which practically paved the way for the study of cardiac electrophysiology as a subspecialty of cardiology. He felt that this electrical force enabled the heart to beat steadily and regulate its own mechanical activity independent of the influences of other parts of the body; an autonomous (self-beating) electrical generator. This is actually true to an extent in that the heart beats independently by itself as long as there is blood supply and can be affected by the body such as when the heartbeat speeds up during a physical activity.

Using a new instrument called a galvanometer developed by a fellow Italian Leopoldo Nobili, he was able to prove that the heart as an excitable biological tissue generated electrical currents. They behaved like what Allessando Volta described as elements in series, which is the electrical cells or batteries of the heart that was connected end to end in form of electrical pathways called the conduction system or wiring of the heart.

This remarkable work led to the discovery by Johannes Peter Muller of Germany that the heart conduction system generated an action potential, which we now know is the characteristic of the electricity generated by each individual cell of the conduction system. This action potential allows the cell to cell generation of electrical current no different than how electricity travels down a copper wire and was compared at the time to how electricity was conducted through the newly developed telegraph lines.

I want to introduce a series of illustrations that refines this discussion of the conductions system. (Fig.25–Fig.27). At this point in our discussion, it's very important to understand these concepts as so much of cardiac disease revolves around pathology within the cellular cardiac conduction system.

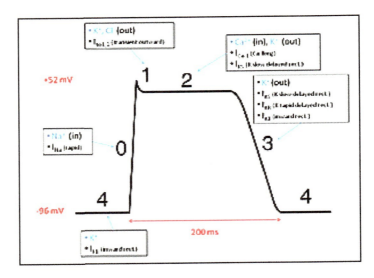

(Fig.25) (en.wikipedia.com) This is a picture of an electrical recording of one cell in the cardiac conduction system made with a very refined type of galvanometer utilized by Nobili.

Hopefully, everyone knows the concept of volts; the more powerful and dangerous is the wire, the more volts in an electrical current. In the case of a cardiac cell, it rests at a voltage of -96 millivolts (mv) or phase four of the action potential when there's no electrical conduction and the cell is at electrical rest. Suddenly, the electrical cell generates a current through three more phases of the electrical spike called phases 0-3 and spike upward. As you can see, the cell generates electricity to +52 millivolts (to the left in red). This is the generated energy that travels through the electrical system before it returns back to phase 4 and goes down to rest at -96 mv ready to conduct again and generate the heartbeat.

These electrical currents and the action potential are generated by the movement of important ions (elements) that are of common knowledge. The initial phase 0 is made possible by the movement of sodium ions that makes up common salt (Na⁺). Next, phase 1 and 2 are made possible by the movement driving into and out of the cell with potassium (K⁺) and calcium (Ca⁺²) ions. These ions move through specific channels in the membranes of conduction cells and are important to understand when it comes to a multitude of cardiac channel diseases such as the most familiar being hereditary and acquired long QT syndromes that leads to sudden cardiac death (SCD) or ventricular fibrillation (VF).

It's also interesting that many athletes become severely depleted in potassium and suffer terminal cardiac arrhythmias and cardiac arrest (not a heart attack). Many of these channel diseases cannot be treated with medicine, but as a lifesaving procedure, require implantation of an automatic implantable cardiac defibrillator (AICD or just ICD) recently developed to shock the heart back to normal if it goes into cardiac arrest or VF.

These conduction cells are also pacemaker cells that generate an action potential repetitively by themselves and called "auto-rhythmic" cells in a resting heart generating 60 beats a minute. By calling it pacemaker, we're simply referring to the fact that these cells are self-contained generators of electricity that are automatic, not dependent on other forces for heartbeats.

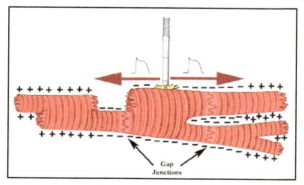

(Fig.26) (www.vhlab.umn.edu) This is a representation of a cardiac conduction fiber in the heart composed of millions of cells. The small probe at the top is inserted into the cells to record the action potential that you can see drawn on the top of the fibers. As illustrated, the cells are separated by gap junctions that connect the cells for cell-to-cell conduction. The cardiac channels can be subject to disease and lead to heart block in which the electricity fails to conduct and an artificial pacemaker will be needed. These cells move from negative to positive as the electricity is conducted one way down the pathway.

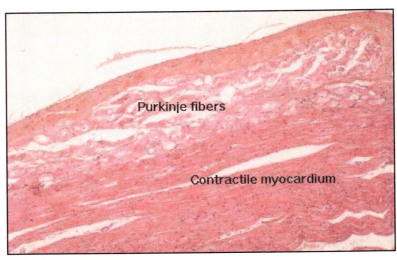

(Fig.27) (Wikipedia) This is a microscopic photograph of a conduction fiber of the heart called a Purkinje fiber. It's just one of the many types of conduction pathways of the heart and is composed of specialized cells that are able to generate an action potential. Notice that it runs next to the contractile cells of the myocardium (heart muscle). It's no different than getting a shock when you touch a live electrical wire. The Purkinje fiber is an electrical pathway that stimulates or shocks the contractile myocardial cells to shorten and squeeze in a rhythmic fashion.

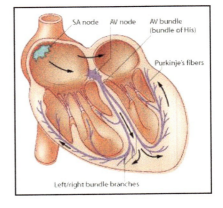

(Fig.28) (medical-dictionary.thefreedictionary.com) This is a picture of the very basic conduction system of the heart. First, note that the top of the picture in the wall of the right atrium is the SA or sinus node. This is a very important structure of the heart because its auto-rhythmic cells go through the action potential.

It's the fastest of all the conduction cells in the heart; thus, it's called the primary pacemaker of the heart. If these pacemaker cells, for some reason, stop their auto-rhythmic function (sinus arrest), then cells down the line from the SA node such as in this picture the AV (atrioventricular node) take over the pacemaker function although at a slightly slower auto-rhythmic rate of firing.

There are several malfunctions of the sinus node, which can lead to both a slowing of the heartbeat (bradycardia) or an irregular heartbeat (sinus arrhythmias) and the most familiar disease of aging called the sick sinus syndrome (SSS). Down the line, pacemaker cells, such as in the AV node, fire too slowly, causing the patient to need the implantation of an artificial pacemaker.

Once the sinus node fires, it conducts cell to cell rapidly through the right atrium and over to the left atrium where it causes the atria to contract and forces blood into the ventricles. Conduction then enters the AV node (AVN), a collection of auto-rhythmic cells in the center of the heart between the atria and the ventricles, where conduction is slowed down or modulated in order to let the atrium complete their contractions. The AVN is a critical area of electrical control of the heart as it also acts as an electrical filter or gate, sort of like a resistor in your computer.

In this function, the AVN acts to slow the contractions and conduction into the ventricles as in some pathological conditions where the atrial starts to beat extremely rapid at up to 300 beats/minute. The AVN filters 3:1, so the ventricle contracts at 100 beats/minute, and you don't collapse. So, in atrial fibrillation where the atrium can chaotically fire 200-300 times a minute, it's the function of the AVN to filter out most of these beats and keep the ventricles from firing so fast that it would lead to cardiac arrest (not a heart attack).

Next in line is the Bundle of His (His bundle) that leads out of the AVN into the ventricles and into the left and right bundle branch. These structures are basically just a specialized electrical pathway into the right or left ventricle that organize conduction for synchronized contraction at the ventricular level. However, these structures can be the source of pathology such as a right bundle branch block (RBBB) and left bundle branch block (LBBB), which can easily be identified on a plain electrocardiogram (ECG or EKG). Although these two conditions can be benign and of little consequence, they can also be harbingers of future heart block and bradycardia that would require a pacemaker implant.

Additionally, the His bundle is an important area where patients with rapidly conducting atrial fibrillation can have a surgery called radiofrequency ablation (RFA). The His Bundle is interrupted to prevent the ventricles from firing irregular and fast and requires a pacemaker implant after the ablation.

Lastly, we come to the Purkinje fibers and the system called the purkinje complex that distributes the electricity to the outreaches of the ventricular muscle. It's interesting to note that pathology in these fibers are not necessarily expressed as block, but in certain conditions, these cells that usually auto regulate at an autonomous rate of 20-30 times a minute suddenly speed up to cause PVCs (premature ventricular complexes). In the worst case scenario, ventricular tachycardia, ventricular fibrillation with sudden cardiac death, or cardiac arrest can occur. This can be both hereditary, and more commonly, a result of a heart attack where the purkinje fibers are deprived of oxygen enough to cause a very rapid or chaotic rate without totally causing cell death.

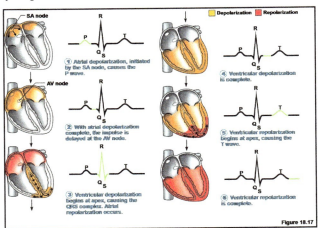

(Fig.29) (www.ryody001.kistory.com) This is the last figure in this group, and it summarizes in a graphic form the lessons we've just reviewed with a few newer concepts to be introduced. One of these are the important concepts of depolarization and repolarization. In this picture, depolarization is orange, and repolarization is represented in red. Basically, after the auto-rhythmic cells goes through their action potentials and the cells depolarize and the muscle beats, the cells get ready for its next depolarization cycle via various ions and gates. This process is called the depolarization-repolarization cycle. After the cell depolarizes, it must repolarize to beat again.

As a new concept that we briefly mentioned before, the electrocardiogram is the way the cardiologist records with electrodes on your chest and arms these depolarization-repolarization cycles. To the left of each pane above, you can see the generation of one beat of the electrocardiogram. Don't worry that you don't completely understand the EKG as we will be covering normal and abnormal EKGs in great detail later in the book.

First, in (Fig.29), the depolarization-repolarization cycle begins in the SA node in the top of the right atrium and depolarization is depicted in the first two frames in red. To the left, this depolarization of the atria inscribes a small initial blip on the EKG called the P wave. In the next 2 frames, the red depolarization wave front move through the AV node and into the right and left bundle branches and finally into the Purkinje fibers leading into the left LV and right RV muscles. The large blip on the EKG after the P wave is called the QRS complex and represents the depolarization and beating of the right and left ventricles.

Interestingly, while the ventricles are depolarizing in orange, the atria are repolarizing in red. Lastly, the ventricles and his-purkinje system repolarize in preparation for the next beat and are recorded on the EKG as the T wave. It's that simple. To me, it's just astounding to understand this remarkable ballet of electricity as it controls basically your life and is designed to last a lifetime. I might add that the long QT syndrome is easily recognized on the EKG as a longer interval between the QRS complex and the end of the T wave. This corresponds to a slowing of repolarization of the his-purkinje system and can lead to sudden cardiac death and a chaotic ventricular rhythm called ventricular fibrillation.

It wasn't until 1875 that Etienne-Jules Marey first documented extra beats originating from the ventricles called premature ventricular beats or premature extra contractions (PVC's) of the heart. Actually, these extra beats can also occur from the atria and are called premature atrial contractions (PAC's). These extra beats of the heart are often described by the patient as palpitations that seem to come and go and often associated with various activities such as during sleep or exercise. Marey did this by actually placing little balloons in the four chambers of the heart in a live horse while recording the pressures on a simple graphic recording device.

What makes this breakthrough so important is that he was able to show that the right and left ventricle contracted simultaneously and that the atria contracted right before the ventricular beat. Also, he showed that when the various chambers of the heart contracted the pressures in the chamber increased. When the muscle relaxed and the pressure decreased, an extra electrical beat such as the PVC would not necessarily cause the ventricle to contract completely. That's because for a time during the relaxation phase, the muscle is "refractory" to contract and is called the atrial and ventricular refractory periods. During this refractory period, the PVC can occur and not cause the ventricle to contract; therefore, the patient feels a very brief sensation like dizziness.

Additionally, he described the chronological order of the heart valves opening and closing and how the beating of the atrium primed the ventricular pressures for their subsequent beat. That established a very important function of the atrial contraction and how the loss of this function with an arrhythmia led to clinical disease. In actuality, Marey was the first practitioner to inscribe the electrocardiogram in the horse's heart utilizing small capillary electrodes that he placed on the surface of the horse's beating heart. He observed that the small P wave of the EKG corresponded in time with the atrial contraction, and the subsequent QRS was associated with the contraction of the right and left ventricles.

As advancements were being made in understanding the various pathways and components of the cardiac conduction system, the EKG for humans was a key development in the study of the cardiac system and cardiac arrhythmias. As an example, the physician was able to record extra beats from the atria and the ventricle, but most importantly, correlate certain abnormalities of the EKG such as a long QT interval that was seen in families and associated with premature sudden cardiac death-the Long QT syndrome.

Actually, the first human EKG was recorded by A.D. Waller of Paris and London in 1897. His main interest in medicine was the study of the electrical phenomenon of the heart. He utilized a machine that was created by Gabriel Lippman in 1873 called the Lippman Capillary Electrometer. Basically, it consisted of mercury electrodes that were mixed with sulfuric acid to create a good conductor of low amounts of electricity and was used to record the EKG (it was called EKG by this time) of animals on a beating heart. However, it was A.D. Waller in May of 1887, in front of a group of doctors at St. Mary's Hospital in London, that Waller placed electrodes on the front and back of a human's chest and recorded two deflections the QRS of ventricular depolarization and the T wave of ventricular repolarization (Fig.30).

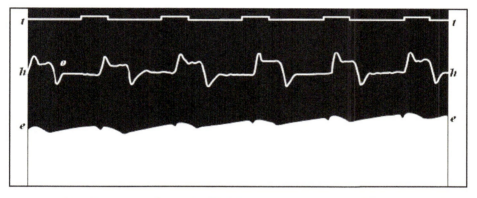

(Fig.30) (www.bem.fi) This is the first surface EKG recorded by A.D. Waller in 1887. The white initial deflection is the QRS complex although it looks very much like the action potential that comes from a single cell. The modern EKG machine processes the QRS into a single sharp deflection. The second deflection after the QRS, which goes down and is negative, reflects the T wave or ventricular repolarization. The previous illustrations of the T wave showed it moving upward. Again, this is how the T wave is processed by modern EKG machines. In the modern EKG, if the T wave becomes negative or downward, this is usually an indication that the heart is ischemic or deprived of blood such as in a heart attack (myocardial infarction). Lastly, note that there is no deflection of the small P wave of atrial depolarization before the QRS as it was too low voltage to record by this initial EKG machine.

At the same time, the German physician, Carl Ludwig recorded the surface EKG from animals and was credited with the first demonstration of an EKG during ventricular fibrillation and ventricular tachycardia (Fig.31). He was investigating the effects of direct electrical currents on the heart and found that they made the heart "fibrillate" and not pump blood. However, it wasn't until quite a bit later that the discovery was made that a direct current to the heart during ventricular fibrillation, which using the paddles on the chest, could convert this rhythm back to normal. Now, portable defibrillator devices called automatic external defibrillators (AED) allow a bystander to deliver lifesaving shocks to individuals who go into ventricular fibrillation in case of an a cardiac arrest.

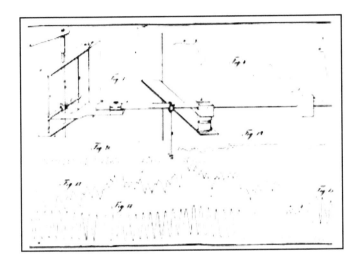

(Fig.31) (www.rcals.com) This is a recording from Ludwig's lab of ventricular fibrillation. The bottom of the illustration is the EKG with rapid peaked waves with no period of rest between the beats. This is ventricular fibrillation or a cardiac arrest where the ventricle is like an empty sack just rapidly fluttering with no time to eject blood. Therefore, it deprives the patient of blood to the brain or body. If not corrected within 5-6 minutes, depending upon the circumstances, the EKG will go flat-line with no electrical activity at all and the patient dies.

However, W. Einthoven was in the audience at St. Mary's at the demonstration of Waller's EKG. The next year, he recorded an EKG from the surface of the human body now called the surface EKG. Einthoven is considered the father of modern electrocardiography although, in his words, he attributed Waller as the first to do a crude surface EKG.

He began his work with refining the EKG machines, utilizing a more precise "capillary electrometer" machine (Fig.31). With this, he identified five distinct points or waves on the EKG that are still used today: the P wave of atrial depolarization, the QRS that are the three short and rapid deflection points that make up the QRS complex of ventricular depolarization, and the T wave of ventricular repolarization (Fig.32). Note the absence of a wave of atrial repolarization as it is too low voltage for the recordings. During this time, arrhythmias of the heart were analyzed through simultaneous pulse and EKG recordings. A true understanding of the cardiac rhythm disorders such as supraventricular tachycardia and atrial fibrillation and identification of cardiac conditions such as a heart attack began with the EKG recording devices of Einthoven.

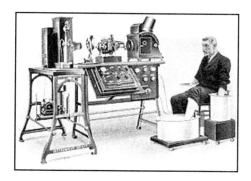

(Fig.31) (en.wikipedia.org) This was the EKG machine utilized by Einthoven in his identification of the various complexes making up the EKG and the diagnosis of rhythm disorder of the heart. He immersed the leg and the arm in a conducting solution, which acted as electrodes similar to the electrodes that are placed on your chest and limbs with modern EKG machines. Although this machine was large, it was very accurate and can be compared to the massive size of old computers in relation to the small handheld devices of today.

Patients were referred to Einthoven with a variety of "palpitations." He substantiated previous work in animals, identifying atrial fibrillation as an "irregularly irregular" rhythm that was often associated with a very rapid ventricular rate controlled with digitalis.

He also validated the clinical diagnosis of PVCs (premature ventricular contractions) and PACs (premature atrial contractions).

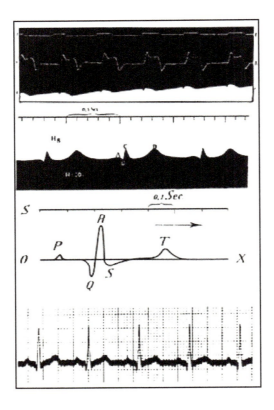

(Fig.32) (www.phuongammed.com) This is a recording of Einthoven, demonstrating the various complexes of the EKG: the third illustration demonstrating the P wave of atrial contraction, the QRS of ventricular contraction, and the T wave of ventricular repolarization. The top plate is the first Waller recording of the EKG, and the bottom illustration is a modern EKG recording that looks exactly like what was analyzed by Einthoven. What's critical about understanding these phases of the EKG is that abnormalities can occur in any part of the EKG and reflect certain types of pathological conditions solely with this inexpensive and simple diagnostic tool. In modern medicine, the EKG is the initial part of most cardiac examinations utilized, for example, in the doctor's office or during an insurance physical exam.

We'll cover all the maladies and the use of the EKG in diagnosis later, but now, I want to cover the immediate diagnosis of a myocardial infarction or heart attack. With the death of heart tissue, a change in the deflection is identified at the start of the QRS complex called a "pathological Q wave" that is longer and deeper than the normal small Q wave deflection. The patient's old EKG recording can be very helpful and lifesaving as any change in the EKG over time is very important. The comparison of acute changes in the EKG in the emergency room can be a critical piece of information in specifically the diagnosis of a heart attack when one has chest pain.

For example, a new EKG may show a pathological Q wave, which was not present on an old EKG. For this specific reason, some people with known heart disease can carry in their wallets a small laminated card with a dated EKG that can quickly be utilized by your doctor for a quick and accurate diagnosis. In this day and age, it's conceivable that a copy of your old EKG can be kept on your cell phone or tablet and can be of remarkable use to the doctor in saving your life. This almost immediate identification of the problem obviates the need for more sophisticated, unnecessary, and expensive procedures while critical minutes tick away.

While we're on the discussion of Einthoven, who was a major innovator in the development of modern day medicine with his EKG machine in my opinion, I think it's appropriate to mention the use of the EKG recording as a guide to the diagnosis and approach to an acute myocardial infarction (AMI). In brief, although we have mentioned the coronary arteries before, there are three major arteries that supply different parts of the heart.

A myocardial infarction is also called an acute coronary occlusion or acute coronary thrombosis. This happens when one of the arteries gets closed off by a clot, which acutely deprives the heart muscle of oxygen and leads to the death of the cells. This event manifests itself in the individual as acute chest pain or pressure and often is associated with profuse sweating (diaphoresis), nausea, vomiting, and shortness of breath (SOB) (Fig 33).

When the paramedics arrive, one of the first things they do is an EKG. It's critical for the cardiologist to be able to do an immediate heart catheterization and break up the clot to save as much of the heart muscle from cell death as possible. Now, the paramedics are able to transmit your EKG directly to the hospital over the Internet or airwaves and get prepared for your arrival. Let's see what the paramedics see and how this simple EKG can save your life (Fig.34)

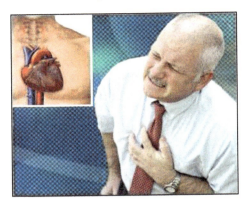

(Fig.33) (www.medindia.net) The chest pain in a heart attack or angina is most often a squeezing pain in the chest that can also be felt in the left neck and the left arm. The pain isn't a sharp pain and doesn't get worse with breathing. The pain can be associated with profuse sweating and usually gets worse, not better, with exertion or your changing your bodily position.

(Fig.34) (www.frca.co.uk)This is the recording of one QRS complex and demonstrates the EKG evolution of an acute myocardial infarction (AMI).

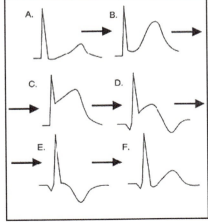

In panel A (Fig.34), this is the normal QRS and T wave. The EKG recording at the end of the QRS complex is at the baseline or origin of the tracing, and this part of the EKG is called the ST segment. It's very important to note that in the normal EKG, this segment that can be fairly prolonged is flat and not elevated above the line as in (ST elevation) or below the line with (ST depression). In panel B, you can see that the ST segment is elevated off the baseline, and the T wave is bigger and more peaked (peaked T waves). These are very early signs that occur minutes after the coronary artery occludes and the heart muscle is not yet dead but is "ischemic" in that the muscle is being deprived of oxygen and is not working correctly.

Thus, when the paramedics arrive, these are the EKG changes that they might see and the accuracy of the diagnosis is greatly enhanced if they have an old EKG for comparison. Next, panel C shows the ST segment being markedly elevated and seems to merge into the T wave, which is somewhat obscured. These changes take minutes to hours to occur and are indicative of a ST segment elevation myocardial infarction (STEMI). If this is transmitted to the hospital, a "code STEMI" is placed in effect. The cardiologist and the catheterization laboratory will be prepared for the patient's arrival as the patient should be taken directly for heart catheterization to bust open the clot and prevent cell death.

There are some EKG conditions that mimic these changes, and if taken to the catheterization laboratory, the coronaries are found to be normal. Thus, an old EKG in the medical records will enhance the accuracy of the STEMI diagnosis. Also, it's fully within your rights for you or your family to ask the physician if there has been a change in your EKG to warrant an emergency catheterization even in the heat of the frenetic events.

In the same light, it's the responsibility of the patient, who's had a previous EKG to at least know that is was normal or had some change, to communicate to the doctor. This will immediately alert the physician, and I assure you that it will immediately improve your level of care rather than just being an ignorant bystander caught in the scheme of events.

Next, panel D shows that the ST segment is coming down slightly. See the inscription at the beginning of the QRS complex a Q wave or a downward deflection. This can occur within 6-10 minutes of the coronary occlusion and signifies the beginning of cell death that can proceed unabated if nothing is done. Some patients have had "silent" heart attacks in the past without chest pain, and the presence of the significant Q wave (Fig.35) on an old EKG is of great use to the cardiologist as he makes a decision to do an emergent verses a planned or elective heart catheterization as an outpatient. As I've stated, an old EKG is priceless.

As the heart goes through a healing process over the next few weeks, one can see in panels E through F that the T wave inverts, maybe permanently, and the ST segment normalizes. Again, there's some variability in these events, but the doctor will refer to this phenomenon as chronic ST and T (ST-T) changes on the EKG. There is no doubt that Eithenhoven noted all these anomalies of the EKG although he wasn't sure of their exact cause. He certainly was able to make the intellectual leap that patients with chest pain or angina pectoris often were seen to have Q waves or ST-T changes and had an ominous prognosis if gone untreated or the chest pain persisted.

If the patient in modern times has an old EKG and presents to the doctor with a complaint of chest pain, any change in the EKG is of great significance for possibly indicating coronary artery disease (CAD) versus the other less dangerous causes such as plain indigestion. If anything, the patient having an understanding of these facts can lessen the anxiety regarding minor chest pain and may support the need for further testing and diagnostic studies such as an elective cardiac catheterization. There is absolutely no question that many cardiologists feel compelled to do a cardiac catheterization based on the uninformed anxieties of the patient who seeks recurrent help for chest pain just to prove to the patient that the pain is not of cardiac origin. This is a very unfortunate situation that occurs far too often.

As I've said, it's frequently compelled by the ignorance and unwillingness of the patient to understand his medical condition and the WIIGS syndrome. It's also the reason for the doctor's perceived fear of an unfounded and baseless medical liability suit in the face of clear evidence that a cardiac catheterization is excessive but still done as an expensive and relatively dangerous procedure with little medical indication. This unfortunate, and sometimes fatal, reality is operative every day in American medicine. Medical knowledge is power, and more importantly, it can save your money as well as your life.

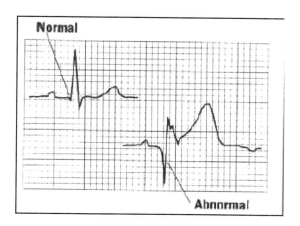

(Fig.35) This is again just one P-QRS-T complex of an EKG. Of importance note that in the top complex at the beginning of the QRS complex is a miniscule Q wave. However, in the second bottom complex there is a very wide and deep initial Q wave that is of great significance to a cardiologist examining the EKG.

First and foremost, the "significant" Q wave suggest that the patient has had a heart attack with muscle damage in the past. In some instances, this could've occurred especially in diabetics without the patient knowing that they even had a previous myocardial infarction. As a single piece of information on one EKG, this finding is useful, but the importance is multiplied significantly if the Q wave was previously absent in the old EKG. If you were to go to an emergency room with chest pain and don't have a significant old or new Q wave but just chest pain, this will make the physician less concerned for true coronary artery disease and to proceed with further less dangerous testing such as a simple treadmill.

However, if one has an old EKG in comparison without the Q wave but now have a new Q wave, then the cardiologist might properly feel compelled to go right from the emergency room to "intervene." He would also do a cardiac catheterization with the idea that the patient may require a "percutaneous coronary intervention" or PCI to open what probably is a significantly closed coronary artery.

I've mentioned about ST-T wave changes on the EKG that is signifying the heart muscle not getting enough oxygen in the evolution of a myocardial infarction. However, in chronic chest pain or angina, there may not yet have been a myocardial infarction but just muscle that has a partially clogged artery. These changes can stay permanent on the EKG, and like the Q wave as an isolated finding on the EKG, ST-T changes has significance. The importance is markedly compounded if these changes were not present on an old EKG. Like the new Q wave, also new ST-T changes may compel the cardiologist to immediately do a PCI from the emergency room or soon after.

Wouldn't the cardiologist be impressed by dealing with an informed patient if you or the family inquired about the EKG changes? The "informed consent" for the procedure would take on significantly more importance as you'll be a truly informed and understanding "consumer" when paying directly or out of your insurance deductible for your medical care. If you're dissatisfied with your previous cardiologist or the one who you first meet in the ER, you are free to inquire or request another physician.

This is especially necessary with the recent trend of using "Hospitalist Care" or shift doctors who never develop a close relationship with the assigned patient because of time and quota restraints. You have the right to refuse this type of superficial care and request a single physician who is not a hospital employee and has the time to explain all aspects of your care in a way that you're able to understand and give you the continuity of care with a personal gain in having a dedicated consumer of his (or her) medical care after your hospitalization.

Furthermore, you are free to ask for a cardiologist and not a hospitalist to be your primary physician. If anything, your own physician may be a source of an old EKG even at 2:00 AM as most now have electronic medical records accessible by the hospital and can afford the ER doctor of all important information.

Using this same argument, the benefit of an old EKG can prove invaluable in the treatment of an emergent treatment of a cardiac arrhythmia. We previously discussed atrial fibrillation, which is a rapid abnormal rhythm of the atrium. It's an abnormal rhythm that has many causes and medical implications, and it's often seen on the EKG of the elderly. The patient may present to the cardiologist or the ER for palpitations, a feeling of an irregular heartbeat and be seen on the EKG, or without any symptoms and incidentally discovered on an EKG during a routine physical or in the ER for a totally unrelated cause.

What I am leading up to, as seen in the case of a heart attack, it is invaluable if the doctor knows that this rhythm was present before on an EKG or it's a totally new finding. Thus, if the old EKG is readily available or if the patient is aware that this is a previous diagnosis, this can be the difference between going home and a possibly unnecessary hospitalization. Unfortunately, in the elderly or demented patient, this is often impossible to ascertain, and it's up to the family to have some of this information or have access to an old EKG. The basic point to be made is that if this is a new arrhythmia in a patient who presents with cardiac complaints, this can be a very important finding and be a strong indication for hospital admission to evaluate the atrial fibrillation or arrhythmia and begin the appropriate treatment.

On the other hand, if this is not a new finding or is found in the asymptomatic patient who just happens to have an EKG in the ER, this may not require inpatient management but rather tests and procedures that can be done out of the hospital or as a hospital outpatient rather than an inpatient. This is a very common reality, and it's critically important that the patient or the patient's representative have an understanding in that incidental atrial fibrillation on an asymptomatic patient can often be a false pretense for immediate inpatient management, which is simply not the case. The physician should be able and willing to engage you in a logical discussion for the need of acute hospital care, and if he cannot or will not, then it's time to get another doctor.

Next, we need to discuss the further investigations and discoveries of this remarkable investigator Einthoven and his wonderful EKG machine (Fig.36).

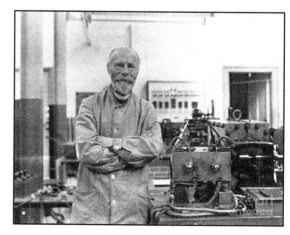

(Fig.36) (medicine150.mdhs.unimelb.edu.au) Einthoven is standing in front of his original string galvanometer, which preceded his more compact EKG machine. I sometimes envy the physicians who lived during this time and the excitement of suddenly discovering useful tool and being able to practice their healing profession unrestrained by ridiculous and stifling medical bureaucracy.

Einthoven ultimately received the Nobel Prize in Medicine in 1924 for his innovative and critical development for the diagnosis of cardiac disease. The term "Einthoven's Triangle" (Fig.37) is named for him and established the all-important basis for a multi-lead EKG recording, which we all experience today when receiving EKG with multiple leads placed on the chest and the limbs.

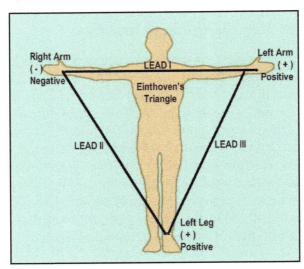

(Fig.37) (general.utpb.edu) Here, we see a depiction of Einthoven's inverted triangle. This is the convention we use to this day and is a reflection of all the leads on your chest, arms, and legs placed with an EKG.

Basically, Einthoven ascertained that the heart generated an electrical field that had a spatial orientation, similar to taking a picture from different angles, so the EKG would look different depending on the orientation of the recording to the heart. He further observed that the leads had a negative and a positive end and fit into the circuit just like a battery with a positive and negative end that must be placed correctly into the flashlight. The leads were placed on the left leg, left arm, and right arm to form an electrical triangle with the recording of three leads with separate "pictures" of the heart: lead I, II, and III. He further refined this to add leads AVF (foot), AVR (right arm) and AVL (left arm). Thus, we had six different leads and EKG pictures, or recordings, of the heart.

Later would come (Fig.38) the addition of six chest leads: V1, V2, V3, V4, V5, and V6. They were directly applied to the anterior chest over the heart from right to left that recorded a "12 lead EKG," which is the standard for today (Fig.39).

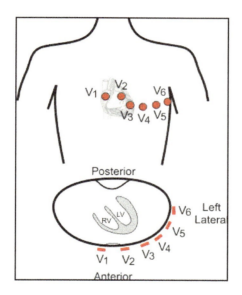

(Fig.38) This is a representation of how the leads (V1-V6) are placed over the chest. Again, these 6 leads are placed on the chest wall with suction cups or sticker's that start from the right of the sternum and end at the left lateral chest. Note that these lead are in around the front of the heart and are a reflection of the electrical currents coming from the RV and the front and also left side of the LV. This EKG road map aids in the interpretation of what part of the heart is involved in a heart attack and which coronary artery is clogged up.

This creation of 12 leads with 12 recordings of the EKG allowed the physician to begin to pinpoint the part of the heart that is most involved with the pathology demonstrated on the 12 lead EKG (Fig.39). For example, one can see that the chest leads V1 and V2 rest more over the right ventricle, and leads V3-V6 lye over the anterior and lateral part of the left ventricle. These leads accurately reflect the electrical activity of these ventricles from an anterior and lateral view, thus specific EKG changes in which leads reflecting in a heart attack what part of the heart was effected and what coronary artery is the "culprit."

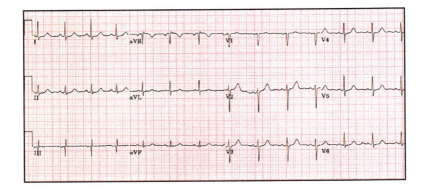

(Fig.39) This is a modern day EKG. It is called a 12 lead EKG as it records all the leads simultaneously: I, II, III, aVR, aVL, aVF, V1, V2, V3, V4, V5 and V6. You can see that the QRS size and orientation are very different in these 12 leads and is a snapshot of the electrical activity of the heart from different perspectives. So, V1 gives you information from the RV, V2-V6, the LV, aVL, and V6, and the lateral aspect of the heart, and II, III, and aVF about the bottom or inferior aspect of the heart. These select leads can be utilized in an acute myocardial infarction to help localize the "culprit" artery that supplies these areas and is the clogged artery that is causing the heart attack or angina pectoris (chest pain). It's an important guide if the cardiologist decides to place a stent to open the artery for your coronary artery disease either during an emergency or an elective cardiac catheterization.

If there is a sudden clotting in the artery to the front of the left ventricle, the left anterior descending artery (LAD), the EKG in leads V2-V4 will most prominently demonstrate ST elevation and the development of Q waves. It is a very important dictum in medicine that if the cardiologist has a good idea of the area involved in the acute event and the culprit artery, then he can do an emergent heart catheterization, which he can concentrate on the intervention such as a stent with the angiogram that confirming what was derived from the EKG (corroboratory evidence).

In more complex terms, if the EKG gives a high probability of the culprit artery being the LAD artery and if this is what he finds on the angiogram, then intervention on this artery rather than other arteries that possibly need later intervention on another day (staged procedure) is done. The EKG evidence is a very important piece of information for the cardiologist to utilize in an emergency cardiac catheterization. It mustn't be ignored by the interventional cardiologist who is doing the emergency percutaneous coronary intervention (stent or PCI). In the same respect, if the patient comes to the ER with right lower abdominal belly pain and the x-rays or CT scan confirm an appendicitis, then the surgeon should just take out the appendix and nothing else he might find such as asymptomatic gallstones during the surgery, which he should not remove during the emergency surgery. In the same light, as in the above example, the interventional cardiologist, in most circumstances, should only do a PCI on the culprit LAD and no other arteries that he may find are clogged at the same catheterization.

Heart Disease-More on the Arteries and Muscle

Now, I would like to back up a little to cover some of the history that we skipped over in while we discussed the electrical system of the heart. It should be obvious by now that the heart is actually three structures in one: the heart muscle itself, the circulation or the coronary arteries supplying this muscle's blood supply and oxygen, and the specialized electrical system of the heart composed of conduction fibers that control the rhythmic function of the heart. The history of these three systems is intertwined and collectively leads up to modern cardiology and the integration of these three systems. The key to understanding these disease states is that when there is pathology of one of these systems, ultimately all three systems are affected.

James Mackenzie (1835-1925) made multiple observations regarding the arteries of the heart, the coronary arteries. He postulated correctly that these three main arteries supplied the various unique areas of the heart muscle (Fig.41). He made the correlation to the previous work of William Heberden, who in 1772 coined the condition angina pectoris or chest pain drawn from the Greek word for strangling. Mackenzie made the intellectual step that angina was caused by obstruction in flow in one or more of these coronary arteries that deprived the specific muscle of the heart of oxygen and created the perception of pain. This was supported by various researchers at the time that made the observation that the patient's heart could be stopped or severely damaged by acute "thrombosis" of the artery with clot with a jelly-like complete plug.

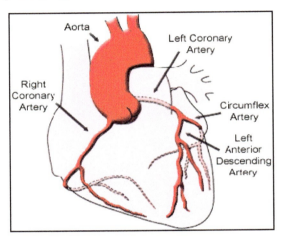

(Fig.41) (www.promocell.com) This is a very important picture to understand and remember. As you can see, there are two arteries that start at the aortic valve on the side of the aorta called the Right Coronary Artery (RCA) and the left main coronary artery (LM). The left main quickly separates into the left anterior descending (LAD) and the circumflex (CX) coronary arteries. It's obvious the RCA supplies a small part of the left ventricle but mainly the right ventricle. Similarly, the LAD supplies the whole front of the left ventricle while the CX supplies the left side, back of the left, and right ventricles. Although not shown in this picture, all three arteries break up into smaller branches to spread the supply of blood: the ramus intermedius, diagonal, posterior descending, and obtuse marginal (Fig.42). All the arteries and the branches are subject to an acute or chronic obstruction by cholesterol plaque and can be the source of angina or a heart attack.

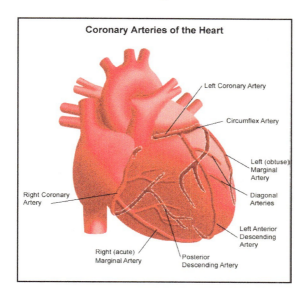

(Fig.42) (www.uchospitals.edu)This is a more comprehensive picture of the coronary arteries including some but not all branch arteries. These smaller arteries can branch into even more miniscule branches were coronary plaque and occlusion can occur. These branches are important to visualize as they supply a much smaller amount of the heart muscle and can be a very questionable target for intervention.

Mackenzie further described these pains as pressure in the chest that could be associated with "radiation" of these pains to the neck, left arm, and back. Also, these pains could occur at rest (rest angina) or specifically with various types of exertion (exertional angina). There are various degrees of clogging of these arteries that can begin at a very young age with 70% clogging of the arteries seen causing angina and a heart attack developing when the obstruction suddenly becomes 100% with an acute thrombosis at the site of the significant obstruction.

It's also interesting to note that it's not unusual for the site of significant obstruction to not be the site of the acute thrombosis but is another remote site when a less significant obstruction or "plaque" suddenly ruptures. This insignificant obstruction suddenly (acutely) grows into a more significant obstruction causing immediate new onset angina and all the way to a 100% closure of the artery and cell death with an acute myocardial infarction. In actuality, this may be the most common circumstance of a heart attack. It raises the questions of the common practice of the interventionalist opening all the clogged arteries at the time of catheterization. When the patient has sudden new angina and goes to an emergent heart catheterization, the invasive cardiologist can find a whole range of obstructions with the challenge ascertaining the right lesion as the cause of the acute event or the culprit lesion. At the other end of the spectrum, the invasive cardiologist may find no significant obstruction in the coronaries during this emergent angiography (heart catheterization).

Let's discuss a term recently coined called the "oculostenotic reflex" to describe the creation of "iatrogenesis fulminans." First, if you look up iatrogenic the definition, it's "disease or complications induced by a physician or surgeon by medical treatment or diagnostic procedures." Fulminanans (fulminant) is defined as "coming on suddenly and with great severity." In case of the oculostenotic reflex, this describes the all-to-frequent practice of the invasive cardiologist doing a stent or an intervention on a coronary or peripheral artery simply because it's stenosed (narrowed) with no consideration of the physiology of the disease or whether or not this is a culprit lesion causing a heart attack or angina.

This simply creates the scenario for many "fulminant" and iatrogenic complications, and in the case of a stent, gives the patient an unnecessary appliance or piece of metal in his heart, which can later clot up and cause further heart attacks. Additionally, this practice may unnecessarily commit the patient to lifelong and very expensive clot preventive medicines that have significant side effects such as bleeding and further requires lifelong expensive and life altering medical attention. The only legitimate need for a cardiac intervention is the need to relieve pain or to prolong life.

As we know, the EKG became important in the diagnosis of heart disease starting with Einthoven. Around 1928, it was observed that the patients with chronic angina pectoris can develop ST-T changes on the monitoring EKG with exercise, which was called the exercise treadmill test, and was a further major milestone. When a normal individual exercises, the oxygen demand of the heart muscle increases and is met with increased coronary artery blood flow to meet that demand.

It was noted that patients with exercise could develop chest pain and further ST-T changes, which suggested significant CAD. This is because when the occlusion or stenosis in the coronary becomes significant the increased blood flow through the coronary artery with exercise is not enough past the obstruction to meet the oxygen demands of the heart. As a result, the patient may develop angina, but almost always, there is the development of EKG changes consistent with the specific area of the heart muscle not receiving adequate blood flow.

These changes of CAD with exercise were depression of the ST segment of 1 mm or more and possibly ST elevation as in an acute myocardial infarction. In angina pectoris where the artery is not totally clotted but only significantly occluded greater than 70%, the early EKG sign is ST segment depression either with exercise or rest (Fig.42 & Fig.43).

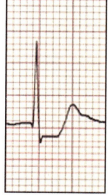

(Fig.42) This is a single QRS complex with the ST segment depression of the line between the QRS and the T wave. Notice that the ST segment is depressed and straight below the baseline. This is called horizontal ST segment depression. This change may be seen in someone with CAD on their resting EKG but is of particular significance if one sees this change with an exercise treadmill test where the ST depression develops with exercise and goes back to normal at rest. This change is referred to as a positive exercise stress test. Although this diagnostic of CAD is not 100% perfect (predictive), there are some causes such as severe hypertension that can cause this test to be "falsely positive" in that the EKG changes develop where there is no significant CAD.

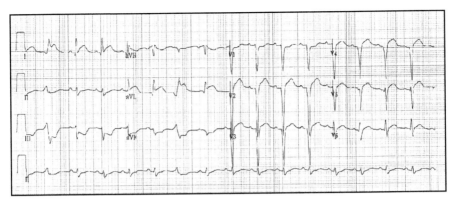

(Fig 43) This is a 12 lead EKG that would be recorded during a treadmill examination or possibly on a patient in the ER with or without angina but with significant CAD. Pay special attention to the leads II, III, and aVF. If you look at these leads, you'll see that the ST segment is noticeably depressed. In most other leads (except I and aVL), the ST segments are normal. If you remember, certain leads take an electrical picture of different portions of the heart. In this example, the leads II, III, and aVF are a reflection of what is occurring in the bottom and lateral parts of the heart and most often the culprit coronary vessel with the stenosis is the RCA or the Cx.

Although this positive test is not infallible and the diagnosis of the culprit vessel may not be precise, this is a very important piece of evidence. In the great majority of cases changes such as this is very accurate and strongly suggest the presence of stenosis in the Cx or RCA, not the LAD, and indicates the need for further testing or immediate invasive procedures such as cardiac catheterization and PCI.

Over the past 10-15 years, the exercise treadmill test has been augmented by the use of radioactive isotopes at a very low radiation level called a nuclear stress test or thallium treadmill. There are also variations of this test that stresses the heart to mimic exercise in those patients who cannot walk on the treadmill: persantine, adenosine, or dobutamine nuclear stress tests. Basically this test injects into the blood stream a radioactive substance such as thallium and takes first an EKG and picture of the heart utilizing a scanner, which picks up a picture of the nuclear tracer that goes to the heart muscle through the coronaries.

Like the EKG, the nuclear scanner takes pictures at various angles and is able to differentiate the concentration of the nuclear tracer in various parts of the heart muscle: the inferior wall, lateral wall, posterior wall, and the all-important anterior wall. In a normal, as well as a heart that has coronary stenosis that at rest doesn't limit the blood flow, the nuclear material distributes evenly throughout the heart muscle. However, if there has been a previous myocardial infarction and some of the muscle is dead and scarred up, that area of the heart will not fill with the nuclear material and show up in the picture as a void where there should've been radioactive activity. This is called an old infarct.

Now, with exercise, the thallium treadmill augments the information gained from the ST depression indicative of coronary ischemia or stenosis. Also, that artery which has a >70% stenosis won't be able to supply adequate blood to its area of distribution. Therefore, on the exercise portion of the nuclear scan, this specific area of the heart will demonstrate a void or markedly decreased radioactivity of the heart muscle. If there are multiple significant coronary occlusions, then there will be multiple areas of the heart that have less nuclear activity in comparison to the resting picture. After exercise is stopped, the nuclear snapshot of the heart returns to normal with all areas perfused homogeneously (Figs. 44, 45, 46)

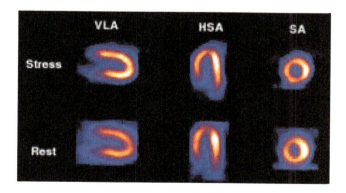

(Fig.44) (www.indiana.edu) This is an image of a normal stress thallium treadmill after it has been processed by a computer. The VLA HAS and SA simply refer to the different "snapshots" or views of the heart to better visualize the distribution of all the three coronary arteries. The images in the bottom show the crescent shape heart muscle, showing that the images with rest and stress are essentially exactly the same. Because the thallium mixes with the blood, these pictures show that with exercise the blood flow through all three major coronary arteries remains the same in both stages. So, there's no major significant coronary stenosis. The computer will generate an automatic report that quantifies the image activity in all the segments of the heart.

Once this report is generated, a radiologist specialist or your cardiologist would "over read" the report with his subjective view of the images. This is where a problem might arise because there is significant room for variation in the reading and visual analysis by various interpreters. They can add various modifiers like "possibly," "low probability," or "high probability" of an abnormality in even a miniscule part of the thallium images. In my experience, this can lead to the computer report of a normal thallium test and the specialist suggesting that there's a "small" abnormality, which frankly has no significance and is called an artifact (falsely abnormal for technical reasons).

It's completely within your rights as the patient to ask the doctor to be given the copy of the computer interpretation and the physician over read or final report. Because all the test results are on a CD, you also have the right to ask for a copy of your test records. I'd strongly suggest that if the computer report differs from the subjective over read, you bring the CD to another practice or hospital for a second interpretation before you proceed with further possible cardiac catheterization. This may cost a bit, but it's worth the satisfaction of a double check before one proceeds with invasive testing and possible dangerous test such as an angiogram.

As seen before, there are studies that suggest that over 30% of thallium images are falsely over read by the interpreter as abnormal and account for a significant number of unnecessary angiograms, which turn out to be normal with no coronary artery disease. This thallium test, which is analyzed as abnormal but in a patient with no stenosis of his arteries, is called a false positive test. It is good to know that as technology increases, the amount of false positive tests is decreasing as read by the computer, but vigilance is key to assuring yourself that the doctor's over read is consistent and accurate.

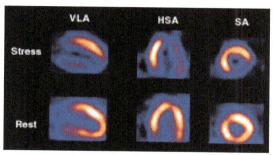

(Fig.45) (www.indiana.edu) This is an image of an abnormal thallium exercise stress test. Note that in the bottom three images at different views of the heart, the thallium is distributed normally like the images in (Fig.42). However, the top images demonstrate in over half of the heart the distribution of the thallium marker in the case of all three images is missing in almost half of the heart. With exercise, the significant stenosis in the culprit artery limits the blood flow to the specific segment of the heart that the artery supplies. It's intuitively obvious that this is a large portion of the heart myocardium. This is a very positive test for the presence of significant CAD, and the chances of this being a false positive test are nearly 0%.

However, the difficulty arises when it's only a very small area of the heart that is "positive" for decreased flow with exercise. For that matter, the area might be so small that the computer reads the test as normal, but the subjective over reader reports "possible" or a "small area" of reversible ischemia. As I have said, in such situations, it's wise to get a second opinion before proceeding with a cardiac catheterization that could most likely be normal and totally unwarrented.

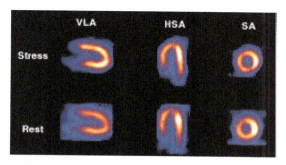

(Fig.46) (www.indiana.edu) Lastly, this is an example of thallium images in someone with an old myocardial infarction. With a heart attack, some of the muscle is dead and scarred and has lost all its blood supply. In these pictures, the rest and the stress images are identical and demonstrate that there is decreased thallium uptake in a significant portion of the heart. Thus, if your EKG has significant old Q waves, this result of a thallium test confirms that there has been a previous myocardial infarction. It may be suggested that in this circumstance, a cardiac catheterization would probably be a good idea even if there is no angina pectoris. In this way, the doctor could confirm the culprit artery that closed and further evaluate life-threatening stenosis in another major artery that could be stented.

It must be pointed out that stress cardiac nuclear imaging is not to be done routinely as part of your screening examination in asymptomatic, low risk patients. By low risk, it's meant having a normal EKG, no insulin dependent diabetes, hypertension, strong family history of a documented heart attack at a very young age, or very high cholesterol levels. This is not a complete list of risk factors, but it's a place to start. Some studies show that such screening as a routine test accounts for 45% of cardiac stress imaging, and evidence from studies doesn't show that the use of this test results in any better medical outcomes for the patient but rather monetary gain for the doctor.

To the contrary, these unnecessary test accounts for a high percent of normal cardiac catheterizations, which in and of itself can cause significant complications, resulting in poorer patient outcomes. Because of these numbers, the patient should make a direct inquiry to the cardiologist why stress imaging is to be done and have the answer to your satisfaction before you undergo any test.

Please check with your insurance company before you undergo myocardial stress imaging studies. First, the insurance company will tell you if precertification is required and what criteria are required for this test. Additionally, as a newer service, many insurance companies will be transparent in telling you the costs and what will come out of your pocket or deductible. Often, they will negotiate a reimbursement with your medical provider to make sure the costs are in line with the standards of practice. Most important, as a newer and much needed added value service, they may have your case reviewed by a medical professional to verify that this expensive test is truly indicated.

Unfortunately, Medicare, as your standalone coverage, doesn't offer such services due to the sheer volume of the tests ordered. However, most senior patients have a co-insurance or gap coverage, which will hopefully provide these very valuable services and offer cost transparency and appropriateness of care. These are new words that describe what is hoped will be an industry-wide practice to prevent 45% of these case that are totally unnecessary. In the case of the patient who has Medicare as their sole coverage, it's a loosing proposition.

Medicare Part B, as an outpatient test coverage, may only pay the physician what he is charging for the test, but ultimately, you'll be paying 20-40% of the technical cost of this expensive test from your pocket. At $1,200-$4,000 a test, this can account for a large part of your budget, especially for an elderly patient on a fixed income. So, if there is no transparency in the costs of your care, it's up to the patient to protect themselves by acquiring adequate knowledge of the test and the appropriateness of your care. These two catch words appropriateness and transparency of care are extremely important to understand in this new age of medical care and cost reimbursement.

It is easy to see that the EKG evidence at rest of a Q wave indicative of an area of heart attack or cell death, which corresponds to the area of no blood flow during the resting portion of the thallium treadmill. This represents strong corroborating evidence and acts to validate the diagnosis of an old heart attack. If these areas don't validate each other, that tends to cast some doubt as to the diagnosis of an old infarction. Of course, any test can be infallible, but it's certainly good evidence to know if it's either positive or negative for an old heart attack.

If the exercise portion of the thallium treadmill indicates a specific area of ischemia and matches the area identified by ST depression during the test, this is good evidence that there's a significant coronary occlusion that should be investigated by further testing or a cardiac catheterization to identify the coronary arteries of the heart that have the occlusions. The cardiac catheterization involves the placement through the groin or arm of a hollow catheter that goes up the aorta and injecting contrast or dye into the coronaries with an x-ray picture of the coronary anatomy and possible stenosis or total occlusion.

An obvious question would be why these non-invasive (no procedure in the body) tests are done at all and not start a cardiac catheterization. Although these non-invasive tests such as a thallium treadmill are getting more accurate because of the remarkable computer interpretation of an immense amount of data, the gold standard for defining the anatomy of the coronary arteries remains the cardiac catheterization. A cardiac catheterization is an invasive test, and as such, requires usually outpatient hospitalization, sedation, and complex introduction and manipulation of catheters in your heart by a highly trained invasive cardiologist.

I mention the term invasive cardiologist in that the procedure for diagnosis is called a diagnostic left heart catheterization. It can turn into a cardiac intervention where the invasive cardiologist finds the culprit stenosis and does an intervention such as an angioplasty or stent to fix the problem at the same time. There is a very critical point that I want to make at this time and one that, I feel very strongly, should not be forgotten.

First and foremost, a cardiac catheterization is fraught with many possible complications some of which may be life threatening or life altering. That's why it's not done as a first line test but only after the non-invasive testing is suggestive of *significant* CAD. This reality is subject to immense variation and interpretation based on the doctor's determination. It's the precise aim of this book to prepare the patient to understand what makes the tests indicate the need for cardiac catheterization or intervention, which will possibly effect the care and prevent an unneeded, expensive, and possibly dangerous procedure. Believe me. As a doctor. I would be very nervous and skeptical about any need for a cardiac catheterization.

For example, I know of an elderly patient who had no angina or any symptoms (asymptomatic) but rather needed a surgery for her carotids. The surgeon asked the cardiologist to evaluate the patient for clearance and for significant CAD, which could affect the risks of his surgery before he proceeded with non-emergent elective surgery. This patient underwent a series of noninvasive tests, which suggested the presence of a coronary occlusion. Notice that I did not say a significant coronary occlusion as the thallium treadmill can pick up very small areas of coronary stenosis in one of those small branch arteries that we talked about.

Now, if you remember, the only reason to fix or do an intervention on a stenosed coronary artery was if there was angina pectoris or that if the intervention would prolong the patient's life. In the case of this patient, when the invasive cardiologist did the cardiac catheterization, he saw no disease in the major bodies of LAD, RCA, or circumflex, but he did find a 90% occlusion in one of the small branches called an obtuse marginal. This lady had no angina pectoris, and in almost no circumstance, is a stenosis in a small branch artery life threatening. The occlusion may have been around for years and would remain that way with the patient never having angina pectoris for many more years.

There is absolutely no validity that a stenosis will advance and cause angina, a myocardial infarction, or death. Quite to the contrary, in studies that look at patients who have known significant coronary occlusions, it was most common for a subsequent heart attack to occur in a less significant area of occlusion that was suddenly newly symptomatic of angina and caused by rupture of a previous small coronary plaque.

However, we talked about the "Oculostenotic reflex" that is present with so many invasive cardiologists that can lead to inappropriate attempts at placement of a stent. For this patient, a stent was placed, so she would probably be on a lifelong blood thinner, and her life would never be the same. Unfortunately for this patient, there was a complication and "iatrogenesis fulminans."

During the stent placement, there was a perforation of her coronary artery which led to bleeding around the heart and sudden thrombosis of the whole major artery from which that branch emanated -the Cx coronary artery. Needless to say, this elderly lady who never needed the stent had a massive heart attack and died on the table. Not only was the family left with a dead relative, but the subsequent medical expenses for a totally unnecessary procedure could have run into the tens of thousands of dollars. This sort of thing happens every day in American medicine where there's lack of feasible medical oversight, and sadly, the death just remains an unfortunate statistic because the family didn't know better. And the doctor lists the cause of death as "coronary artery disease."

It's not my intent to frighten the reader with such a stark reality, but it should alert one to the fact that cardiac catheterization is not a benign or completely safe procedure. Although many physicians will just brush over the complications for your consent, this isn't a procedure to be taken lightly. I suggest, if a loved one or yourself has no angina pectoris but is subjected to a diagnostic cardiac catheterization as an elective outpatient procedure prior to a major surgery, demand the cardiologist to discuss the precise reason for it with the patient or the family before the procedure and establish guidelines for the possible placement of a stent.

Remember that it's totally within your rights as the medical consumer to ask the cardiologist that you want to be consulted before any intervention is contemplated. The cardiologist may try to make excuses why this is not feasible, but I would, without equivocation, reject any such argument and become extra vigilant of this doctor's medical care. There is no other way that I know of that the patient can protect their interests. Any faith that the system would prevent such a problem is just a pipe dream as the "system "is frankly run by the exact organizations that are creating the problem. I'm sincerely hoping that you will defend against such a disregard for a life.

There's one more warning or caution that, I feel, must be made at this time. Again, it's not to scare the heck out of the reader but rather encourage you to be a prudent and cautious consumer of your medical management. It is a very common practice in America that a cardiologist, who just does cardiac diagnostic procedures and not stents or interventions, does your initial cardiac diagnostic procedure.

If a significant culprit lesion is identified, an invasive cardiologist must be called in to do the intervention. This can be done as a cardiac procedure as an outpatient at the same time but usually entails some delay as the invasive cardiologist must come to the catheterization laboratory. In the worst case scenario, the diagnostic cardiologist tells the family or patient that the intervention will be done the next day. Although, there are some valid reasons for this type of delay and the need for a second procedure the next day, these reasons are few and far between. One that is often given is that the kidneys have to recover from the dye load, so the doctor wants to wait another day. This excuse has absolutely no physiological or demonstrated basis in a multitude of studies. This is, I might add bluntly, an excuse based on the interventionalist's schedule.

Not only does this behavior double the patient's risk as another procedure is necessary, but it also doubles the medical expense. And Medicare may not pay for this duplication of medical care. As a common practice, it's possible with Medicare audit and rejection that there is significant financial burden to the patient. Subsequently, the hospital will bill the patient for the total care! This has happened, and with new Medicare rules, this rejection of payment to the hospital and the physician may become an all too frequent reality. As a firm guideline, a cardiac catheterization should never be done by anyone but an interventionalist and who can do a PCI during the same procedure.

I would like to elaborate on another issue that we reviewed. It's also a common practice for the diagnostic or interventional cardiologist to own their own free standing catheterization laboratory that may also be joint owned by the hospital. The issue of whether cardiac catheterization should be hospital based or in a separate and freestanding catheterization laboratory has been the subject of much debate by cardiologist, medical ethicists, and even insurance companies. There is extreme concern about this site not being attached the hospital and is rarely equipped to do anything more than a diagnostic catheterization and not an intervention. If a culprit lesion is found that is deemed appropriate for intervention, then the patient must be transported to the hospital that is equipped for the intervention and any complications with this transportation that might ensue.

If this does not ring up a red flag, then I should. It's astounding to me that Medicare puts up with what I consider overtly dangerous practices. This type of arrangement results in double billing and endangers the life of the patient if there is a complication of the diagnostic procedure in the separate catheterization laboratory. Also, the transport of the patient could mean a threat to his life if the diagnostic catheterization finds an unstable situation. I do feel that Medicare will soon stop this practice, but for now, be aware that there's almost no circumstance where one should go for their diagnostic catheterization to an unattached, freestanding outpatient surgicenter.

More insidious is that if the patient is transferred to the hospital for what was essentially an outpatient procedure, the patient is may now be considered a full admission to the hospital as a transfer rather than an elective outpatient procedure. The billing implications for Medicare Part A&B are staggering and exponentially increase the patient's bill and the expense to Medicare. It's a threat to your life and your pocketbook. It simply increases the profit for those that own or have an interest in the freestanding clinic with no regard for what is in the patient's best interest. If you're a patient in an area where you have no choice but a freestanding clinic, make it very plain to the doctor that a cardiac intervention is to be done on another day at a hospital as a scheduled outpatient procedure of your choosing.

Before we proceed with this history of cardiology, there is another expensive loophole that I'd like to cover. This affects the patient's pocketbook rather than his life, but it does bear mentioning. If a patient has a thallium treadmill at a private cardiologist's office, the expense may be approximately $1,500, which covers the professional fee of the doctor and the procedural or technical fee that pays for the equipment and the nuclear material. However, if the procedure is done in the hospital, then the exact same procedure may cost $4,000-$5,000. Medicare justifies it by stating that the hospital bares the expense to pay for care of the uninsured.

In some cases, I feel that it can be justified if the equipment is more up-to-date and the interpretation is done by an independent cardiologist or a specialist radiologist. The physician who will possibly do the intervention that is subject to the interpretation of the significant abnormality with some possible bias will be eliminated from the equation. The principal point to be made is that the hospital-based test can be 4 times the expense for the exact same test as one done in the office setting. This is a loophole.

If you go to an outpatient clinic such as one in a shopping mall, and if this freestanding clinic is owned by a hospital corporation, which it usually is, then they're allowed by Medicare and the private insurance companies to bill as if the patient was having the procedure in the hospital. In general, this may be mentioned in the fine print of the consent, but I consider this deceitful and dishonest. There may be no way around this loophole as even private cardiologist are being bought out by corporate entities, and the same test the next day in the same office with the same equipment can be quadrupled overnight! There's no way to combat this situation other than to seek out, for such a procedure such as a chest X-ray, a privately owned emergency care center in your neighborhood.

It's a further interesting point is that in this billing scheme for a thallium treadmill, the professional fee for the cardiologist or radiologist interpretation may be the same as the corporate paid physician who may actually be paid less for the interpretation. It's actually the technical fee for the equipment, and staff that takes a marked increase. As said before, all the staff are now employed by the corporation, and this set up only increases the marked profit for the medical corporation at the patients expense. To make matters far worse, Obamacare only perpetuates this abuse as it favors corporate medicine because it's the only entity with the infrastructure to manipulate the amazing complexities of reimbursement under this onerous system. So contrary to the advertised savings to the patient, Obamacare actually may actually triples or quadruples your medical expenses.

CARDIAC CATHETERIZATION

At this juncture in the discussion of the history of cardiology, I would like to temporarily take a leap back to the early 1900s. Let's take a look at cardiac catheterization as a diagnostic and therapeutic tool. This technique drew upon all that was known about the heart until this time and led us into a new era of the understanding of normal and abnormal cardiac function in humans. According to Andre Cournard in his Nobel lecture in December 1956, the cardiac catheter was the "key to the lock" in understanding disordered functions of the heart.

According to Cournard, cardiac catheterizing was first performed and given the name by Claude Bernard in 1844. We briefly mentioned his name before, but in his case, the subject was a horse, and the catheters were introduced into both the right and left ventricles. Claude Bernard's careful attention to scientific technique allowed him to demonstrate the enormous potential for cardiac catheterization in the management of heart disease. These included the use of the catheter in the left ventricle to measure the cardiac output, which is a measure of the strength of the heart. Now, it's utilized in modern catheterization in humans to assess the damage to the heart muscle and in the management of congestive heart failure.

Werner Forssmann is the first doctor credited with passing a catheter into the human heart. Amazingly, he did this in his own heart passing a catheter through his arm artery to the heart utilizing a fluoroscope! He refined this technique with multiple catheterizations of his heart and received the Noble Prize in Medicine in 1956. After that, he went on to become a urologist. However, his work was invaluable and led to the direct injection of medicine into the heart, which was utilized in the injection of epinephrine with a long needle directly into the heart in patients with a cardiac arrest. As a fellow in cardiology for a few years, I used this technique which today, in very special circumstances, can still be successfully utilized for intra cardiac injections of medicine in the heat of a cardiac arrest.

Further developments in this exciting time of discovery was the technique of transseptal catheterization developed in 1959. Now, there's newer techniques of radiofrequency ablation of atrial fibrillation and in the ablation of certain types of supraventricular tachycardia that utilize transseptal access to the left atrium. Transseptal technique is also utilized extensively in procedures for valvular heart disease and for mitral valve repair "clipping" for leakage of the mitral valve. Basically, transseptal is a technique in which a catheter is placed from the right atrium into the left atrium through the wall or septum that separates the two chambers. This is the only reliable way to enter the left atrium. In certain places, this wall is very thin, and in the beginning, this technique was guided by the x-ray landmarks.

In a modern day technique, one uses echocardiograms from inside the heart to aid in its safe application. The lesson to be taken from this technique is that there's much room for serious complications as it takes a great deal of experience. The most serious complication is when the catheter inadvertently enters the high pressure aorta and causes what can be life threatening bleeding around the heart in what is called a pericardial effusion and cardiac tamponade. When one goes for radiofrequency ablation of atrial fibrillation, this technique is one of the factors that make this a highly perilous procedure and usually warrants an inpatient admission.

In 1970, Drs. Swan and Ganz at Cedars Sinai Hospital developed the "Swan Ganz" catheter, which is a tube that's placed often when the patient is in the ICU or the catheterization laboratory to be kept in for days to facilitate monitoring of the heart function. Also, this technique can be quickly done at the bedside and without the assistance of x-ray guidance in skilled hands. I have firsthand knowledge of it as I trained to be a cardiologist under these two men. This technique is rather safe and is often critical in the monitoring of the heart function in congestive heart failure or an acute myocardial infarction.

As a side note, I'd like to say that these two men were some of the most gracious and humble individuals that I have ever known. It cannot be stressed how important this tool has become in the care of an acutely ill cardiac patient.

However, with any new development came the abuse of the technique. Specifically, there are well-defined indications for Swan Ganz catheterization in the acutely ill CCU patient or in the patient with cardiac surgery. It's often placed by a cardiac fellow in a teaching hospital such as Cedars Sinai under supervision, and in my experience, it's generally done safely and for the right reasons. The problem becomes in the unskilled hands or for the non-acutely ill patient at the bedside. There can be complications or even death. After the techniques development, it became a rapidly accepted and widely-used modality.

Only after its development, medical studies looked at the use and complications of the procedure. They confirmed that its use should be reserved for the acutely sick cardiac patient, post myocardial infarction patients in heart failure, and post cardiac surgical patients. What's not intuitively obvious is that these studies showed that the complication rate is higher when the catheter is used as a standard protocol in even the minimally complicated cardiac situation. Thus, the recommendation was made for its specific use in the ill cardiac patient rather than as a standard procedure in the patient with a heart attack that is stable and without complications.

Next, the technique of coronary artery catheterization was first performed on a human being by Dr. Mason Sones at the Cleveland Clinic in 1958. There's no doubt that this was a very important milestone in the practice of cardiology because it gave us a means of visualizing the coronary arteries in a beating heart to assess the amount of pathology and the possible need for treatment. Although it has many more applications in the diagnosis and treatment of heart disease, we'll focus on its use in the diagnosis and treatment of coronary artery disease for now.

More recently, we saw the development of catheter based interventions. The first was angioplasty introduced by Andreas Gruentzig in 1974 when he did the first peripheral human balloon angioplasty. Basically, angioplasty (remodeling of the vessel) or percutaneous transluminal coronary angioplasty (PTCA) involves introduction of a balloon into the coronary stenosis where the balloon is inflated to compress the atheroma and open the artery.

Throughout this period of time, the technique was refined, and new systems of guide wires were introduced to help the invasive cardiologist steer the catheter into the coronary artery.

Within the coronary artery, it allowed the interventionalist better and more successful access to the stenosis for angioplasty. Simultaneously, devices were introduced to allow the operator to actually try to eradicate the atheromatous collection in the artery by laser vaporizing them. Another device called a "Rotablator" was introduced, and it worked like a little roto-rooter that spins and actually cuts the atheroma in a procedure called a rotational atherectomy.

At the same time that Gruentzig was developing PTCA, investigators in Germany were administering a clot busting medicine call streptokinase to patients, and more recently, tissue plasminogen activator (TPA) through the catheter to open the artery in the acute phase of a myocardial infarction. Although this technique is used rarely in the 2014 era, as a doctor, I'd give this agent and watch as the ST elevation of the EKG normalize with the application of these agents that could be done at the bedside. For me, this was a transformational experience as it was done in the CCU at Cedars Sinai. When the acute heart attack was stopped in its tracks and a human life was saved, the medicine was dissolving the clot. It was at that time that I realized how exciting it was to be a cardiologist. However, as I have said, the use of TPA has been essentially been replaced by PTCA/stenting as studies have showed superior short and long time survival with these newer acute stenting techniques.

Like all the advances we've discussed, the advent of catheter based interventions was a miraculous tool to relieve angina, improve lifestyle, and prolong one's life in many cases. However, the possibility of misuse and overuse of the technique became widespread. As in the case of the "oculostenotic reflex" we talked about, just because there is a stenosis in the artery, it doesn't mean that this is the culprit artery and that intervention will have any benefit. Most importantly, the intervention itself may introduce adverse effects that could negatively affect your life. So, I will attempt to point out the opportunities for misuse and how you as the patient can protect yourself as best you can. I must stress again that the most important protection you have for your medical care is knowledge.

To continue, the major advance was the coronary stent called the Palmaz-Schatz Stent, which was named after the pioneer in the technique and introduced in 1994. It involved placing a stainless steel support device that's permanently implanted within the coronary artery and acts to compress the stenosis and open it so that blood flow could be restored. Into the present, this technique has expanded to become the most widely used coronary intervention as the stent was refined and became coated with a drug to prevent clot from developing on the stent, which was a foreign body introduced into the body.

There is no doubt that with the introduction of PTCA/stents interventional cardiology has become the dominant field within cardiology as its remarkable efficacy in prolonging the quality and duration of life has been demonstrated in multiple studies. The techniques of diagnostic angiography in the evaluation of disease have continued to evolve, but the actual simultaneous interventions are now more often accomplished. The evolution of catheter-based intervention will continue to evolve into the 21st century and beyond as the usefulness of this technique to replace cardiac surgery is taking on remarkable proportions. At the present time, these catheter techniques are now being utilized to replace the aortic valve, close an atrial septal defect, cure the leaking of the mitral valve(mitral regurgitation), and lessening the consequences of congenital heart disease.

In addition, interventional cardiologist and interventional radiologist are using these techniques in a truly staggering evolution in the treatment of vascular disorders other than in the heart-peripheral interventions. Some of these include PTA (percutaneous transluminal angioplasty) to open the arteries in the brain in an acute stroke, fixing malfunctioning shunts for dialysis patients, PTA of the legs and arms in patient with pain in these limbs (claudication) or critical ischemia, opening arteries in the intestinal system, and opening the pulmonary vein in the heart which can become stenosed as a long term complication following ablation of atrial fibrillation.

Undoubtedly, these catheter-based interventions will rise as this technique is used more frequently. These applications are just but a few, but the future holds the amazing promise of more interventions that will both improve lifestyle and prolong life with improvement in survival. I truly hope as the reader of this book that you are as excited at these prospects for the future as I am. There is simply nothing that compares to a patient coming back after one of these procedures and reporting how much better their lives have become.

In addition, potent antiplatelet agents (platelet IIb/IIIa receptor antagonists) are taken orally and were developed to prevent the long-term stent clotting. To prevent in stent restenosis (ISR) these agents can be taken for one month, one year, or lifelong after the placement of a stent. This must taken into consideration when the decision is between PTCA of the occlusion and the further addition of a stent. This decision is often based on the anatomy of the lesion itself, but there's room for consideration of one technique over the other in many instances. However, there is no doubt that the short and long-term efficacy are superior with the use of a stent.

CORONARY CATHETERIZATION PROCEDURE

At this time, we'll discuss the technique of coronary visualization by coronary angiography and the various possible interventions. There are many indications for catheterization itself, a few that I have touched upon, and when we come to these individual disease states, it's well established that cardiac catheterization is the technique for diagnosis and treatment. But because the use of catheterization in the management of coronary disease is the predominant use of catheterization, we will now delve into this procedure in its entirety.

INDICATIONS

Coronary catheterization is recommended to confirm the presence of coronary artery disease, its anatomic severity and position, and determine if there's any other anatomic factors that may affect the decision for an intervention in the patient. The most common indication for coronary catheterization without debate is in the "Acute Coronary Syndrome" (ACS) that requires an invasive cardiac procedure contemplated with a PTCA, stent, or cardiac bypass surgery. This is also unequivocally true for a patient with an acute heart attack by EKG or an acute heart attack identified by a blood test, which is a high called troponin or cardiac markers.

The patient with ACS often has a new or existing coronary stenosis that suddenly, for multiple known and unknown reasons, "ruptures" and is open to the rapid blood flow. It further collects platelet deposits and closes more causing a heart attack or new or increasing angina pectoris. The patient presents to the ER after the paramedics are called or from the doctor's office where he identifies an ACS. Contrary to what many cardiac interventionalist use as a justification for their interventional procedure, ACS is a specific syndrome that is acute and not chronic such as in chronic angina pectoris over a longer period of time.

Although the patient may tell the cardiologist that the pain is increasing in severity or frequency, this often is not ACS but what is called "Crescendo Angina." This may not require an emergency catheterization without further noninvasive confirmation of disease such as a nuclear treadmill. In the case of true ACS, the syndrome characteristics and identification are such that the cardiologist may immediately resort to the catheterization without the need for further confirmatory tests except for an EKG and blood tests to look for cardiac damage. It's not uncommon for the patient in the early stages of ACS to have a normal EKG and blood tests, but if there is an old EKG to compare, there are very major changes that further confirms ACS.

This comparison can be a very important clue to the true diagnosis of ACS. Without the often subtle changes in the EKG, there's an increased possibility that the ASC isn't the result of CAD but of other causes such an acute ulcer. Nevertheless, it's usually in the best interests with this circumstance of an ASC that the patient takes faith in the cardiologist's correct decision to proceed with emergent (unscheduled or non-elective) cardiac catheterization, which is always done in the hospital as there is simply no ASC that should be done outside the hospital in a free standing clinic. Thus, there is a major distinction between crescendo angina, which is more chronic and subacute, and true acute ACS in both its recognition and management.

I can assure you that Medicare and most insurance companies are now reviewing charts when submitted for payment, and the proper distinction of the real situation can have significant implications on the proper charges and reimbursement for the procedure. Also, in the future, it may have significant impact on the patient's financial responsibly. In the case of a Medicare patient, the review and added financial burden for the patient may not be evident for even a year after the hospitalization. The patient can suddenly be presented with an additional bill one year after the procedure, which was improperly billed as an inpatient procedure and ACS rather than an outpatient stable or crescendo angina.

A very real example of this problem revolves around Medicare review of the procedure in a "retroactive" review for the appropriate hospital and doctor payments. As of 2014, this is being done as a more active process, and recently, new rules came into effect by Medicare that will result in possible draconian cuts or even the lack of reimbursement if the review is in significant conflict with documented facts of the case. Note, that I use the word document very specifically. It's the responsibility of the doctor and the hospital to document every pertinent facts of the case as it relates to the specific situation. If it's not documented, as far as the reviewer is concerned, it didn't happen. Additionally, if the doctor's handwriting is unreadable by the reviewer, it's outright rejected.

The goal of cardiac catheterization is to identify the culprit lesion for the ACS and intervene with either a PTCA or a stent. Although this may seem logical and rather obvious, it is actually complex in many situations. Often, the interventionalist finds multiple possible lesions in the coronaries. The true art of the procedure and the doctor's experience with clinical excellence dictates what artery is subjected to intervention. As discussed, the EKG in the ACS or acute heart attack will often give the cardiologist a hint at what part of the heart and what coronary artery are involved. Most often however, the interventionalist may feel inclined to intervene on multiple vessels or lesions when he is doing the intervention for an acute heart attack or ACS because of the oculostenotic reflex.

Although there's a few debatable reasons for this relatively common practice, this multi-vessel intervention is dangerous and adds time and complication rates to the procedure. The patient, who is acutely ill, or the family should ask the doctor, either before or after the procedure, what he plans to do or what he has done. I have no doubt that most family members will be uncomfortable questioning the doctor unless they are loaded with the type of knowledge that we are discussing in this book. As I've said, "knowledge is power."

The second broad indication for performing cardiac catheterization is in patients who are stable enough to be scheduled as an elective or planned outpatient procedure versus an emergency catheterization. In one common circumstance, heart catheterization is done when there is a patient with chest pain of an obscure etiology. This is usually the patient seen by the doctor in the office with chest pain that results in a borderline, equivocal thallium treadmill, or an EKG that has minor abnormalities. It's difficult to outline all the reasons that arise with chest pain that doesn't warrant a cardiac catheterization, but it's important to recognize and be vigilant to the overutilization of heart catheterization for this reason.

As an example, if you are less than 50 years old, have a normal EKG, a negative thallium, a normal blood pressure, and no significant documented (not hearsay) history of a first line relative having a heart attack at an early age, or other reasons for chest pain, you must be examined before one resorts to an invasive heart catheterization with its concomitant risks. This becomes an even greater dilemma if you're in the hospital admitted for chest pain and possible angina. The admission itself has little merit when the EKG and treadmill are negative.

Often, because you are in the hospital already, the doctor feels compelled to do the catheterization at this admission rather than schedule it as an elective planned procedure in the future. This practice is done because of the WIGGS (What If I Get Sued) syndrome and has become an all-too-common practice. The problem with this scenario is that if the case is opened up for Medicare or insurance company review, and if it determined that it was unwarranted at the time, the patient may end up with a significant monetary liability. Furthermore, if it results in a two-midnight stay and the doctor converts you to inpatient, Medicare might deny the inpatient classification and significantly reduce the reimbursement to the hospital. As of 2014, they may actually deny all payment to the doctor, and this opens the patient up for a substantial monetary liability.

The third and very important intuitive indication for catheterization is this. If the doctor suspects a significant coronary artery disease although there is a normal stress test and normal EKG with no supported family history but in conjunction with a history of an angina "equivalent" or questionable angina, he may try to warrant the catheterization with the expectation of needing an intervention such as a PTCA/stent or open heart surgery. This opens up a gigantic problem in catheterization being done to a totally asymptomatic patient or the patient with a symptom such as shortness of breath, which is not chest pain but felt by the doctor to be an angina equivalent. I want to reiterate that a good rule of thumb, and one that is supported by numerous clinical research studies, is that the only reason to have an intervention or surgery is to relieve the symptoms of true angina or to prolong life.

Based on these numerous studies, this is the standard of medical care for the cardiac interventions. The oculostenotic reflex, which compels many doctors to do an intervention because it looks bad and in a patient with an angina equivalent, results in interventions that are generally unsupported and unneeded. In a large medical research study published in a world-renowned medical journal, inpatients with minimal to tolerable symptoms and no specific culprit lesion identified, medical therapy such as diet change with control of cholesterol and blood pressure in addition to exercise may actually lead to a better survival!

Additionally, this doesn't even approach the unique and unequivocal fact that the vegan diet can actually reverse the stenosis. In many cases, it cures the patient of coronary disease. This simple truth is something that organized medicine greets with skepticism as they don't want you to know the facts because it would significantly reduce the highly reimbursed interventional procedures that are, to be blunt, the mainstay for so many physician's incomes.

Thus, there are multitudes of clinical research studies as well as published standards of care by the large cardiology associations that precisely outline when a PTCA/stent is indicated in most of the types of lesions seen in the coronary arteries. For example, a stenosis in the LAD when it comes off the aorta is called a proximal or ostial occlusion. Intervention on this lesion greatly increases survival and can overt a large and often fatal heart attack or cardiac arrest.

If a culprit lesion for chest pain, identified as one that matches the area suggested by the thallium, or the EKG, it's definitely indicated to intervene on the lesion. The problem arises when the treadmill was negative and the cardiologist did the catheterization because he suspected the chest pain was for angina and finds a lesion. Thus, if it's unknown as to the true consequence of the lesion for survival, and there is absolutely no assurance that a PCI can cure the chest pain in light of the thallium or EKG being negative, it is very questionable if a PCI should be done at all. As usual, a PCI is most often done, and in some studies, it's estimated that under these circumstances, 80% of the patients aren't relieved of their symptoms because they were simply not caused by the incidental stenosis.

In a similar circumstance, and one that is of great concern because of its prevalence, catheterizations are often done in totally asymptomatic patients who are scheduled for elective surgery for another problem. The surgeon wants the patient cleared for surgery as he may have a history of previous heart attack or a known previous stent. In this case, the cardiologist often orders a nuclear treadmill and even though the patient is asymptomatic, if the treadmill or the EKG are positive, then the patient is scheduled for a cardiac catheterization. More often than not, a stenosis is identified that cannot fit into the category of a life limiting lesion during this procedure and the patient is completely without angina. Because of the lesion being present, the interventionalist does a PCI and subsequently clears the patient from a cardiac point of view for the elective surgery.

This procedure is outside of the proper standards of care, which subjects the patient to the risks of the PCI and commits the patient to lifelong antiplatelet medications that can complicate the contemplated surgery due to bleeding. There's an added risk of a heart attack if the antiplatelet medicine is stopped for surgery. Often times, the elective surgery needs to be postponed for one month to a year before the antiplatelet medication can be safely stopped. Also, there's the risk of future occlusion of the stent, which can be greater than 25% and up to 50% in five years. The cause of this statistic is multiple but includes the patient stopping the antiplatelet medicine voluntarily. Unfortunately, the older patient on a fixed income with the dwindling Medicare pharmaceutical coverage under Obamacare can no longer afford to pay for this expensive medication and must make a decision between eating or continuing their medications.

The serious problem now is that this totally asymptomatic patient that was treated contrary to the standard of cared will most likely develop angina pectoris as the in stent stenosis is usually more critical than the original obstruction. An even more serious problem is that the patient may now develop a myocardial infarction. The truly downside of this situation is that the original occlusion could've been managed by simple diet and medicine with the cardiologist clearing the patient for surgery without any cardiac intervention. But again, because of the WIGGS syndrome combined with the oculostenotic reflex and the ignorance or lack of desire to conform to the standard of care, the cardiologist is unwilling to take this approach in the totally unfounded probability of a cardiac problem during the elective surgery. Additionally, the families, who may also feel the entitlement to have a procedure, are uninformed and ignorant as to the dire consequences.

The question now becomes how the patient or family can approach this problem. It's compounded by the fact that it's estimated in research studies that over 60-70% of cardiac PCI in America is not within the standard of care and not indicated. Also, in the case of PCI being done on the minimally symptomatic or totally asymptomatic patient, it's inappropriately done in over 90% of the cases. These are truly astounding numbers and accounts for the remarkable monetary costs to the health system, and more importantly, to the patient who has to pay the bill.

In some of these cases, the insurance pre-approval process for an elective catheterization would deny coverage to the procedure. The unfortunate consequence is if such a review is done after the procedure. If the insurance company or Medicare (Medicare does not yet have a preapproval review) decides not to reimburse the hospital or physician, then who will be left over to pay the bill? I know of no other way for the patient or the family to approach this problem other that full transparency in the process with the physician and the hospital and the educated patient discussing the procedure with the doctor before the catheterization.

The problem arises if the physician only gives lip service to this request or if they are either ignorant of the standards of care for these situations or unwilling to deviate from the way he has been doing it in the past. This is when the family and the patient should insist that the interventionalist comes out to the waiting family to discuss his plan for intervention and make a convincing argument for the contemplated PCI.

Before we proceed with next section, I'd like to summarize as best I can some of the reasons why the interventionalist may tend to do a PCI with a clinical situation that doesn't meet the standard of care. I truly feel that if the patient's family displays their knowledge of the situation and conveys that to the physician, he'll feel far less threatened by the possibility a lawsuit and the WIGGS syndrome. The unfortunate reality in American Medicine is that most doctors are convinced of a possible malicious or unfounded lawsuit. They think a lawyer can convince an uneducated jury by just showing a picture of a stenosis of an artery that it should have been fixed. This insanity occurs every day in the court system.

The real tragedy is that Obamacare does absolutely nothing to bring about tort reform, and in its misguided attempt to improve medical costs, just perpetuates the over utilization of resources that we have talked about. The leaders of our country, and in its worst manifestation in the form of Obamacare, there is simply nothing done to stop this utter waste of manpower and money. We will talk about this later. Thus, in the long run, the patient must protect himself and develop a rapport with the doctor that is based on mutual trust out of knowledge and understanding.

TECHNIQUE OF CORONARY CATHETERIZATION

In the technique of cardiac catheterization, a long, flexible, and thin tube or catheter is put into the blood vessels leading to the aorta through the groin or arm (Fig.47) and (Fig.48). In the case of a coronary angiogram, this catheter is placed in the coronary arteries and a special type of dye is injected into the coronary arteries to visualize the artery utilizing an x-ray. You're generally awake for the procedure and can see the pictures of your coronary arteries as the doctor visualizes your heart (Fig.49). Being awake, you can talk to the doctor and take instructions from him as he does the procedure. You'll be given an anti-anxiety medicine that will calm you down and help control some of the inevitable fear during the procedure. Catheterization is generally painless, but the doctor will inject some local anesthesia in your groin or arm to numb the area when he places the catheter in your arteries for access to the aorta and into the coronary arteries.

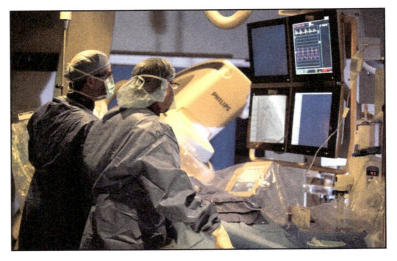

(Fig.47) (www.enloa.org) This is a picture of the cardiac catheterization laboratory where the procedure is done. Note the large x-ray machine over the patient under the sheets that is utilized to take the x-ray pictures during the procedure. The newer machines such as in this picture use far less radiation than the old machines. The amount of x-ray that you're exposed to is minimal in a normal procedure, which may last ½ hour to 2 hours. On the right, you can see the digital display screen that the doctor looks at during the procedure. If in this picture the patient looks to the left, they can simultaneously view the pictures of the catheterization.

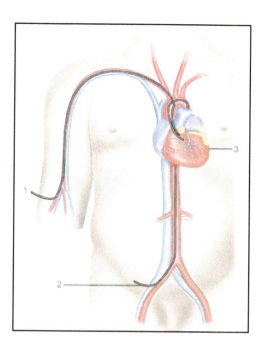

(Fig.48) (www.nhs.uk) In this illustration, one can see the catheter as it is inserted either in the groin or the arm up the aorta to the heart an inserted it the coronary arteries at the aortic valve origin.

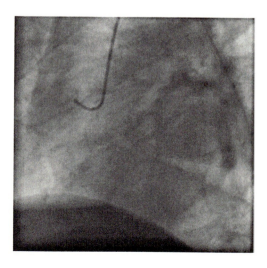

(Fig.49) This is the x-ray picture of the catheter going up the aorta and placed into the orifice of a coronary artery. When you're having your catheterization and look over at the display screen, this is what you'll initially see. On the right, you can see the catheter going up the aorta. It turns at the aortic arch to go down to the aortic valve and into the origin of the coronary arteries for injection of contrast material and visualization of the coronary artery.

The access to the aorta and into the coronary arteries is done from the groin (femoral approach) or the arm (radial or brachial approach). The arm approach is newer, and the choice of the site is based on the experience and familiarity of the cardiologist with either approach. There is some suggestion that the arm approach is safer since it general avoids some complication of the femoral approach, but both access sites are appropriate. If I were given the choice, I'd choose the radial approach.

The complications from this stage of the procedure are multiple, but I'd like to cover the salient points. First, when the artery itself is entered, the needle for entrance access can penetrate completely through the artery and cause bleeding behind the artery with the loss of blood. This is a hidden complication but can explain some loss of blood after the procedure. This complication is diagnosed either by a CT scan of the groin or a form of echocardiography called a duplex scan of the area. Secondly, when entering the artery, the needle can cause a tear in the artery or a separation of the lining of the artery, which is called a dissection.

Again, this complication can cause loss of blood, but more importantly, it can cause the artery to close with some jeopardy to the blood supply to the limb. If this occurs, the doctor will often stop the procedure and do a duplex or CT scan of the artery. This complication can cause a swelling at the site of the needle entrance called a hematoma, and a more serious consequence results in bleeding from the femoral artery into the back of the lining of the intestinal cavity called a retroperitoneal hematoma. Again, this is diagnosed by either a duplex or CT scan of the groin. These complications can heal themselves but can also require emergent surgical intervention.

The last important complication involves the aorta. When the catheters are thread up or across the aortic arch, it can also cause these same complications in the aorta, which have far more dangerous consequences. Thankfully, these hitches are rare but can occur more in the elderly (>80 years old). These complications require immediate surgical interventions and can be life threatening. A more common but still rare complication is when the catheter goes up or across the aortic arch and the catheter breaks off an atheroma or cholesterol deposit resting in the artery and the resultant "embolism" that can travel to the legs or arm and more importantly to the brain and cause a stroke. Again, this is much more common in the elderly and should be food for thought before a catheterization is done in any patient over the age of 80.

As we've already discussed, the procedure is mostly done in a hospital. The reason that in general the hospital is fully equipped for an intervention such as a stent and prepared for any emergency complication. This includes a cardiac surgeon if an emergency cardiac bypass is required. Also, as I have previously said, one should avoid a catheterization by a cardiologist who's not specially trained as an interventionalist who can place a stent or angioplasty if required. If this isn't the case, the use of two cardiologists often leads to the need to come back the next day for a second procedure and intervention. This only leads to a double chance for serious complications and a double bill for a procedure that should've been done in one day.

Based on the two-midnight rule, the second day might result in your being placed as an inpatient with the resultant change in your Medicare billing that may result in a higher bill for the patient. Furthermore, Medicare may question the legitimacy of the two-midnight stay for a procedure that could've been done in one day. These rules may actually result in a denial of payment to the doctor and possibly the hospital for the procedures and significant financial exposure to the patient.

Before the procedure starts, the physician will have you sign the consent form. Like most consents for a medical procedure, they're overly complex in their wordage for an average person to understand. So, I'd like to give you some pointers. First, contrary to the usual habit, most patients listen to the doctor explain the consent, but it's often quite cursory. You're then given the consent form to sign, and it's critical that you read it. This document tries to list off all the complications that can ensue.

There's no doubt that it's impossible to anticipate all that can go wrong and the consent doesn't necessarily protect the doctor or take away your rights, but you should prepare for anything that concerns you. Review with your doctor the exact indication for your cardiac catheterization, and discuss what he plans to do. Before he places a stent in your heart during the catheterization, ask him to do a brief explanation during the procedure or reach out to the family in the waiting room. You may be somewhat sedated but should aware enough to think and make a decision. Hopefully, you'll use the information from this book and be able to respond with insight.

The most important suggestion from this book is that every consent that you sign as of 2014, and especially after the new Medicare rules of September 8, 2014, should include a clause that any charges for the doctor's fees that are denied payment by Medicare will not be passed on to the patient. This clause will protect you from what will undoubtedly be more denials of Medicare payment for hospital procedures and admissions that Medicare deems unnecessary or not indicated. Ensure that your demand be added to the consent for hospitalization when you're admitted to a hospital. The doctor and the hospital will try to avoid these clauses, but there is nothing to prevent you from writing in the clause yourself as you sign the documents. This clause should read, "Any charges denied to the hospital or the doctor shall not be passed on to me."

At this time, we should discuss the various contraindications to do the cardiac catheterization especially when it's a planned, elective procedure versus an emergent procedure where the doctor has little choice but to do the catheterization in a timely manner. First, hypertension should be controlled when it's severe before and during the procedure. If it cannot be controlled, the high blood pressure significantly effects the safety as well as the efficacy of the procedure, so the procedure should be avoided until the blood pressure is controlled. Unfortunately, this contraindication is often ignored or overlooked. Other conditions that should be controlled before the procedure are significant anemia, heart failure, febrile illness, and low potassium.

Another controversial contraindication to the procedure is anticoagulation. In actuality, this is a very complex problem that has to be individualized in every unique situation, but there are some general guidelines to direct the physician. Most problems arise when a patient is on warfarin for atrial fibrillation for a history of vein thrombosis or pulmonary embolism or for having a mechanical heart valve. In the case of atrial fibrillation, much depends on whether the patient has had a previous stroke. If not, all of the organized cardiology groups have endorsed the safety of being off the warfarin or other newer anticoagulants for one week.

Thus, if the physician chooses to do the catheterization off the warfarin, the drug can be safely stopped at home and the thinning for the blood can be checked at the doctor's office with an INR test before you go to the hospital for the procedure. As of 2014, this scenario is rarely followed, and the doctor will have the patient admitted to the hospital a day or even two days before the procedure to go off the blood thinner. In the case of atrial fibrillation, this is not only unnecessary, but Medicare and most insurance companies will simply deny payment for these days—and the patient will again be exposed to excessive financial liability.

If necessary for "convenience" issues out of distance from the hospital or advanced age, the patient can simply check into a hotel close to the hospital for the appropriate outpatient testing before one is admitted to the hospital for the catheterization. There is absolutely no reason the doctor cannot check your blood thinning in the lab before you go to the hospital. Your blood may be too thin, and the procedure postponed. If you're kept at the hospital, payment for simple "custodial" care will be denied, especially if the doctor has you taking up a room waiting for your blood thinning to correct. It's purely out of convenience of the doctor that he doesn't send you home immediately and asks to come back for the procedure in one or two days.

In the case of anticoagulation for a mechanical heart valve, this becomes a much more challenging problem. In this case, there is a significant danger to be off the blood thinner for more than a day during the procedure due to the risk of a blood clot and a possible stroke. Additionally, many interventionalist are choosing to do the procedure with a degree of anticoagulation due to the relative safety demonstrated in various research studies. Nevertheless, I feel it is important to be continuously anticoagulated and the most prudent and cost effective manner is to stop the warfarin and to be placed on a drug that the patient can easily and simply be injected under the skin called Lovenox.

The Coumadin is stopped for a week before the planned procedure, and the patient is given a prescription for the Lovenox to be injected under the skin twice a day until the procedure. On the day of the procedure, it's stopped, and after waiting for 4-6 hours, the procedure can be safely done, minimizing the risk of bleeding. Once the procedure is done, the Coumadin is restarted. The Lovenox is continued at home for a short time, perhaps 2-3 days, while the Coumadin blood thinning takes effect.

This scenario seems simple enough, and although many cardiologists have learned to adopt this approach, there are many who have not. First, the argument is that the patient cannot afford the expensive Lovenox, and there is a need to admit the patient one or two days before the procedure to take them off the Coumadin and start an intravenous blood thinner called heparin. Other arguments against Lovenox is that the patient is too old to give themselves their own shots or that the patient lives too far away from the doctor to come in for a check that the Coumadin has worn off before the procedure while the patient is on the Lovenox.

The problem with these arguments is that recently Medicare may not approve the IV heparin approach, and in some circumstances, just deny payment for the patient who was admitted days before the procedure for its administration. Medicare does not recognize these fallacious arguments for IV heparin, and I assure you that the cost and financial risk to the patient for a denial is far greater than the cost of the Lovenox. I wholeheartedly agree with this Medicare judgement. Also, if the distance is too great, the patient can get a hotel room in proximity to the doctor. If the patient is too old, they can get home health care to come to the house twice a day to administer the Lovenox before and after the procedure.

If the doctor holds the patient in the hospital for 2-3 days after the procedure to use IV heparin instead for the subcutaneous Lovenox, the policy is being pursued to also deny all the days of hospitalization as well as possibly the procedure. I imagine that in many cases, the doctor assumes that even if the days are denied, he has his "protocol" to do as taught as the safest for the patient and is unwilling to change his ways as he feels he will still be paid for these denied days. I consider this argument to not only be invalid, but frankly, dangerous and narrow minded thinking.

As of September 2014, the doctor will no longer be paid for his services on the denied days, and there's the risk that he will try to pass this cost to the patient. Thus, it's very important for the patient or the family to be aware of this problem and discuss it with the physician. If he insists on doing it his own way, it's critical that he documents in the chart the exact reasoning behind his decision, so that if it is logical and makes sense, the days won't be denied.

PROCEDURE

Once the patient finally goes to the catheterization laboratory, the cardiac catheters are introduced into the aorta and up to the coronary artery orifices or ostium that are at the aortic valve. The doctor will inject some dye into the blood through the catheters into the coronary artery (Fig.50) and (Fig.51). You may feel flushed or warm with this injection, but this is normal. The dye utilized by the doctor for the visualization of the coronary arteries is a special solution that is opaque to the x-ray and outlines the stenosis. This dye is generally safe, and through the years, it has been improved upon to cause the least side effects. It has iodine in it, so if you're allergic to iodine, such as allergic to shellfish, tell the doctor. He can give you medicine before the procedure to minimize your chances of having an allergic reaction to the contrast material.

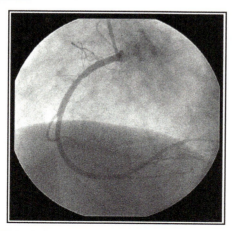

(Fig.50) This is a screen shot during a catheterization after the dye is injected into a normal right coronary artery. Importantly, notice that the artery looks smooth and does not appear to have any obstruction or stenosis.

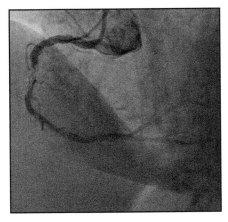

(Fig.51) This is a screen shot of an abnormal RCA. You can obviously see that although the dye does get through to see the whole artery meaning that the obstruction is not 100%, it is fairly obvious that the artery is irregular with cholesterol build up, and there is a severe obstruction in the middle of the artery. If this is the culprit artery, the doctor will proceed with a PCI and stent.

The important point about this contrast solution is that it can actually cause acute kidney injury, and in some cases, complete failure of the kidneys. This is more common in the patient who had previous renal disease or failure, one kidney, or had a renal transplant. This situation often resolves itself in days, but in the worst case scenario, it can lead to temporary or permanent dialysis. It's extremely important that the doctor is aware of this situation, and he will admit you to the hospital 6 hours prior to the procedure in order to give you intravenous (IV) fluids to prevent this reaction.

The doctor used to admit the patient the day before the procedure for IV fluids. However, it's totally unnecessary as the studies clearly demonstrate that there is no benefit to hydrate more than 6 hours before the catheterization. Furthermore, most insurance companies, especially Medicare, will no longer pay for 24 hours of unnecessary pre-hydration.

Not only is the use of contrast material itself a risk of renal injury, but the actual amount of contrast utilized during the procedure is a critical determinant of the chances of renal damage. In this respect, the doctor does his best to limit the amount of contrast, but this can be significantly compromised if the procedure takes more time and more pictures of the coronaries. Thus, this presents a major problem when the interventionalist proceeds to intervene on more arteries than are identified as the culprit lesion. It's perfectly reasonable to stop the procedure after this culprit single lesion is approached and schedule a second procedure in future as a "staged" intervention. In this manner, the kidneys can recover after the first catheterization before the next percutaneous coronary intervention (PCI).

Similarly, when the diagnostic test is done at a freestanding clinic and transferred to the hospital for a PCI, this essentially two procedures that could have been done in one day utilizes excessive unneeded contrast to re-visualize the arteries for the PCI and only adds to the increased and unnecessary risk of contrast-induced toxicity to the kidneys. Also, it's my hope that some insurance companies may ask for a pre-approval of a second procedure and have the situation reviewed by a second cardiologist to assure that the second intervention is medically indicated and within the accepted standard of care. I wholeheartedly condone such a practice.

Some cardiologist feel compelled to keep the patient in the hospital to let the normal kidneys recover to do the second staged procedure. This is an absolutely ridiculous practice and exposes the hospital to coverage denial and inappropriate inpatient services. If the patient is stable and the PCI is not emergent, it's appropriate to discharge the patient and readmit as a staged procedure at the future time. It's better to have two appropriate procedures at different times than one multiple-day procedure that will be denied. With a staged procedure, if the patient's angina goes away after the first procedure, the second staged PCI may be avoided, deemed as unnecessary, and be suggested to be treated with medication and diet.

One of the very good consequences of Obamacare is that it has fostered the formation of medical organizations called Accountable Care Organizations (ACO). This is a group of doctors and possibly a hospital that is paid a basic lump sum by Medicare to care for a group of patients who then pays for any procedure out of their lump sum for any hospitalization or procedure. It's in their benefit to keep the patient healthy and avoid expensive intervention. In the case of a staged procedure, it would greatly benefit the ACO, as well as to the patient, that the second staged PCI is reviewed by one or a group of cardiologists who are part of the organization or an outside service hired to do the "appropriateness of care review" before the second or third procedure is done.

They would decide if the intervention is indicated, if the patient can be treated by medication, or recommend the efficient application of diet and exercise for the proper future management. We shall see how this plays out in the future, but I see this as a very positive step in the proper, safe, and cost-effective approach to medical care. As I've said, it would be significantly more profitable in many situations for the ACO to place the patient in a managed program administer by the ACO for proper diet, exercise, weight loss, smoking cessation (it is possible a smoker could not join an ACO), and compliant cholesterol and hypertension management.

This approval process by the ACO would additionally give the patient an estimate of the cost of the proposed and appropriate procedure called "transparency in care." This is a very important advance, which is in contradistinction to the current rage for some insurance companies and internet companies that charge for their assessment to give employers and patients the ability to estimate a cost of a proposed procedure or hospitalization. The true absurdity of these tools is that they're not only a rough estimate without anticipated complications in the care, but they're complex to use and absolutely do nothing to approach the problem of whether the procedure is appropriate to be done in the first place.

This true transparency of care takes doctor-to-doctor discussion (peer to peer), and the insurance companies and the employers may not utilize this service as it's too "expensive," or there is no infrastructure or procedures in place to accomplish this task. Let's truly hope the spread of ACO type of care structures approach this problem correctly to finally afford safe and cost-effective cardiological care.

Once the interventionalist identifies the culprit lesion, he will then proceed to a PTCA or a stent. If he's not sure of the lesion's significance, he may do a procedure before the intervention call a FFR (fractional flow reserve) that can help identify if the lesion is severe enough to cause angina and need the PCI. I have found that many times, if the procedure is done by a cardiologist who isn't an interventionalist, he'll stop the procedure here and justify his actions to study the lesion on a second procedure to measure the FFR and possibly do a PCI.

If the FFR is not significant in the second procedure, the patient has been exposed to the extra risk of the procedure and the dye load for no PCI with absolutely no medically supportable reason. Again, as we have seen, Medicare has the potential of denying the whole procedure as excessive, especially the second procedure, which was not indicated and more importantly expose the patient to double the danger.

Once the lesion is considered significant, then the doctor will proceed with the PCI or even recommend coronary artery bypass surgery (CABG). Each PCI takes an additional dye load and will be one of the variables determining if the doctor proceeds to do more than one PCI or recommend CABG. We have also discussed this situation, and it always becomes a huge problem if the interventionalist decides to do multiple PCIs without adequate proof that the further PCI procedure will extend one's life or is responsible for the patient's symptomology.

So, the PCI is done, and a PTCA or stents are placed (Fig.53). It may take more than one stent to fix one long stenosis, and it's not unreasonable for a long lesion in a major artery such as the LAD, RCA, left main, or circumflex that the physician could actually use three or four stents. There is no doubt that this may be the proper approach. In the same respect, in a small branch artery, it's truly incumbent upon the interventionalist to demonstrate and prove that any PCI on such a small artery can prolong life or cure angina.

For instance, if the thallium test done before the procedure demonstrates a possible lesion in the anterior part of the heart but the small branch lesion supplies the back of the heart, then it's very unlikely that a PCI on this small lesion will cure the chest pain, and even more unlikely, that intervention would have any effect on life span. In actuality, this procedure may cause deterioration in life style and shortening of predicted life span with the implant of a totally unnecessary stent!

The real problem, and ethical issue that is becoming a real problem in American medicine, is when the patient demands treatment even though the doctor makes it very clear that the PCI would not benefit the patient or even has the potential to cause long-term harm.

The practice of entitlement and the absolute demands of the patient or the family creates a real problem for the doctor who strives for ethical care but has to deal with potential conflict with the demanding patient. This is actually the subject of much debate within the medical community and an issue, which is only becoming more important to approach with the entitlement mentality reflected in Obamacare.

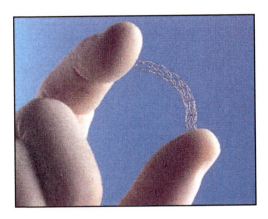

(Fig.53) (www.heart-specialist.org) This is a picture of a coronary stent. It's very flexible, so it can be placed in the coronary artery and is made of a metal such as stainless steel that consists of wires woven into a mesh that fits into the coronary artery. These stents can be coated with a clot preventing material and is called a drug eluding stent (DES) in contradistinction to a non-drug coated bare metal stent (BMS). The difference in the use of these two stents may be technical or have the need for a relatively anticipated major surgery in the case of a BMS, which only needs blood thinners for one month.

An interesting statistic is that on the average over a five-year period, a stent (Fig.54) costs $9,500 more than just diet and lifestyle changes. As of 2004, the cost of stents was up to 40 billion dollars for the year and predicted to be over 150-200 billion dollars in 2015. That makes it the single most expensive cumulative procedure in medicine. This is truly an astounding cost especially as 50-70% of these stents may be unnecessary and Obamacare only perpetuates.

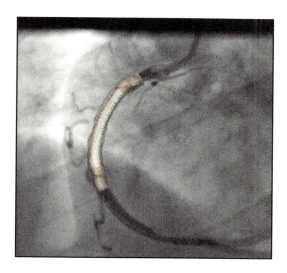

Fig.52 (galleryhip.com) This is a depiction of a stent deployed in the right coronary artery. Note that the stent is long and is guided by a wire in the coronary artery over which the stent is guided into the correct position.

You're probably wondering how the difficult situation with PCI and stenting of small branch coronary arteries can be true. When a stent is placed, there is the risk of at least 25% within one year and 50% within five years that the stent will close-this is markedly higher in small branch arteries. As we have previously mentioned, this may create angina where there was none before. Also, there is the added risk of more PCIs and the added probability of stent "restenosis" that can cause a new myocardial infarction.

Before we proceed, I would like to mention one very exciting prospect for the use of stents and especially the long-term use of blood thinners. There is the development of stents called "biosorbable scaffolds" that are basically nonmetallic stents out of a material, which is drug coated and is actually reabsorbed in the blood system and leaves the artery opened over a period of time. In this way, after a defined period of time, the blood thinners can be discontinued and there is reduced incidence of restenosis.

I predict that, as studies confirm the safety and efficacy of such stents, they will become the standard of care. In this same respect, the use of laser catheters, which basically vaporize the lesion, may be shown in studies to add to the safety and efficacy of a PCI procedure and obviate the need for a stent and long-term blood thinners. However, remember what I have stressed. A procedure or new stent may look logically better or more effective, but there are always long-term consequences. It's only after medical studies confirms their efficacy will they be accepted as the new standard of care.

STENT

A stent is deployed to the appropriate culprit lesion. In actuality, the deployment of a stent is a relatively safe procedure. It's delivered to the appropriate spot over a balloon catheter around the balloon, the balloon is inflated, and the stent expands to into the artery. The physician chooses the right size stent both in diameter for the vessel and in length to cover the whole lesion. Because of the long length or complexity of the some lesions, the interventionalist must may use two or three stents to cover the culprit lesion. It should be mentioned that the use of multiple stents will increase the risk of restenosis of the stents over time because there are more stents to close.

As we have repeatedly stated, this situation can be compounded by the interventional cardiologist feeling compelled to put stents in multiple lesions in the heart based on the oculostenotic reflex, which haven't been identified as the culprit lesion.

Sometimes, this practice is justified if the physician has seen multiple areas of ischemia on the prior nuclear treadmill. Also, the second area may be a critical area of ischemia based on the large size of the artery or if deemed life threatening. Nevertheless, the stenting of multiple unrelated lesions has been studied recently. The consensus is that it may be more prudent to do only one lesion which is associated with better long-term results based on the high incidence of contrast induced kidney failure due to the extra contrast needed as well as the increased restenosis rate. So, in patients with angina, the culprit lesion should be done first. The patient should be observed over time for recurrent or persistent angina and even undergo a repeat stress test after the first procedure.

It has been shown that the medical management of angina after the main culprit lesion is fixed has the same or better long-term survival than second stent. If medical management is unsuccessful or the angina is severe and interferes with one's lifestyle, the second lesion can be stented after the kidneys have recovered from the first intervention and contrast load. At the same time, the use of percutaneous coronary interventions in patient with extensive occlusion on angiogram , a very positive stress, and have extensive multi-vessel disease on the angiogram may have a better chance of long term survival with coronary bypass surgery rather than multiple use of stents for multivessel revascularization. There have been many case reports, and there is an excellent documentation on this subject which we shall soon cover.

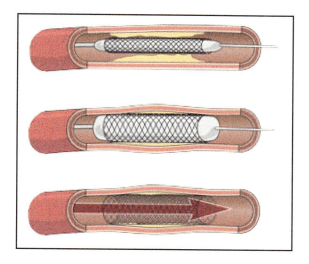

(Fig.54) (intermountainhealthcare.org) In this picture, the lesion or the cholesterol buildup in the artery is the plaque. The catheter is directed to the plaque, and the balloon is inflated, which expands the stent. The balloon is then deflated, leaving the expanded stent in place. The balloon and the stent compress the plaque and open the artery. Before the advent of the stent, when a stent is not used, then the procedure was just the balloon inflating and compressing the plaque. This is called a percutaneous transluminal coronary angioplasty (PTCA).

COMPLETE TOTAL OCCLUSION

The last subject to be covered before moving on to bypass surgery is complete occlusion of a coronary artery. For example, a patient with chronic stable angina develops worsening angina and referred for a nuclear treadmill that demonstrates a large area of ischemia in a culprit vessel. So, the patient undergoes a coronary angiogram, and an artery is found to be 100% occluded. In over 90% of these cases, the doctor finds that collateral have grown into this artery past the total obstruction and feed the distal artery.

In some cases, there was ischemia on the treadmill, and these collaterals are not sufficient to meet the metabolic demands of the heart especially with exertion. In over 50% of these cases, attempts at opening the chronic total occlusion is unsuccessful or associated with significant complications such as a tearing or dissection of the proximal coronary artery. In such case, the procedure is abandoned, and the patient is treated with diet and life style modification.

The acute, complete closure of the artery is an absolute indication for PCI. However, chronic total occlusion (CTO) is defined as complete or nearly complete (95-99%) closure of the artery for more than three months. At times, it's hard for the interventionalist to ascertain the chronicity of the CTO, but there are signs such as calcification that shows its chronicity. The majority of these patients have collaterals that have grown into the artery and can be insufficient to supply the myocardium with blood specifically under exertion. It's absolutely critical that the doctor perform a nuclear treadmill before attempting at PCI in these situations.

Therefore, if a CTO is found during a catheterization and there no preceding nuclear stress test quantifying the degree of ischemia or if there was only a small degree of ischemia, PCI shouldn't be done (contraindicated) in the case of chronic exercise related angina. If the treadmill demonstrates that the area of the CTO is already dead and there is no reversible ischemia, PCI of this area is absolutely contraindicated, and unfortunately, is not always adhered to in the practice especially with the less-trained interventionalist.

There is significant controversy as to whether a CTO should be subject to PCI verses CABG. If there are multiple, large artery occlusions (multi-vessel disease) then the indication is unequivocally for CABG. The controversy exists when there's a branch vessel disease that doesn't show up on the nuclear treadmill. Then PCI may be the best option if the angina is stable. There have been many inconclusive studies that have tackled this problem, and the general consensus is that each case is individual and that survival may be better with PCI. But the amount of repeat procedures is greater with PCI and may favor CABG after all.

The bottom line is that the doctor has the responsibility to discuss CTO with the patient and the family before any intervention. CTO is never emergent, so it can be done as an elective outpatient procedure, not part of a multi-day admission. Often, the PCI on CTO can only be done in specialized centers with a great amount of expertise and experience. It's essential that the patient or the family queries the doctor about his experience with it, how many he's performed, and to document specifically what he says for your records.

I feel that if the doctor hasn't performed over 50-100 CTO procedures, then CTO PCI should be done at a specialized center that probably has done over 500 such cases. Every hospital keeps an accurate record of the amount of CTO PCIs performed. These records can be requested by the patient, and one should be beware of the hospital that refuses to show or claims that no such record exists. Since CTO PCI is almost never emergent, there's always adequate time to make the appropriate decisions without being coerced or rushed into it.

HOSPITALIZATION FOR ANGINA PECTORIS AND MYOCARDIAL INFARCTION

I'd like to elaborate on the hospitalization for angina pectoris and a myocardial infarction to add to our previous discussion of cardiac catheterization, the manifestations of chest pain, and a heart attack. Angina and a myocardial infarction are one of the most common causes of admission to the hospital and deserve special mention.

First, the most common presentation of angina can be the new onset for the first time or angina that's been present and already evaluated by a cardiologist but is getting worse and occurs with less exercise or at rest. As previously mentioned, it's often hard to differentiate true angina from just chest pains, which can have many causes as muscle pains, chronic pain, gastrointestinal problems such as an ulcer or esophageal disorders, and muscle strain from lifting. Nevertheless, one ends up in the emergency room with this chest pain, and the first thing the ER doctor will order is an electrocardiogram.

Note that chest pain is the most common cause of ER visits in the United States. This electrocardiogram may be very revealing for a new heart attack, and in this scenario, you may be taken directly for a cardiac catheterization for a possible angioplasty and stent. It's important to know that even if the EKG is very suggestive, the angiogram may be normal and not demonstrate any coronary artery disease in up to 10% of the time. This is especially true in females, who have a sudden extremely stressful situation and the EKG and blood test are positive for a myocardial infarction. They are taken for heart catheterization where it is found the arteries are totally normal but the heart function is abnormal. This is called stress syndrome or Takatsubo's syndrome. In this scenario there are numerous false positive readings of the EKG, or the clinical suspicion is very high that it warrants an immediate cardiac catheterization that ultimately turns out to be normal.

The point is that in case of a normal cardiac catheterization, the admission should almost always be classified as outpatient or observation. There are many doctors who try to write a certified or not certified admission as inpatient, but that's totally incorrect. The patient and the family must be vigilant in recognizing this error and seek its rectification. It's not necessarily your right to know your admission status, but the physician will have no choice but to answer and explain his reasoning if asked directly. Nevertheless, if the angiogram is normal, the physician may insist on a further barrage of tests in the hospital to determine the true nature of the chest pain.

Usually, this is done out of convenience for the doctor or the family. It may result from the WIIGS syndrome and the family who requests an immediate further evaluation or work up in the hospital. However, this circumstance and further tests are simply unrelated to the initial diagnosis. And as of 2015, Medicare will deny the charges and further hospital care.

These further tests are usually done as an outpatient such as a colonoscopy or a tube down the stomach to look for an ulcer or inflammation of the stomach called gastritis as a cause of the chest pain.

These interventions are one-day tests done in outpatient clinics, not in the acute care hospitals. This information can save the patient a great deal of money and headache as these further tests have no business being done in the acute care hospital in most cases. So, if denied by Medicare or the insurance company, the patient may be responsible for a potentially large financial responsibility even after a year of the discharge!

Just imagine getting a hospital bill for $5,000-$10,000 or more a year after your discharge. It's all for chest pain with normal coronary arteries that resulted in two or three more excessive hospital days due to further tests that were unrelated and should've been done in the outpatient setting. This reality is certainly in the realm of a possibility and can only cause substantial financial and social hardship if not a very negative effect on your credit rating if unable to pay. These rules relating to unrelated procedures are covered in great detail in the CMS.gov website under provision 541 and CY 2015 if you're up to a complex read. This section of my book is a good substitute for trying to wade through the incredible complexity of these two rules. As of 2015 the writing and management of CMS.gov may become more readable and palatable to the general public to digest.

If the patient is transferred from another institution that cannot do the catheterization with the high suspicion of a heart attack, it's no different. Observation or outpatient status is appropriate for those with normal coronary arteries. However, the situation may be different for a true heart attack or angina that requires an emergency intervention such as an angioplasty or stent. It's completely within the realm of a possible two-midnight stay, which is well outlined in the CMS.gov website and warrants an inpatient admission status. This takes the proper orders to occur, and the doctor may feel that you could be discharged the next day. If the intervention was done on an emergency basis with a true heart attack with muscle damage rather than unstable or acute angina, the two-day expectation of admission is very possible and should be properly documented in the orders or the medical record.

As of CY 2015, the expectation can either be in the orders as a certification as we have discussed or ascertained from the doctor documentation in the chart.

Now, the circumstance of the hospital admission may be very different if the presentation to the ER is possible angina and the ER doctor feels you might require hospital admission. Under ideal conditions, the cardiologist would come to see you and determine if the admission to the acute care hospital was required and the evaluation could've been done in his office with a nuclear treadmill and an echocardiogram. However, a doctor coming to the hospital in the middle of the night is becoming a very rare scene, and an inappropriate acute care hospitalization is very common. Often, it's driven by undue family or patient concerns or anxieties and the WIIGS syndrome.

In this circumstance, the doctor would rather take the easiest expediency and admit the patient. It's not completely out of the question that a 45 year old with a normal EKG and negative blood tests for heart disease is admitted and taken for a heart catheterization out of anxiety of the patient and the family. In addition, it includes the doctor's fear of lawsuit although the angiogram is totally normal and the patient didn't require the hospitalization in the first place. It's conceivable that the whole acute care hospitalization is deemed inappropriate and not indicated under 541 and CY 2015.

In the future, the patient could be financially responsible for a good portion of the hospital bill; however, it'll be up to Medicare to enforce the rules already on the books to save money and benefit the patient by preventing undue, expensive, and often, dangerous tests. The problem is that the government has a terrible habit of ignoring the rules on the books that could potentially help solve the situation and the dysfunctional American medical system.

Lastly, if the patient is actually admitted to the hospital for chest pain in the middle of the night, it takes up one useless hospital day. The first thing in the morning, either the doctor will elect to do an angiogram or a nuclear treadmill with a possible echocardiogram. When the doctor sees the angiogram as unnecessary, can't fit it into his schedule, or doesn't want to waste a hospital day that results in custodial care for a day, the patient can be discharged on the same day or early the next morning as an observation admission and not with inpatient status.

It's my fervent hope that private insurance companies such as United Health Care, Blue Cross, or Aetna, as well as Medicare, adopt a strategy to review these cases to save themselves money, and more importantly, foster proper and safe cardiological care. I think it's happening, and the Medicare creation of Accredited Care Organizations (ACO) does quantum steps in creating this optimal situation and will hopefully spread under Obamacare for the remarkable benefit to all those involved: the insurance provider, hospital, and the patient.

The provisions for ACOs under Obamacare and the new CMS rules are a wonderful development and could lead to a significant money-saving situation, which will improve patient care, ultimate medical outcomes, and will foster and perpetuate a free enterprise system rather than a form of socialized medicine.

CORONARY ARTERY BYPASS SURGERY (CABG)

At this time, we'll review some of the history and techniques of CABG. It's important to recognize that it's a complex and difficult decision to have a bypass surgery for coronary artery disease over PCI. As of 2014, the indications and techniques of CABG are evolving rapidly, but the exhaustive subject is beyond the scope of this book. Nevertheless, the consultation with a cardiac surgeon when bypass surgery is contemplated is a time to ask many questions and assure yourself of the need for bypass surgery.

In my opinion, the cardiac surgeon is one of the most skilled of doctors and will always give a forthright opinion. I think it is very important to weigh the risks of bypass surgery versus the benefit. Again, this may take exhaustive discussions both with the surgeon as well as your cardiologists regarding the use of PCI in the less complex cases as the better alternative. This is certainly true in discussion regarding CTO PCI verses surgery.

A bypass surgery is basically a surgical procedure performed to relieve angina pectoris and reduce the risk of death from coronary artery disease. Arteries or veins from other parts of the body are used to sew into the diseased artery past the obstruction to improve the blood flow down to the myocardium. As of 2014, a "hybrid" procedure is done at times where not only is the artery "bypassed" but the interventionalist does a PCI upstream or even downstream from where the bypass graft is sewn into the coronary artery. It requires an amazing coordination between the surgeon and the cardiologist and can be a very times consuming and complex procedure. Hybrid techniques can be a very effective option in centers that are equipped for it.

This surgery is usually performed when the heart has stopped and requires the use of a cardiopulmonary bypass machine, which takes over the pumping function of the heart while sewing in the bypass grafts. Usually, the bypass machine requires a full sternotomy where the central sternum is separated to allow access to the heart. However, in the case of the bypass of only one or two major arteries, the surgery can be done off the bypass pump on a beating heart and be "minimally invasive" without a sternotomy but with an incision in the lateral chest. This technique requires a very skilled surgeon and may be done in only large specialized centers. Recently, in an even more amazing and possibly more effective technique, the minimally invasive CABG utilizes robotic techniques whereby a robotic arm does the sewing into the beating heart arteries.

There are various terms utilized to describe the bypass graft surgery: single vessel, double vessel, triple vessel, or quintuple vessel bypass, which refers to the number of arteries that are bypassed. Usually, the LAD is bypassed in a single vessel bypass, the LAD or circumflex/RCA is bypassed in a double vessel bypass (Fig.55), and the LAD, RCA, circumflex are bypassed in a triple vessel bypass, and the diagonal branch off the LAD is included in a quintuple bypass. Note that the number of arteries that are bypasses doesn't imply the level of risk or illness, but is just the number of arteries that are diseased. The most common use of bypass surgery is involving the left main coronary artery that gives rise to the LAD and the circumflex, which may be one of the most life threating of all cardiac conditions and requires a double bypass into the LAD and the circumflex coronary arteries.

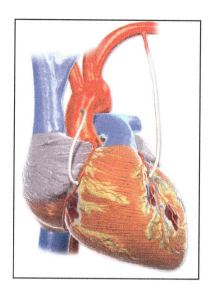

(Fig.55) (commons.wikimedia.org) Double bypass. Off the aorta and a major artery off the aorta are the veins utilized to sewn into the coronary arteries of the heart past the significant obstruction. Up to five grafts can be sewn into the various coronary arteries and branches if an extensive amount of disease is present, and specifically, if the nuclear treadmill and catheterization demonstrate multiple culprit arteries.

An important point regarding coronary bypass grafting is that two of most influential cardiology groups—the American College of Cardiology and the American Heart Association—published in 2004 the most accepted guidelines and preferred treatment modality for CABG.

1. Disease of the left main coronary artery (LM)

2. Disease of all three major coronary arteries (LAD, Left Circumflex, and RCA)

3. Diffuse disease not amenable to treatment with PCI.

4. Preferred treatment for patients with several high risk comorbities (disease) for PCI such as those with much damaged ventricles or severe diabetes mellitus.

An additional indication as of 2014 is that minimally invasive bypass surgery can be contemplated with critical stenosis of the top (proximal) LAD alone when the use of PCI is difficult due to the particular anatomy of the artery.

There are some additional points to understand about CABG. First, there have been multiple studies that looks at patients with a multi-vessel disease. A patient with multi-vessel disease can be basically understood as those individuals who have involvement and critical lesions in more than two arteries and their large branches. Uniformly, the long-term survival and freedom from adverse cardiac events and strokes in multivessel disease are far better with CABG than with PCI. It's partly due to the need for multiple PCI procedures, the concomitant cumulative risk of adverse complications, and the degree of restenosis events such as a second heart attack.

I think there is no doubt that each patient's case is unique and that there may be reasons for doctors choosing to do PCI for a multi-vessel disease. However, if the catheterization is a planned intervention rather than an emergency procedure, much discussion must be established and the doctor must provide a satisfactory reason for choosing PCI over CABG. CABG is a very complex and serious surgical procedure with better long-term survival but a definite short-term risk in terms of multi-vessel coronary disease where the interventionalist is talking about 3-4 stents in multiple arteries that isn't an emergency. I've found cardiac surgeons, as a group of doctors, to be very forthright and complete in their consultations with patients. So, it'd be prudent to seek out a surgical consultation for CABG regarding your individual circumstance.

There is some controversy regarding the use of CABG and PCI for the treatment of CAD, specifically in the class of patients that have "stable" angina pectoris. If it's chest pain from CAD that isn't necessarily increasing, and additionally, cardiac catheterizations demonstrates no involvement of the proximal part of the LAD or the left main coronary artery, multiple studies on CABG grafting have failed to demonstrate that CABG may improve short-term survival (< 1 year) or reveal any benefit in long-term survival (>5 years) over medical therapy. Thus, the CABG, as well as PCI, can alleviate the chest pain temporarily but don't necessarily increase longevity.

The partial reason for that is the vast majority of heart attacks and acute coronary obstruction don't originate in the present significant obstructions but rather come from the rupture of a small plaque that immediately becomes the culprit lesion. Thus, the aim of true therapy for this disease is to lower the creation of new plaque in the coronary arteries. A safer, and more effective treatment of stable angina, as well as the patient with lower risk, is to do daily exercise, quit smoking, control hypertension, closely control glucose levels in diabetes mellitus, lose weight, and drive cholesterol levels down to prevent blood clotting and the formation of new plaque in the coronary arteries.

With the Vegan diet, there's no doubt that it can lead to regression of established lesions in the heart and the control of stable angina pectoris. Thus, longer term behavioral and medication treatment may be the only way to avoid coronary artery disease and general vascular disease in the arteries of the legs that can lead to loss of limb and disease of the brain arteries that inevitably leads to premature vascular decline in mental function and "vascular dementia." It's my strong personal feeling that there's no patient who smokes that doesn't need intense counseling as they're ingesting a poison, which is a slow suicide. The denial of this reality is astounding in our society and must be addressed to prevent premature death or disability with inevitable mental decline as well as remarkably high medical costs.

HISTORY OF CABG

Now, let's move on to the history of CABG, which can be very interesting. The first coronary artery bypass surgery was performed in the United States on May 2, 1960 by Dr. Robert H. Goestz and a team of cardiologists and thoracic surgeons at the Albert Einstein Hospital in the Bronx. Since then, there have been advancements in the technique that includes the use of one of the chest arteries—the internal mammary artery—that is grafted primarily into the LAD. Many of these advances were introduced at the Cleveland Clinic Hospital.

To regress, a successful CABG was made feasible by introduction of the heart-lung machine by Dr. John Gibbon. This machine basically allowed the surgeon to stop the heart while the machine takes over the circulatory function of the heart muscle. One large shortcoming of the machine that still exists today is that it doesn't prevent what appears to be the inevitable creation of small even microscopic "emboli" or clots that travel to the brain although the blood is thinned to prevent large clots.

Also, there's a short period of time in the process of hooking up to the machine that the brain is deprived of adequate oxygen, and this leads to, especially in the elderly, to acute or chronic mental decline. This factor should always come into play when considering CABG especially in patients greater than 80 years of age or those with previous cerebrovascular disease such as a stroke or vascular dementia. In this sense, it is often an option, especially in left main or LAD disease, to discuss "off pump" CABG, which is done on the beating heart and can be done without opening of the sternum but rather a smaller lateral incision between the ribs.

Further interest in off pump coronary bypass surgery (OPCAB) had resurgence in the 1990s when Benetti and others published their remarkable results with OPCAB in 2,000 patients. OPCAB takes a remarkable amount of technical skill on the part of the surgeon and was only offered at major medical centers in the beginning. Primary benefits of this technique where significantly lower end organ damage such as to the kidneys and cerebrovascular vascular accidents (CVA or strokes) with fewer short and long term cognitive deficits, lower transfusion rates, and reduced incidence of infection. It must be understood that in contradistinction to specifically the use of PCI of proximal LAD disease, OPCAB doesn't require the lifelong commitment and risk of expensive and possibly dangerous antiplatelet agents.

ELECTROPHYSIOLOGY

Now, we come to the part of the book that is closest to my heart (pun) as I'm an electrophysiologist which is a subspecialty of cardiology. I deal with the conduction system of the heart, the subsequent arrhythmias or dysrhythmias (irregular or abnormal heart bests), and their treatment. In order to truly understand these diseases, which can be complex and not intuitive, is to be familiar with the history of electrophysiogy and its evolution into modern diagnosis and treatment.

First, I'd like to give you a taste of what it takes to become an electrophysiologist. As you can guess, I've been an electrophysiologist for 35 years, and as such, was practicing this specially at the beginning of its inception as a functional subspecialty of cardiology. At the beginning of electrophysiology, there were no more than 100 electrophysiologists in the country. At that time, these electrophysiologists, who were mainly self-taught, formed the society of the North American Society of Pacing and Electrophysiology (NASPE) in 1979. The name was later changed to the Heart Rhythm Society (HRS), which was supposed to reflect its growth and diversity.

Nevertheless, the original name was most appropriate in its reflection of the special place electrophysiology had as the subspecialty of cardiologists. There is no doubt that these original pioneers were regarded as the smartest group of doctors in the country (humble). Electrophysiology, at that time, was a highly intellectual specialty that drew upon all the previous historical knowledge and applied it to the understanding of the electrical diseases of the heart. In their early stages as subspecialists, the electrophysiologists didn't have much at their disposal to treat these maladies, but the remarkable advances in the understanding of these disease states heralded incredible and rapid advances in treatment that came later.

Ever since the recording of the first electrocardiogram by A.D. Waller in 1897, it was understood that the human heart gave off an electrical field that reflected the electrical control and rhythmic beat of the heart muscle. However, this was preceded by many anatomic descriptions of specialized heart tissue and given names although the exact function of these structures wasn't completely understood. These structures opened the way for these original electrophysiologist to ascertain the mechanisms of many arrhythmias of a heart and their importance in disease and survival.

In 1845, J.E. Purkinje recognized the specialized fibers in the myocardium and hypothesized that these specialized tracts of Purkinje fibers were responsible for the spread of electricity throughout the ventricles. He reconfirmed the presence of the main divisions of the electrical pathways called the left and the right bundle and recognized that these specialized Purkinje fibers were the distal spread of these major branches. (Fig.56)

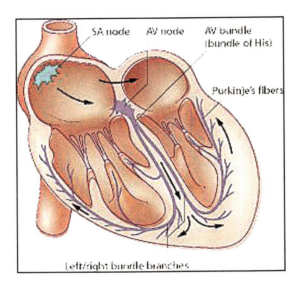

(Fig.56) (medical dictionary.thefreedictionary.com) This is a basic diagram of major branches of the cardiac conduction system as it branches out into the heart muscle. Note the central importance of the AV node and His bundle. They electrically connect the atrium to the ventricle, leads to the left and right bundles, and spread throughout the ventricles as the Purkinje fibers.

In 1893, W.J. His Jr. identified the all-important His Bundle structure named after him and the AV node. These structures play a major role in the development of arrhythmias of the heart and heart block that require artificial pacemakers. In 1907, L. Aschoff discovered the sinus node (SA node) that was recognized as the main "pacemaker" that controlled the heartbeat. The heartbeat impulse first arises from this structure, and the structure is the principal control of the heartbeat initiation and propagation throughout the heart. It was these first 100 electrophysiologists in NASPE, who truly started to analyze these structures as they related to electrical disease, arrhythmias, and conduction disease, which heralded a remarkable era of cure and prolongation of life.

Now, we enter what is possibly the most fascinating development in modern medicine, which was the advent of interventional electrophysiology. As the interventional cardiologists are able to do a PCI on the coronaries, the interventional electrophysiologists are able to do procedures that diagnose and treat many of the electrical diseases of the heart. The interventional electrophysiologist can place catheters in your heart that act as recording electrodes to record the electrical activity of many of these electrical structures. Utilizing this technique, the electrophysiologist can figure out the mechanism of the exact arrhythmia or heart block, and may ascertain the appropriate treatment including the use of ablation treatment for arrhythmia. Although we have yet to talk about ablation that is a way of the electrophysiologist to eradicate the arrhythmia and actually cure the patient. All of these innovations came about from these 100 electrophysiologists, who were innovators and visionaries.

In 1969, Dr. Benjamin J. Scherlag, Ph.D. and colleagues were the first to describe the intracardiac catheter recording of the His bundle. I can't describe the importance of this discovery, but as far as invasive electrophysiology is concerned, this one seminal act opened up the whole modern era of electrophysiology and the cure of many heart rhythm diseases.

I'd like to elaborate about Dr. Ben Scherlag. After meeting him, I've been given the privilege to refer to him as Ben, and I do consider him a personal friend (Fig.57). I first met Ben when I visited University of Oklahoma for classes on radiofrequency ablation taught by Dr. Warren (Sonny) Jackman, whom we'll discuss in a moment as he's another remarkable innovator in the field of cardiac ablation.

This was a time of new discovery as the use of curative radiofrequency ablation was still in its infancy. Dr. Scherlag and I realized we had a common interest in some of the more hypothetical aspects of cardiac electrophysiology. This common interest was centered on the arrhythmia called atrial fibrillation. With Ben, I collaborated on the publication of an article that detailed my results and experiences with a novel form of radiofrequency ablation for atrial fibrillation. We'll go into detail about this procedure for the possible cure of atrial fibrillation further in this book, but for now, I'd like to say that Ben is one of the true greats in the evolution of electrophysiology and in its application to modern medicine.

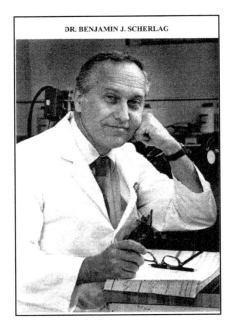

Fig.57 (by permission of Dr. Scherlag) This is a picture of Dr. Scherlag in his laboratory.

Dr. Scherlag was the first individual, as I have said, to record the electrical potential of the His Bundle utilizing intracardiac electrode catheters. At first glance, this may seem like just a small step in the big scheme of things, but in actuality, it was a truly pivotal discovery that ranks among the most important in modern medicine.

(Fig.58) and (Fig.59)

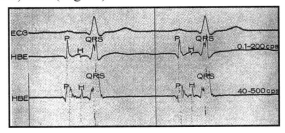

(Fig.58) (by permission of Dr. Scherlag) This is a picture of the first clinical recording of the His Bundle in a man with an intracardiac electrode. Note the first deflection labeled P, which is the intracardiac electrical recording (electrogram) of electrical contraction of the atrium that corresponds to the P wave on the surface electrocardiogram. The last big deflection is the QRS electrogram of the ventricular contraction as we've seen on the surface electrocardiogram. However, there's a deflection labeled H, which is the electrogram recording of the electrode next to the His bundle in the heart, in between these two electrograms on the intracardiac recordings.

This technique with catheters in the heart (Fig.59) was immediately accepted with the danger of making a budding electrophysiologist out of the reader. If the patient has a very slow heart rate and one records the P and the H without the following QRS, it makes sense that the electrical pathways are blocked and a disease is in some place of the conduction system anatomically below the His Bundle. In this case, the slow heartbeat would be arising in the conduction system after the his bundle. If you refer back to (Fig.56), you can deduce that the block is either in the common bundle below the His or in the left and right bundle branches, and the heartbeat comes from fibers below these structures. There, now you're all bourgeoning invasive electrophysiologists!

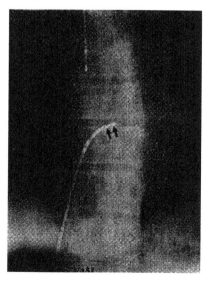

(Fig.59) (permission of Dr. Scherlag) This is the actual x-ray picture of the electrode catheter in the heart on the side of the right atrium and positioned next to the anatomic site of the His Bundle. It was through this electrode that the His Bundle electrogram was recorded. It must be emphasized that these electrode catheters are metal covered by Teflon or plastic coating that are good electrical conductors in contradistinction to the hollow catheters used in coronary angiography.

Soon, Dr. Hein Wellens and Dr. Dirk Durrer in the Netherlands were the first to perform programmed stimulation of the heart. This technique had its roots in the concept that one could record the His Bundle and the potentials of the atrium and the ventricles. With this technique, the budding electrophysiologist could deduce the mechanisms of many common arrhythmias based on "reentry" that were then treated with individually designed pharmacological therapy. Two of these common arrhythmias were seen in a syndrome called Wolff Parkinson's White syndrome and a very common form of paroxysmal supraventricular tachycardia (PSVT) called AV nodal reentrant tachycardia (AVNRT tachycardia). With this newly found knowledge, specific drug actions could be applied directly to treat these arrhythmias without the hit and miss techniques of the past.

When Dr. Wellens would present his data at the yearly meeting of NASPE, all ears and eyes would be glued to his every word in order to understand and apply his techniques in their practice of programmed stimulation techniques. Thus, we had the dawning of the modern era of tachycardia management that became the treatment of various serious and life-threatening arrhythmias that were initiated in the ventricles such as ventricular tachycardia (VT). The recording of the action potential of the His Bundle and within the atrium and ventricle substantially changed our understanding of the mechanisms of drug effects, specifically in sudden cardiac death and the arrhythmogenic basis of these life threatening arrhythmias.

ARTIFICIAL PACEMAKERS

We'll now jump ahead to discuss a very important development in electrophysiology, the invention of the artificial pacemaker. Utilizing the previous investigations, it was discovered through programmed stimulation of the heart that there were a multitude of electrophysiological mechanisms and basis of a slow heartbeat or the development of "heart block" in the various pathways making up the cardiac conduction system. Basically, an artificial pacemaker is a device implanted under the skin with electrodes placed in the heart that take over the rhythmic function when the heart pathologically slows down or the electrical impulses are blocked at various sites along the electrical pathway system.

Some pacemakers have a single electrode in the atrium or the ventricle while others have two or three electrodes in the atrium and the right and left ventricle. These pacemakers can be checked and programmed through devices that communicate through the chest-wall skin, allow the electrophysiologist to program the pacemaker for different functions, and check the integrity of the electrodes and the pacemaker generator. A pacemaker with two electrodes is appropriately called a dual-chamber pacemaker, and a newer device that has a third electrode over the left ventricle is called a biventricular pacemaker. These newer devices control the heartbeat, have another capacity to treat serious heart failure, and have added a remarkable capacity to the treatment modalities available to the electrophysiologist.

The history of pacemaker development in cardiology is truly interesting. The use of electricity to affect the heart is called electrotherapy which means the use of an outside source of electricity to stimulate the heart tissue for a beneficial therapeutic response. The evolution of electrotherapy over the past 50 years set a milestone with the cooperative efforts of the doctor, chemists, and engineers. The doctors who advocated electrotherapy were often looked at with scorn as it was felt to be outside the bounds of reasonable therapy. Now, this disdain has turned in to great respect due to the great benefits of these new devices. The field of pediatric surgery for congenital heart disease benefited because many of these diseases and their surgical corrections are associated with heart block and the use of a pacemaker in these patients was truly lifesaving.

Aristotle saw the heart as "the source of all movement, since the heart links the soul with the organs of life." It was Hippocrates who made the observation that those who have frequent and strong faints without warning were prone to die suddenly. Interestingly, these two observations were amazingly correct and was one of the strong impetuses to the development of modern electrotherapy. In 1580, Geronimo Mercuriale formulated the hypothesis that fainting, which he he called "syncope", was associated with a slow heart rate.

In 1775, the Danish physicist, Nicolaev Abildraard, discovered the first effects of electrical energy when applied to the body. He found that when he placed electrodes and shocked a hen's head, he could cause the animal to fall dead. He then tried to apply shocks to various parts of the body with no effect to revive the animal until he applied the shock over the animal's chest and caused the animal to reanimate. Thus, he "defibrillated" the heart, which was a truly incredible observation at the time that had profound consequences for modern CPR (cardiopulmonary resuscitation).

Abildraard's discovery was fundamental. There is no doubt that the application of electricity to the head, which stimulated the whole body as well as the heart, didn't always result in the hen to fall dead. We now know that the electricity must be applied to the heart when it is "vulnerable" to this consequence in order to make the heart fibrillate and cause a cardiac arrest. This is during the repolarization of the ventricular muscle on the T wave of the cycle called "shock on T wave". Also, when you shock the heart or defibrillate it back to normal rhythm, it must be done during the QRS complex, not on the T wave. At this time in history, electricity was being used in transmission lines, and golf clubs were being made out of metal, so the physicians were aware of a lineman being shocked or a golfer shocked by lightning usually, which usually but not always, led to death due to a cardiac arrest.

Luigi Galvani, an Italian physician, made a fundamental contribution to modern electrophysiology when he found frog muscles and hearts gave off an electrical field and acted as an electrical generator. It's the first time that it was recognized that the heart not only had intrinsic electrical activity but that there were pronounced effects on the heart when electricity itself was applied to this muscle. This demonstration had profound effects on modern electrophysiology.

During the French Revolution, Marie Francois Xavier Bichat experimented on decapitated human bodies. As a generator of electricity, he used a large "battery" that had been developed by Allessandro Volta that put out direct current measured in volts. He found that if the decapitated bodies were fresh, the heart could be reanimated to beat by the application of direct current. As a next logical step, he utilized this technique in bodies with heads that had apparently "died" when brought to the field hospital. It was the rudimentary beginning of CPR. In 1872,

Duchenne de Boulogne actually resuscitated a child who drowned by applying current through the leg and the chest.

An important breakthrough came in 1882 when Hugo Von Ziemssen of Prussia had a patient, who had their sternum removed through an industrial accident with only skin covering the heart. Unfortunately, this patient suffered from collapsing or syncopal spells, and during one of these spells, the heartbeat was very slow. So, they applied rhythmic electricity to the actual heart and observed that it sped up the heart and the pulse and the patient woke up! Thus, this is a milestone in the development of a crude external artificial pacemaker.

In 1834, William Stokes described "apoplectic" loss of consciousness caused by loss of cerebral blood flow, which is caused by a slow heartbeat that he called "bradycardia." This was simultaneous with another Irishman Robert Adams finding bradycardia and syncope. The syndrome that's known as "fainting" or "Stokes-Adams" attacks has persisted in modern electrophysiology.

As we have previously discussed, the electrocardiogram became in generalized use during the late 1800s to early 1900s. Utilizing this modality Woldemer Mobitz described various types of blocks between the atrial P wave and the QRS; in modern parlance, a 1st and 2nd degree AV block. They also substantiated previous clinical observations that the impulse time between the P and the QRS of R wave could be prolonged when associated with a long PR interval or 1st degree AV block seen on the EKG. The readers must familiarizes themselves with these terms as they have important implications in modern day cardiology and electrophysiology.

1st degree heart block is a common normal finding on an electrocardiogram in athletes. However, it's also fairly common in the elderly and can be due to a pathological block in essential parts of the conduction system below the His Bundle (infrahisian block). The only way it can be verified is by an invasive electrophysiological study. With these invasive studies, if 1st degree block is associated with Mobitz 2nd degree infrahisian block, then a pacemaker is definitely indicated especially if the patient is having syncope or episodes of extreme weakness.

The problem arises because many electrophysiologist incorrectly find Mobitz 1st degree block and make incorrect assumption that a patient who is usually over the age of 80 needs a pacemaker without an electrophysiological study first. It's made more complex because it takes an expert to differentiate Mobitz 2nd degree block from 1st degree block. When a pacemaker is inappropriately placed, it will have no useful benefit. Unfortunately, this occurs repeatedly in the modern practice of cardiology and electrophysiology in the elderly. It may take some expertise by the family to assure themselves after a close discussion with the electrophysiologist regarding the true necessity of the pacemaker as a result of informed discussion.

It's even more important to engage in this discourse with the physician if the patient is over the age of 80 or if they have advanced dementia. Various studies have shown that patients with dementia in nursing homes often have bradycardia or even Mobitz 1st or 2nd degree heart block on their EKG. In that case, it's paramount for the family to query the doctor regarding the necessity of a pacemaker—especially if the need is more of a kneejerk response to the EKG or if a pacemaker will have any meaningful effect on the patient's quality of life, longevity of the 90-year-old, or a patient with advanced dementia.

There is no doubt that in some elderly with early dementia that bradycardia or episodic heart block may be contributing itself to episodes of reduced supply of blood and oxygen to the brain and resulting in a speed up of the process of dementia. This is often attributed incorrectly to "Alzheimer's Disease." Such is an incorrect assumption and is generally made of expediency. The really difficult decision comes about when considering the quality of life of the patient; furthermore, if the family or the patient wants the expense and complexity of an artificial pacemaker for prolongation of a life for the 90-year-old, who may be disabled due to other disease.

I think these decisions are very difficult with the availability of such wonderful instruments such as a pacemaker, but the use of this modern technology must be regulated by the reality of life itself. Most cases demand a face-to-face and open discussion with the electrophysiologist on the benefits versus the risks of such interventions. This is a crucial step that is sadly left out of modern "hurry up" medicine. After reading this book, I hope that the readers understand to demand such discourse as this philosophy should be remembered whenever a modern life prolonging intervention is contemplated.

Also, it's not callous to consider the part of the equation that is the remarkable expense of these interventions. I've been involved with families that consider it heartless to deny an intervention just because of its cost. But with such expensive interventions in modern medicine, I want to assure the reader that it must be considered when offered such a large expense as a pacemaker ($20,000-$40,000). It's not cold; it's reality. For a 90-year-old confined to a nursing home, bedridden with dementia, and not able to feed themselves, contemplation of a pacemaker because their heartbeats are slow can border on the ridiculous. In my opinion, the family should be alerted to such medical absurdity as it is an everyday occurrence.

Guilt can be a very strong emotion and will usually result in a very poor decision. Quite often, the physician offers a pacemaker due to the WIIGS syndrome because he assumes the family will want or demand a pacemaker due to a slow heartbeat. I'll keep reiterating throughout this book that the patient or the family must assure the doctor that they're aware of the options and are making an informed decision with appropriate knowledge. I think the decisions for the utilization of modern day miracles, such as a pacemaker, is driven by an unholy sense of entitlement that has only exponentially increased under Obamacare. In this sense, the family or the patient may think they've the right to have a pacemaker no matter how ridiculous a decision it may be.

Obamacare has simultaneously fostered this disease of WIGGS by offering nothing in terms of tort reform. There is no doubt that Obamacare has done more to set back medicine to prehistoric times than any modern day legislation. In this respect, the patient feels that the government will pay regardless of the absurdity of a decision. The concept of Obamacare has only made this type of thinking an epidemic of cataclysmic proportion. The patient or the family may think they have a "God Given Right" to these interventions no matter how ridiculous they may seem. I further feel that this modern day atmosphere in our society is actually one of the strong motivators of those who came up with Obamacare in the first place.

With that said, let's get back to the history of electrophysiology. We've previously talked about Einthoven, who was one of the innovators of the modern electrocardiogram. But I'd like to expand this history further. Another interesting fact about him is that he'd record an electrocardiogram of a patient in the hospital and over the telegraph lines of the day to transmit this signal, which was of the electrocardiogram, to his physiology lab over a long distance for his analysis.

Thus, this can be thought of as the beginning of telemedicine that is just now becoming into vogue. Now, when the paramedics get to the scene of a cardiac event, they're able to transmit to the EKG to the ER for interpretation and for them to prepare for the patient's arrival. Einthoven was greeted by widespread skepticism by the medical community, but he persisted with his work and was awarded the Nobel Prize for Medicine in 1924. It is noteworthy to mention that commercial and semiportable versions of the electrocardiogram machine weren't developed until the late stages of World War II for the need by the field doctors for a way to help diagnose the wounded, especially in the heart.

In 1932, Albert Hyman in the United States developed what is considered one of the first external pacemaker machines. His interest started with the observation of epinephrine being directly injected into a stopped heart that was partially effective in reestablishing a heartbeat. This was utilized until the 1970s, although he had come to the conclusion in the 30s that it wasn't the drug that was working, but it was the needle setting up a current in the heart. This led to the first working external pacemaker used for "stopped hearts" in the ER by placing a needle that acted as a bipolar electrode into the atrium through an insertion point between the ribs. Using a hand cranked device, he generated heartbeats at regular rates. But his work was viewed with great skepticism again, and he unsuccessfully enlisted the government to utilize his "Hymanotor," an external pacemaker to revive dying servicemen during World War II. Such was the fate of the early pioneers of electrostimulation of the heart.

In the early 1950s, Grass Manufacturing Company produced the first commercial stimulator designed for intracardiac stimulation. These devices were used to restart the heart in cardiac surgery patients. When I started practicing as an electrophysiologist, the Grass Stimulator was considered state of the art for intracardiac electrophysiological testing.

Paul Zoll in the 1950s is credited with numerous innovations in cardiac pacing technology. However, he is most known for the development of a percutaneous pacing machine that stimulates the heart through skin placed electrodes called the Zoll External Pacemaker, which is used to this day in patients who are being monitored overnight in the hospital for backup pacing while waiting for a permanent pacemaker implant in the morning.

The late 50s and early 60s were heralded by a multitude of revolutionary thinkers and devices. In 1950. Earl Bakken, whom I had the honor of meeting, started Medtronic corporation that developed the first externally-worn, battery-powered pacemaker for patients with bradycardia and complete heart block at the level of the His Bundle. He was an engineer by training but worked in hospitals, repairing and designing electrical equipment and developed relationships with doctors who told him of the need for a pacemaker in many untreatable patients.

The next important advance was the result of a cardiac surgeon, C. Walton Lillehei, who was a leading cardiac surgeon that developed techniques, especially in repair of congenital heart defects in the neonatal and pediatric population. However, many of the structural problems of these tiny hearts were associated with a multitude of conduction and arrhythmia problems, and he saw the need for an internally implantable pacemaker system. Lillehei developed an electrode catheter covered by a Teflon sleeve that could be implanted in the right ventricle through an introducer in the vena cava. He had to enlist the help of Earl Bakken for a miniaturized pacing device that could be permanently implanted in these children.

The first devices developed by Bakken were external transistor battery-powered miniature devices but permanently implanted intracardiac electrodes. This was a very important breakthrough as the newly developed transistor allowed miniaturization of the unit (Fig.61). A story goes that Bakken delivered one of his new devices to Lillehei to use on a lab animal with surgically produced heart block. Two hours later as Bakken was walking past the neonatal ICU, he saw his device hooked up to a baby with the new Lillehei internal catheters. When asked, Lillehei remarked that the baby would've died had it not been for this new device!

At the time, there were new stimulant drugs such as atropine, adrenaline, and isoproterenol that would act as temporary solutions, but obviously, the baby couldn't leave the hospitals with intravenous drug heart rate support. The morality of Lillehei was the patient comes first. Compare this to the modern day FDA run by a cohort of pencil pushers who squashes the basic principle of medicine that places the life of the patients before the interests of the multibillion dollar companies that only promote such decadent behavior. Lillehei's remarkable lifesaving work is a "feat that is unlikely to ever be repeated" given the labyrinth of regulatory requirements that you now have to go through for the introduction of a new device. Please try to open your eyes to the true motives of these wonderful innovators in medicine that put their patients' wellbeing before anything else-the life of a human.

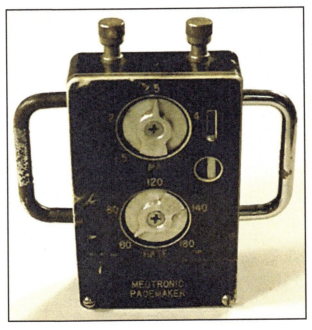

(Fig.61) (galleryhip.com) This is a picture of the first miniaturized transistor-powered external pacemaker by Medtronic Company. This piece of equipment was placed with a cord around the neck of the baby or adult patient and was designed to give life. That was realistically impossible before this remarkable device that was developed unbridled by the ridiculous and onerous rules of the FDA. To them, these children's deaths is just a statistic with a sterile comment in a register. I had the honor of meeting Mr. Bakken before he died and visited the remarkable museum where these devices on display at the beautiful Medtronic Headquarters in Minnesota. Medical historians regard this device as the first application of transistor technology to a medical device, and after 1957, we saw the explosion of such technology in a variety of life-saving medical devices.

The next bold step was the production of a miniature transistor-powered pacemaker that could be implanted under the skin with a self-contained mercury battery, which allowed the patient to leave the hospital with the device implanted. However, the exposed leads out of the body resulted in serious infections.

On October 8th, 1958, the first implant of a completely self-contained subcutaneous pacemaker with leads was performed in Sweden on an engineer named Arne Larsson. This case was done in the dead of night to avoid publicity. The first units were rather complex, but relatively compact and employed mercury batteries and conduction technology from the development of field telephones used in battle. They were encapsulated by an epoxy material developed by Ciba-Geigy and didn't result in allergic reaction to their implantation in the body (Fig.62).

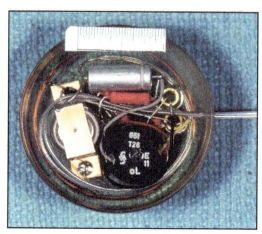

(Fig 62). (www.siemens.com) This is a picture of a replica of the first pacemaker implanted in a human being. Note the epoxy water proof enclosure and the miniaturized battery with wires instead of printed circuits, which weren't developed until more than 10 years later.

Here's another true story regarding a patient's pacemaker that is part of medical lore. Arne Larsson had Stokes Adams Attacks 30 times a day with fainting but lived a great deal of time in a hospital bed. His wife was a very insistent lady who pleaded at night to the surgeon, Dr. Ake Senning of the department of thoracic surgery at Karolina Hospital in Stockholm, to place an implantable pacemaker that she read about in the newspapers. Her husband was dying, and there was no other option to save him. He had to give up his hobby of sailing and couldn't be allowed back to his beloved boat.

The first pacemaker was implanted and lasted for only three hours. Senning later commented that he though he damaged the connections since he waited hours in the operating room until a new unit was delivered with no backup. He said, "In the 1950s we did not have any liability problems. The patient and relatives were happy if the patient simply survived." Wouldn't that be a wonderful situation if it existed today? Now, the family, if they were so inclined, would hire an unscrupulous lawyer who advertised on T.V. to sue for product liability and malpractice because the first pacemaker didn't work and risked his life. Although they saved his life in the long run, this is the reality of 2014, and it'll only get worse and squelch creativity in medicine without meaningful tort reform.

However, Arne Larrson out-survived all the surgeons and engineers that were involved with his lifesaving pacemaker implant. Later, he required five new lead systems and 22 pacemakers of 11 different models. He died of cancer in 2000 at the age of 86, but was able to enjoy his love of the sea and of his wife for many years (Fig.63).

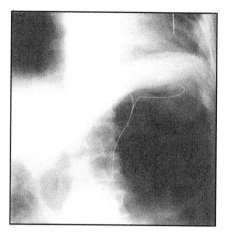

(Fig.63) A chest X-ray of Arne Larssen's first pacemaker implant. Note the leads going into the heart and the pacemaker generator connected to the leads implanted under the skin beneath the sternum and ribs.

Over the ensuing 20 years, the pacemaker evolved into a small device with reliable leads run on lithium iodine batteries and microchip technology. Since 1960, over 4 million pacemakers have been implanted, and the average lifetime of a pacemaker is between 5-15 years. The leads have steroid eluding tips that make the contact with the heart more reliable, and the pacemakers can be fully programmed through the skin. These pacemakers can also be checked from home via the phone or the Internet and allow the patient convenience who has trouble with ambulation or transportation.

The newer pacemakers since 2014 are no larger than a fifty-cent coin. They're almost invisible under the skin and less prone to inflame the skin or erode through the covering, exposing skin to the air. Titanium cases were developed that made the pacemaker basically impervious to leakage and infiltration of body fluids, and their safety from malfunction while becoming nearly 100% reliable. Each pacemaker has memory that stores cardiac events such as an arrhythmia. Furthermore, the pacemakers were given artificial intelligence to sense a change in the patient's conduction parameters and automatically adjust to the new pacing needs; special computer algorithms and sensors that could sense motion and exercise, which made the pacemaker a thinking autonomous machine.

Lastly, the year 2000 saw the introduction of the biventricular pacemaker. Almost as important as the development of the transistor in 1949, these new pacemakers opened up a totally new indication for the use of pacemakers that has turned out to be a truly life-altering event for many patients. The biventricular pacemaker uses an extra lead that is implanted from the veins through a structure called the coronary sinus, which goes over the left ventricle rather than inside of it as does the right ventricular lead. Being at the inception of this technology, I witnessed some truly innovative and talented electrophysiologists who saw the promise of this technique and risked their careers and the threat of liability. These devices extended their patients' lives and immediately improved their overall lifestyle and feeling of wellbeing in patients with disabling congestive heart failure and shortness of breath.

Basically, the biventricular pacemaker with the use of an LV lead allows the device to synchronize the contraction of the RV and the LV in a normal fashion (CRT or cardiac resynchronization therapy). In a healthy heart, the LV contracts slightly earlier than the RV during normal pumping of the heart. In congestive heart failure, the patient often develops block in the left bundle branch or its ramifications in the purkinje system to cause the LV to contract later than the RV. In heart failure and with the common leakage of the mitral valve in this disease, the dysyncrony of the LV and the RV becomes even worse.

With the biventricular pacemaker, the device in pacing both ventricles allows the programming of the pacemaker to make the RV and the LV contract simultaneously or at an interval that can be optimized by the appropriate programming and coordinating of the ventricular contractions with the atrial stimulation. This can be a very complex undertaking, but by using cardiac echocardiography, this resynchronization can be optimized to afford the greatest efficacy of the pacing system. This optimization of ventricular contractions is very effective in relieving the symptoms of heart failure and can bring immediate wellbeing to a patient suffering from shortness of breath and fluid in the lungs.

More importantly, CRT therapy can actually lead to an improvement in the contractile efficiency of the heart in a measure called the ejection fraction of the LV during pumping of the blood. This number, which is usually greater than 50%, is usually measured by echocardiography or nuclear scanning techniques and is a very important measure in the diagnosis and treatment of heart failure or a damaged heart from a heart attack or cardiomyopathy.

Another use of CRT therapy is for patients who suffer from pacemaker syndrome. This syndrome is far under diagnosed by contemporary electrophysiologist due to the ignorance of the electrophysiologist to understand the amazing versatility in programming of the new pacemaker systems. However, it's obvious that because the dual chamber pacemaker system utilizes a pacing electrode in the RV that the RV will be first to contract with the electrical impulse spreading from the RV electrode to the LV. Thus, this situation creates an iatrogenic (artificial and self-caused) form of "cardiac dysynchrony" and can cause symptoms of heart failure and fatigue. In the early pacing systems that used just one lead in the RV and were not so versatile in their programming, up to 50% of patients would end up with some form of pacemaker syndrome.

Frequently, when a patient with a pacemaker system is admitted to the hospital for symptoms of heart failure, the cardiologist or electrophysiologist enlists a barrage of diagnostic and therapeutic modalities like a cardiac catheterization and medications when it's simply the pacemaker syndrome. In many cases, this syndrome can be reversed by proper programming of the pacemaker system and replacement of the dual chamber pacemaker with a CRT device in some. This seems to escape the contemporary clinician simply because they aren't trained to recognize this condition and rely upon technology rather that proper diagnostic thought.

I think it's very important for the patient with a pacemaker or the family to keep in mind that it's just pacemaker syndrome most of the time and that should be considered before the physicians offers a barrage of invasive and unnecessary procedures. In my experience in a 90-year-old with a dual chamber pacemaker system, the development of extreme weakness and fatigued was common, especially if the patient had an ejection fraction of less than 35%. In this select population of the elderly, it's completely appropriate to suggest the implantation of a biventricular pacing system to improve the quality of life (not disabling dementia) and let them continue with active lifestyles.

Additionally, there's a class of patients where the degree of intrinsic bradycardia or heart block is so severe that the pacemaker is basically taking over for every beat of their heart. This is called complete pacemaker dependency. It's not common when the pacemaker is first put in at a younger age, but the degree of pacemaker dependency almost always increases as the patient ages. Once the patient is 100% dependent on the pacemaker for the heart to beat, then the incidence of pacemaker syndrome can approach 80% or higher. In this scenario, the treating cardiologist or electrophysiologist must recognize the diagnosis and suggest very early on the upgrade of their older single or dual chamber pacemaker with a biventricular device.

As I have said before, this is frequently unrecognized by the doctors, and I want anyone experiencing this situation to be keenly aware of their therapeutic options. 100% pacemaker dependency takes five minutes to diagnose with interrogation in the office or hospital of the pacemaker. One of the algorithms present in all modern pacemakers accurately reports the percent of the paced heartbeats. Anything over 90% is essentially a pacemaker dependency. A lot of cardiologists do a cardiac catheterization under the pretense of looking for other causes of new onset heart failure in the elderly patient with a permanent pacemaker when they are only dealing with pacemaker syndrome and first deserve a trial of pacemaker reprogramming before doing further invasive testing or looking for "ghost" coronary artery disease.

An interrogation of the pacing system would've led to simple reprograming of the system, and the suggestion of a CRT device would've sufficed rather than the far more dangerously invasive and often unproductive cardiac catheterization. Whether the cardiologist admits it or not, the risks of adverse consequences of a simple heart catheterization such as renal failure or perforation of an artery in the patient over 80 years of age can reach 20-30%. At the same time, upgrading to a CRT device has significantly fewer, if any, rare side effects or complications.

Lastly, the use of CRT pacemaker therapy has taken on a large indication in the treatment of atrial fibrillation. We have yet to talk about atrial fibrillation in its entirety, but atrial fibrillation can lead to the very high heart rates that are very difficult to control even with a multitude of medications. Once the electrophysiologist has exhausted all relatively noninvasive maneuvers, he's faced with the option of radiofrequency ablation of the arrhythmia. This can be a very complex and difficult procedure, but the ablation of the arrhythmia itself is sometimes ineffective and shouldn't be done in patients over the age of 80 because of untoward complications.

However, in this age group, there's a very good option. Simple ablation of the AV node and the His Bundle completely severs the connection between the fibrillating atrium and the ventricle. This leads to complete AV block and the heartbeat of the ventricles to be about 30-40 beats per minute. Thus, a pacemaker is needed, and it is absolute indications for a CRT implant rather than a simpler single chamber device (a dual chamber device is not used as the atrium is fibrillating and cannot be paced) because the patient with this slow heartbeat will be completely pacemaker dependent.

First, I can't mention the amount of physicians who incorrectly and illogically place a dual chamber device as the atrial lead will never be able to pace a chronically fibrillating atrium. It's mind boggling why this totally irrational procedure is done. Nevertheless, the proper thing to do would be to place a single chamber device or a biventricular system. Many electrophysiologists rationalize the single chamber system over a biventricular device either because they don't do biventricular pacemaker implants or it's reasonable to try the simpler single lead system first to see if it works well. This logic is incorrect, and if the physician suggests AV nodal ablation for the refractory rapid atrial fibrillation, the patient and the family should insist on a CRT device, not a single or even sillier dual chamber device (the doctor makes more money with the dual chamber device).

If the doctor says he doesn't do biventricular devices, then go to someone else. In my experience, some insurance companies may not approve the CRT device over a single chamber device because of the increased cost of the biventricular pacemaker. One can still appeal as to the determination and present a cogent argument. This maneuver will compel them to act appropriately and seriously consider the rationale. Another option is to find an electrophysiologist who feels the CRT implant is the correct choice, and who'll be your advocate if the insurance company balks at its approval.

It must be stressed at this point that just a slow heart rate doesn't necessarily require the placement of an artificial pacemaker. The decision to place any type of pacemaker must be tempered by how permanent is the bradycardia or heart block in the whole clinical scenario. When many cardiologists see any hint of bradycardia or Mobitz type I heart block, they immediately think of placing a pacemaker. This is something akin to the oculostenotic reflex we discussed with cardiac PCI and compels the cardiologist to choose a pacemaker without considering numerous other options or consequences.

First, slowing of the heartbeat is an almost natural consequence of aging. The real clinical expertise comes into play when one has to decipher if a pacemaker is required. Often, this may not be an immediate decision, and in my experience, takes a very good electrophysiologist who can consider all the variables. In the elderly, the critical question is how slow is normal for the patient and are there any extenuating circumstances slowing the heart that can be reversed before the decision to place a permanent pacemaker. There is no question that a bedridden or severely impaired patient may not need the faster heartbeat to meet the demands of the body.

A rather bogus diagnosis that is often used to justify a pacemaker is "chronotropic incompetence." This simply refers that the heart rate doesn't increase sufficiently to meet the oxygen demands of the body although the resting heart rate may not be significantly slow enough to require a pacemaker that has an algorithm that speeds the heart with exercise or movement. The fallacy of such a diagnosis is that it takes significant testing to accurately assess this certainty, and it's often used as an initial and completely bogus pretense in the elderly patient. The error of this diagnosis is that many of the elderly don't exercise enough to justify the pacemaker!

Also, the physician may place a holter monitor on the patient and make the patient to wear it for days to record the heartbeat and that the heart rate doesn't increase. This may be true, but the error lies in the fact that at no time did the patient in his log book for the holter report that he was unduly fatigued or short of breath. Thus, the physician is simply responding as a reflex to the slow heartbeat rather than thinking of the physiology behind the true need for pacemaker implantation.

Also, it is important to take into consideration that the heartbeat normally slows during sleep or inactivity. This observation is also much more pronounced in elderly and athletes. First, some researchers feel that obstructive sleep apnea is much more common than previously estimated. Obstructive sleep apnea is the phenomenon of when the patient simply stops or slows breathing during sleep to the point, causing oxygen deprivation to the body and the brain. It's often characterized by snoring but not necessarily a precondition. The important thing to note is that an apnea (stop breathing) leads to slowing of the heart beat and probable heart block.

It's my opinion that most minimally obese, if not morbidly obese, have a component of sleep apnea, and this explains the preponderance of pacemakers placed in patients with higher weights. Sleep apnea is also frequently seen in the elderly due to the natural aging of the brain reflexes that control breathing. For those patients, rather than the reflex placement of a pacemaker, a trial of continuous positive airway pressure (CPAP) to alleviate the bradycardia should be considered. The consequences of sleep apnea are multifold, but there's no doubt that it's a leading cause of early dementia and now is known to be a very important cause of atrial fibrillation. It can lead to permanent bradycardia and heart block due to a damaged heart conduction system with episodes of hypoxemia (low oxygen in the bloodstream). It can be argued that the cause of a patient dying in his sleep is the result of sleep apnea and stopping of the heart due to hypoxemia.

The last topic in the pacemaker has to do with the incidental finding of bradycardia or heart block in the asymptomatic individual when they go into the hospital for an unrelated and planned elective procedure. The continued hospitalization may be recommended by the electrophysiologist or cardiologist because the bradycardia will require a pacemaker. However, the slow heart rate was an incidental finding aside from the coincidental hospitalization for a totally unrelated condition. If there are absolutely no adverse symptoms that can be related to bradycardia or possibly indicated after further testing such as an electrophysiological study or form of continuous outpatient rhythm recordings, then a pacemaker won't likely be necessary. Thus, the lesson to be learned is that slow heart rate is slow doesn't mean there's need for an immediate pacemaker implant.

The reason this is so important to understand is that Medicare, as of 2015, is clamping down on second unrelated procedures being done at the same time, resulting in a two-midnight stay when they're non-emergent and not medically related to the primary reason for hospitalization. It's more appropriate to evaluate the patient as an outpatient. If a pacemaker implant is found to be truly indicated, it can be done during another hospitalization. Let's say you were admitted for a gallbladder removal and then have a pacemaker implant, Medicare can deny payment to the hospital and the doctor for a non-emergent pacemaker implant that could've been done during another hospitalization as an outpatient procedure and was even not necessarily indicated in the first place. This means possible financial liability for the patient.

AUTOMATIC IMPANTABLE CADIAC DEFIBRILLATOR (AICD or ICD)

The next important milestone in electrotherapy of the heart was the development of the ICD. As far as I'm concerned, this singular advance has done more for the sparing of human life than any previous milestone-period. The genius and motivations behind its development make a very compelling story. Since I was around as a young man, I witnessed it firsthand this remarkable unfolding evolution of its development and its ever-expanding use as a lifesaving tool. This was a quantum leap in our therapeutic armamentarium.

The prime innovator in the development of the AICD was a physician named Mieczyslaw (Michel) Mirowski who was born on October 14, 1924 in Warsaw, Poland. The story of this man is nothing short of incredible, and he endures as one of the greatest innovators in the history of modern medicine. Before we delve into this fascinating story, let's review the subject of Sudden Cardiac Death so that we may understand what Dr. Mirowski did to change the face of electrotherapy of arrhythmias and in many ways the fabric of modern medicine.

SUDDEN CARDIAC ARREST (SCA OR SUDDEN CARDIAC DEATH)

Once, SCA used to be the leading cause of death among adults of the age of 40 in the United States and other countries. The introduction of the AICD dramatically reduced the incidence of the third leading cause of overall death of adults over the age of 40. In the United States, over 400,000 people of all ages experience emergency medical assisted (EMS) out of hospital SCA per year. This is an amazing number and equates to 1,000 events a day, and nine of the ten victims die. The number of people who die each year from SCA is more than the combined deaths due to breast cancer, firearm deaths, colorectal cancer, diabetes, HIV, house fires, and motor vehicle accidents. With bystander assisted CPR and the use of the portable ICD, this number of deaths could be reduced to four of ten victims.

What exactly is SCA? SCA is the sudden pulseless condition that is a result of the abrupt cessation of the pumping function of the heart. When blood stops flowing to the brain, the person suddenly collapses. The principal cause of SCA is the arrhythmia called ventricular fibrillation, but equally common is sudden bradycardia and complete standstill of the ventricle or arrhythmias called ventricular tachycardia and Torsades de Pointes.

These cardiac arrhythmias can be the result of multiple conditions with the most common one being a heart attack itself. In the beginning of the heart attack, the patient is almost always aware of the problem as they experience chest pain. However, as a result of the sudden loss of blood supply to part of the heart due to the coronary occlusion, the heart may then fibrillate and the patient will collapse with no forewarning (prodrome). While a heart attack can lead to SCA, there are many other conditions that can lead to SCA. These conditions include:

1. Abnormal thickening of the heart muscle called Hypertrophic Cardiomyopathy that runs in families.

2. Arrhythmogenic Right Ventricular Dysplasia and Catecholiminergic Ventricular Tachycardia both running in families.

3. Brugata Syndrome and Long QT Syndrome that are EKG abnormalities that can lead to SCA and can run in families or be the first in the family have the disease.

4. Various heart rhythm disorders such as Wolff Parkinson White Syndrome that can lead to ventricular fibrillation and recurrent sustained ventricular tachycardia.

5. Recreational drug use especially with smoking cocaine which can cause terminal cardiac arrhythmias. This also includes acute alcohol toxicity.

6. Electrocution seen commonly in individuals hit by lightning or linemen working on high voltage cables.

7. Commodio Cordis when, usually in a child, when they are hit hard in the chest by commonly a pitched baseball, in a car accident, or football trauma. This may not happen on the first episode of trauma, but there can be an initial change in the EKG called a left bundle branch block (LBBB) that can herald the possibility of a future occurrence of a SCA.

8. Lastly and probably most importantly, is what is called a cardiomyopathy of the heart. This condition can come about with no specific cause and called idiopathic cardiomyopathy, or it can be due to a virus infecting the heart (non-ischemic cardiomyopathy-NICM), post-partum, various inherited muscular diseases, and most commonly, ischemic cardiomyopathy (ICM) due to coronary artery disease. These are all characterized by the decrease pumping efficiency of the heart with what is called the ejection fraction of the LV (EF) that is measured by an echocardiogram or nuclear study and less than 35% (normal greater than 50%). This can also be measured by a cardiac catheterization, and an EF of less than 35% is a very strong indication for implant of an AICD.

It is interesting to note that there is a significant race adjusted difference in the incidence of SCA. It may be a combination of the genetics of the race or environmental factors. In the United States, incidence of SCA per 10,000 adults is 10.1 among blacks, 6.5 among Hispanics, and 5.8 among whites. One can only hope that this discrepancy in race will lessen as everyone can afford the same healthcare and possibly prevent SCA.

It is also compelling that in athletes, 56% of SCA is due to preexisting cardiac disease, which is often some of the familial causes we have just mentioned. The true catastrophe of this number is that adequate prescreening for athletes at any age can reduce this number significantly. Why resistance to prescreening in these individuals by organized medicine simply boggles my mind. The sheer insanity and ignorance of the liberal minded politically correct numbskulls have this fantasy that they somehow can overcome death- unfortunately death is irreversible and not debatable.

However, there still is a high incidence of SCA in normal hearts during very heavy training or competitions that is usually cause by the sudden loss of potassium and magnesium as one over exerts themselves without replacing these electrolytes and subsequent ventricular fibrillation. The incidence in females is 1/3 that of males, but recently, the discrepancy has lessened as more females became involved in competitive sports.

Over the past 10 years, the use of the portable automatic external defibrillator has had a marked effect in the successful revival of people with SCA. Unfortunately, over that past few years, we're seeing less of these units readily available because of budgetary cuts. Basically, they are a portable device (AED) that delivers a defibrillating shock to the pulseless individual with SCA. Because of the design, the use of these units on a collapsed individual who doesn't have SCA can't harm anyone other than wake them up with the sudden shock to the chest!

AEDs can commonly be found in airports, train stations, on an airplane, and at the ballpark. They're very easy to use with large visual instructions inside and basically involves placing sticky electrodes on the chest and pressing a button. That's it! There's no danger to the operator and no legal liability based on the Good Samaritan Laws in every state. Even if you don't know CPR, the use of the AED is an absolute lifesaver. Just remember that the new guidelines for CPR just call for chest compression and don't entail mouth to mouth air exchange.

AICD HISTORY

Now, we come back to the development of the implantable AICD. As we previously mentioned the story begins with the amazing creativity and foresight of one man, Michel Mirowski. I met Dr. Mirowsky before he died at a NASPE meeting, and I was awed by the humble nature of the man, who basically changed the course of medicine and the treatment of SCA.

Dr. Mirowsky was born in Warsaw, Poland. The story of his early life is nothing short of amazing and is one of remarkable bravery and strength. He grew up in a large Jewish family in Warsaw, and his life took on a dramatic turn with the rise of Nazi Germany and World War II. With the invasion of Poland in 1939, the atrocities against the Jews in Germany had already spread to Poland. Michel knew he couldn't remain in Poland and continue his education as a physician. In his memoirs, he wrote that he was convinced the Germans had no intention of allowing any Jew to survive.

He made a very bold move at the age of 15 to flee with a friend from Poland to Russia. Although the Russians were also intent on sending Jews to labor camps in Siberia, because of his intelligence, he somehow escaped the camps, worked in Russia to finish his early education, and house himself with his friend. He was able to avoid the disease and starvation that was so common in Russia at that time and became convinced he wanted to be a doctor as he spent many hours volunteering to aid the sickly Russians.

After spending five years in Russia and the war ended, he returned briefly to Poland to find that he was the only survivor of his immediate and extended family, who were all exterminated by the Nazis. He entered a period of depression but soon went to Medical School in Lyon, France in 1947. Despite not knowing any French or English and being subjected to the oppressive anti-Semitism in France, he finished Medical School and met his wife, Anna. It was at this time, in Medical School, he knew he wanted to become a cardiologist. It simply attests to the power of the human spirit to see a man overcome so much death and anti-Semitism and be able to continue his quest.

Upon graduation from medical school in 1954, he worked initially in Tel Aviv, Israel and pursued further specialty training as a cardiologist in Mexico City, Baltimore, and Staten Island. As a cardiologist, he set up a private clinic in a small community hospital in Israel.

His new boss, Professor Harry Heller, became his inspiration and influenced the work of Michel and basically change the face of modern electro therapy of the heart. Dr. Heller began to have episodes of ventricular tachycardia that was documented by EKG and soon died of SCA. Apparently, Michel took this very hard as he had firsthand knowledge of his friends disease and death and was absolutely helpless as a doctor to save his life in the face of a fatal arrhythmia. It was with Heller's death that Michel first conceived of the idea of an implantable defibrillator, which would constantly monitor the heart through leads like a pacemaker. If a fatal arrhythmia was sensed, the unit would defibrillate the heart back to normal rhythm.

In 1968, Dr. Mirowsky was recruited by the famed Jewish hospital in Baltimore, the Sinai Hospital. It was there that he was given the directorship of the newly conceived coronary care unit that cared for the very ill cardiac patients with heart attacks and significant arrhythmias. He was given time to do research as a director, and the hospital also had a newly formed animal laboratory and engineering department.

In July of 1969, in conjunction with another cardiologist, Dr. Morton Mower, Michel began work on an implantable, self-contained AICD. Within a month and with the help of the engineering department as well as the new development of transistor technology, they produced the first ICD that was implanted in a dog but utilized small external defibrillator paddles. He had yet to devise the appropriate lead technology.

They published a paper on this research but were met by remarkable skepticism and ridicule by the cardiology community. Frankly, to this day, I'm not sure of the origin of such scorn and bias to the old ways. Faced with adversity, Michel plowed on with his dream in his usual strength of character. There is no doubt that the pain of his friend's death and the anger about the Holocaust had much to do with the framing of his character. After personally speaking with Dr. Mirowksi, one cannot help but wonder within this remarkable humble man, there was not a part of him that hoped his ICD would make up in part for the sheer barbarism of Nazi Germany. It's also intriguing to contemplate if similar emotions drive the modern day Israeli to be one of the top innovators in medical technology for the advancement of the whole of mankind.

Mirowski and Mower eventually obtained the support of a major pacemaker company in 1970, but after two years, the shortsighted company decided that there was no market for such a device and dropped support. It's amazing how utterly wrong they were in their decision. It is interesting that once the ICD became generally accepted, this company joined the fray. However, their device was and remains technologically inferior compared to others. Such is the world of medical devices.

In 1972, with the aid of a physician and electrical engineer, Dr. Stephen Heilman, who started a small medical equipment company, put his company engineers at the disposal of Mirowski and Mower. Heilman and his company, Medrad, were very excited about the concept and prospects for an ICD. This partnership was amazingly fruitful, and the first AICD prototype that was small enough and with internal leads was implanted in a dog. It's a now very famous footage that I saw for the first time in 1975 at a meeting in Chicago. In it, a dog was walking and had a small shock and fell to the floor in cardiac arrest. After about 20 seconds, the dog shook with a larger shock and got up and walked away!

Within that moment, this development catapulted Mirowski to the forefront of cardiac research overnight. There's no way that I can convey to you the utter awe that I had as a young electrophysiologist seeing this amazing demonstration-basically rebirth. Having been in practice for a very short time, I had already experienced the pain of having patients, with whom I had very personal medical relationships die of fatal arrhythmias. They died suddenly, and it was out of my control to prevent their SCA. The pain of such loss to a doctor is very hard to describe, but I can only reflect on the pain of Michel when he lost his friend and mentor.

Instantly, I became a firm supporter of the AICD, and over the ensuing years in my practice, I implanted hundreds of ICDs and saved countless lives. For as long as I live, I will never forget the face of the first patient of mine, Albert or Al, who was successfully shocked and saved from SCA. In subsequent years, I ate many a barbecue at his house to his and his wife's ever-grateful hospitality. I have and always will consider him a wonderful friend.

At Medrad, Mirowski and Mower eventually made a unit refined for human implant, and it was approved for human use by the FDA in 1980. Immediately, they enlisted the support of the cardiac surgeons at Johns Hopkins Hospital. The original surgeon, Dr. Myron Weisfeldt, and the electrophysiologist, Dr. Philip Reed, successfully implanted the first human ICD implant using leads that were placed on the surface of the heart by open chest approach. This unit was large at 225 grams, and the leads could only be implanted by open thoracotomy over the surface of the heart, but it was very effective in its limited scope to defibrillate.

I can personally attest to the fact that the first implants were fraught with a great amount of anxiety and fear on the part of the surgeon and electrophysiologist during their implantation. In order to assure that the unit was effective, once the leads were placed, the patient's heart was shocked into ventricular fibrillation and SCA. Then they waited, for what seemed like an eternity, for the unit to sense the arrhythmia and automatically shock the heart back to normal rhythm. Sometimes, it had to be done multiple times to assure the proper placement of the leads, and the whole procedure certainly drained me physically and emotionally as I waited for the unit to work.

The next few years, there was a very rapid advancement in the technology of the ICD. The first ICDs were designed to just shock the heart during ventricular fibrillation. Newer models, which also got considerably smaller, had computer algorithms added. This allowed them to sense ventricular tachycardia, which is a very rapid and dangerous ventricular rhythm that can deteriorate to ventricular fibrillation and is considered in the class of arrhythmias as SCA. In addition, the ICD could rapidly pace (overdrive pace) and terminate the arrhythmia without the shock. This was very useful as it made the ICD a more versatile tool.

Soon followed the ICD with the capability of acting as an independent pacemaker—thus the name ICD-pacmaker. And ICD was permanently added to the vocabulary of electrotherapy. In late 1980, true to Mirowski's early vision, came the development of specially designed shocking leads that could be placed like pacemaker leads through the veins into the RV; thus, these leads were implanted without a thoracotomy and the associated risks of major surgery.

In the late 1980's Mirowski was diagnosed with multiple myeloma and succumbed to the disease in 1990. However, his legacy will always remain the ICD, and even more important the attention he drew to the medical problem of SCA.

NEWER ICD TECHNOLOGY

Unlike the early ICDs, the newer models became much smaller, and many were 90 grams, the size of a large pacemaker (Fig.67 and Fig.68). They had a much longer longevity and could last up to 8 years before the need for change out. Remember that the change out just required a simple surgery as the leads are nearly permanent. Unfortunately, there were rare recalls of the leads or the generator unit. These were mandated by the FDA and alerted the electrophysiologist to a possible malfunction of the lead. This could easily be checked by the programmer because they worked with a magnet and sensing head applied over the unit.

Often, they just required additional scrutiny by the physician. However, this sometimes required replacement of the RV shocking lead. At first, the old lead was left into place while a new lead was implanted. The old lead was capped and had no function. But over the past 10 years, the electrophysiologists gained the new technology to use a laser to remove the lead. Thus, the lead could either be removed by pulling it out, which was often fruitless, or enlist the use of the relatively safe laser assistance extractor.

As we saw with pacemakers, we've recently seen the development of ICDs with the addition of a LV lead called a biventricular ICD or a CRT (cardiac resynchronization therapy)-ICD. This was also a great leap forward as in most patients with an ICD, the EF is less than 35%, and the patient may have a component of severe congestive heart failure. If the patient has a LBBB or used the pacemaker function of the ICD, more than 90% of the time, the addition of a LV lead could actually alleviate the CHF and pacemaker syndrome. Therefore, they actually would lead to an improvement in the EF and health of the heart.

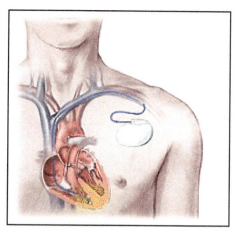

(Fig.67) (www.heart-disease-and-prevention.com) This is a drawing of one of the new ICDs that is composed of the smaller pacemaker size shocking and pacing unit. It's under the tissue in the left shoulder with the lead advanced through the left subclavian vein into the RV where it can sense the arrhythmia and shock or overdrive the tachycardia back to normal rhythm.

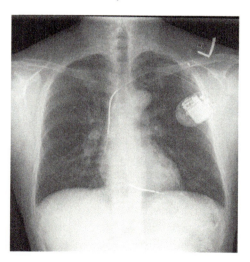

(Fig.68) (en.wikipedia.org) This is a chest x-ray of a patient with a single lead ICD. Note this unit is a little lower in the chest, and there is one lead attached to the unit through the subclavian vein into the right ventricle with two white electrodes in the RV apex and at the RV inflow.

The ICD is impervious to x-rays but not to the magnetic field of a MRI (magnetic resonance imaging) machine. This can be a problem if the patient needs an MRI, where only a CT (computerized tomography) can be done. However, as this book is being written, there's a whole new generation of pacemakers. Soon, ICDs where the circuitry is protected against an MRI and is MRI safe will be developed. It's only a matter of time when this same technology is applied to the more complex ICD to make MRI safe.

Whether to place an ICD is a very complex decision, and most medical decisions require close interaction with your electrophysiologist. There is much room for the considerations of various variables that can affect the emotional decision whether to accept a life prolonging device. For example, in the elderly, especially over the age of 80 or with a component of advancing dementia, the decision to implant an ICD must be tempered with the patient's or the families desire to see productive prolongation of life.

In general, it's not good to place an ICD in such cases, and many cultures in the world do not implant an ICD in patients over the age of 60-70. In the US, there are guideline that direct the use of an ICD in patients over the age of 80 which mandate strong physician documentation of the need for the ICD. Unfortunately in America, this is often neglected and could be cause of Medicare denying payment for the procedure in the very near future. Further, the guidelines by Medicare and organized cardiology and electrophysiology societies for any ICD in any age, are very precise, and all physicians must adhere to the insurance companies and Medicare parameters in determining if the ICD was appropriately indicated.

If the doctor doesn't follow the guidelines and doesn't document the appropriate qualifying criteria and ICD indications in his office or hospital chart, this data can and will be reviewed by the payer and the post procedure payment could be denied. Unlike a lot of procedures in electrophysiology, the guidelines are also used by the Department of Justice in ICD implant audits. Unfortunately, the electrophysiologist often fails to follow through for ICD implant timing specifically in proximity to previous procedures such as PCI or CABG. For example, an ICD implant shouldn't be done within 60 days of a PCI or CABG. It can be grounds for Medicare's denial of reimbursement, and often, they'll demand the hospital repay the amount received for the procedure. It remains to be determined if these circumstances will result in the financial liability for the patient.

For example, a very common scenario is the interventionalist ascertaining if the patient is a candidate for an ICD during a PCI. The intervention is done, and the patient is kept in the hospital for another day to undergo ICD placement the next morning. Under the these circumstances, the placement of the ICD is not only unrelated to the PCI procedure, but the ICD being placed within one day of a PCI is absolute grounds for Medicare denial let alone a DOJ audit for being completely outside the bounds of the established standards of care. Without question, the family or patient must take on a proactive role in such situations. In this scenario, it's totally appropriate to tell the electrophysiologist that the ICD implant is to be deferred for 30-90 days unless he can adequately document in the chart a need for an emergency ICD implant. Again, these exceptions to the DOJ rules are also well defined, but take the appropriate physician documentation in the chart to validate the placement of an ICD within days of a PCI or CABG.

There have been some very important medical studies that specifically addressed the need and the indications for an ICD implant. These studies are the basis for the ACC/ HRS (American College of Cardiology/Heart Rhythm Society) guidelines that have been established as the absolute standards of care for the placement and indications for an ICD. These protocols have been incorporated in a set of guiding principles established by Medicare in National Coverage Determinations (NCD).

Over the past few years, these guidelines have been used by the Department of Justice (DOJ) to recoup payment for ICDs that were improperly planted and contrary to the standards of care. Government scrutiny of ICD implants has been vigorous over the past 5 years based partly on the fact that an ICD implant costs $30,000 to $40,000, and the prevalence of improper ICD implants is so high. Thus, the government takes these drastic actions, and Medicare is serious about conforming to the Standards of Care.

Basically, the ICD is implanted as primary or secondary prevention of SCD. I will explain these terms. Secondary prevention means that the ICD is implanted after a patient has survived an episode of SCD. So, the patient is identified to be at high risk for a second SCD event, and the ICD is implanted to prevent certain death. It was hard to do a study to test the efficacy of such treatment to extend one's survival because the efficacy of the ICD in prevention of SCD was intuitively nearly 100%.

However, some basic studies were done, and the use of the ICD for secondary prevention of survival turned out to be an absolute indication for an ICD implant. Note that I specifically "truly" documented episode of SCD. This is where some significant variability lies, and it's because there is a clause in the standards of care that allows some interpretation and lead way by the electrophysiologist in determining the cause of an apparent SCD episode.

First and foremost, just because a person passes out, the paramedics are called, and they do CPR or defibrillation, it does not automatically qualify as an SCD episode. For example, a young or very old patient may have a "fainting" spell where the heartbeats slow. In this slowness, the heart may be very vulnerable to an episode of ventricular fibrillation, and when the paramedics arrive, it's the arrhythmia they see and transmit to the hospital and start CPR. However, the initial event was not a spontaneous cardiac arrest for ventricular fibrillation that the ICD would've converted. In this case, bradycardia led to the appearance of a primary episode of SCD.

In this instance, the electrophysiologist has the option based on the standard of care of documenting that he feels this was truly a primary SCD without equivocation and thus a candidate for an ICD. The proper management of in this young or old is to first do a cardiac catheterization to rule out coronary disease as the primary cause of the event. It's important to do as the electrophysiological study involves placing catheters in the heart and as they try to reproduce and document that using well-defined stimulation protocols if they can make the heart go into ventricular tachycardia or ventricular fibrillation. If they can't do this, then ICD is not indicated in my opinion.

The problem lies in the fact that the electrophysiologist insists on the placement of an ICD even in the light of this negative evidence and when there's no definitive substantiation of a primary episode of ventricular tachycardia. In this case I've outlined, the primary arrhythmia was bradycardia possibly compounded by exercise-induced low potassium (hypokalemia) which heralded SCD and not the unprovoked emergence of ventricular fibrillation. A young person, say 40 years of age, could end up with an ICD that never shocks for the next 20 years because the ICD wasn't indicated in the first place. Also, when it's time for a replacement, the electrophysiologist, partly driven by the WIGGS syndrome, blindly replaces the unit rather than checking if a replacement is truly necessary.

For example, let's say a patient has an ICD implant for 10 years that never shocks, and the heart function improves to the point where the ICD is no longer indicated. The doctor appropriately removes the ICD only to have the patient abuse his body for 10 years and die of SCA and an acute heart attack. At that point, the grieving family sees a TV ad from some unscrupulous (in Jewish, we call it shyster with no morals or ethics) malpractice lawyer, who argues for a large insurance settlement based on the argument that the patient wouldn't have died if he still had the ICD. Such ridiculous abuse of the legal system is prevalent and is a reflection of how our malpractice tort system is in this country.

The more difficult dilemma is the primary prevention placement of an ICD for the treatment of SCD that has *not* yet occurred but will probably occur, let's say, in the next 5 years. The issue of whether a patient should receive an ICD for primary prevention is a far more complex issue in this case. Implantation of an ICD has risks. First, a device can be recalled and may subject the patient to the prospect of a possibly dangerous laser lead removal, which can lead to putting a hole in the heart. And the ICD could become infected, which is a catastrophic event that requires the complete removal of the device, six weeks of IV antibiotics, and the patient wearing a complex "shocking vest" called a life vest for a six-week period before a new device is implanted.

Lastly, the ICD placement can result in inappropriate shocks when a young person jogs and his heart rate gets high enough that the ICD misinterprets as a SCD arrhythmia and shocks him. Devices are also expensive and may require multiple replacements. There is also the commitment to lifelong expense on a specialized doctor or medical center for long-term follow-ups.

The most important risk factor for sudden cardiac death for primary prevention is an impaired LV ejection fraction with the risk for ventricular tachycardia or ventricular fibrillation increasing markedly as the ejection fraction drops to 30-35%. The measurement of this ejection fraction can be done in various ways such as echocardiography, cardiac catheterization in ventriculography, or by nuclear techniques. Significant room for variations can occur in these methodologies, and it's wise for the patient to be aware of the fact that the echocardiogram interpretation of EF is subjective and may vary from reader to reader. In general, the nuclear techniques and ventriculography rely on computerized numbers, so they're more accurate and reproducible.

Unfortunately, it is common for the physician to rely on the lowest ejection fraction that may be that of the echocardiogram. When the time for replacement comes around, the EF is suddenly normal at 55%. So, there is a valid question as to the wisdom of ICD replacement especially if the device has never shocked the patient over the lifetime of the first ICD.

Nevertheless, the risk of SCD with a reduced EF is also dependent on the cause of the low EF: coronary artery disease, a previous heart attack, an idiopathic, or no ischemic cardiomyopathy due to coronary artery disease but rather where the low ejection fraction may be due to an old virus attack on the heart, or is purely speculative. If the EF is low due to coronary disease, the patient is at a higher risk than those with an idiopathic cardiomyopathy.

The major clinical trials of ICDs for primary prevention were all positive with reductions of overall death of 30-50% over a two year period. These studies include the *MUST* study and the SCD-HeFT trial where it was calculated over a two year period, that one in every 14 patients with an ICD lived who statistically should have died. This is a remarkable number and attests to the incredible efficacy of the ICD in prolonging your life.

Very importantly, it was found that if the ICD was implanted before waiting one month after a heart attack, the patient did worse and more likely died. This was the basis of many of the breaches of the standard of care found by electrophysiologists in the DOJ audits of inappropriate ICD implants. For some reason, the doctors ignore the fact that the EF can improve with healing of the heart attack, and if the patient has an event such as a cardiac arrest within one month after their heart attack, the physician may feel compelled to immediately place an ICD. With this knowledge, the patient and the family should be vigilant for any decision to place an ICD before one month after a well-documented heart attack.

Similarly, the EF can improve significantly after coronary artery bypass surgery (CABG). A routine placement of an ICD right after or within 3 months of a CABG conveyed no benefit for prevention of SCD as demonstrated in the CABG-PATCH trial.

The decision to place an ICD in a patient with a newly discovered idiopathic non-ischemic cardiomyopathy is more difficult. It's because the EF can improve to better than the benchmark 30% and obviate the need for an ICD implant with proper and established medical protocol treatment of the weak heart. The EF can improve significantly with the proper medical therapy of a non-ischemic cardiomyopathy; standards of care mandated for these patients to undergo the well-documented medical therapy from 3-9 months before ICD implantation.

The difference in these numbers is based on different studies, but the benchmark is at least three months of proper therapy. This requirement is where the problem lies as the documentation by most practitioners is very poor. If a patient visits the electrophysiologist for the first time, there probably is no assurance that there has been this three months of properly documented therapy. This challenge has been the basis of the greatest breach of standard of care that the DOJ found as up to 90% of the ICDs for non-ischemic cardiomyopathies were placed without adequate documentation of the three-month benchmark.

It's astounding that all the physician has to do is document somewhere in his chart that there's been three months of maximal medical therapy for the cardiomyopathy but doesn't. Of course, if audited, somewhere in the charts or the doctor's office notes there must be a notation of the various medicines that were utilized for treatment to assure that there was adherence to the proper guidelines for optimal medical therapy. Also, the thing about the criteria for 3-9 months of optimal medical therapy is that the patient doesn't have such a severe cardiomyopathy and congestive heart failure (CHF) that renders the patient bedridden. This is called Class IV heart failure, and is an absolute contraindication to placement of an ICD.

Unfortunately, the roots of the non-adherence by physicians are multifold. I think the most prevalent is the sense of entitlement as well as the WIIGS syndrome. First, the entitlement is that the patient or the family has very limited knowledge of the ICD and demands the ICD irrespective of the doctor's recommendation for the three-month therapy. The doctor might recommend that the patient wear a life vest for three months, but the family, after being told that the patient is at risk for SCA, demand immediate ICD implant to avoid wearing the life vest for 1-3 months. The prevalent environment of entitlement and the lack of tort reform have significantly fostered this attitude resulting in rampant abuse of the system.

In my opinion, these attitude have led to a significant amount of inappropriate ICD implants because the patient simply expresses their "God given option" to have the immediate ICD implant. This is further driven by the politically correct mentality of "patient driven care." The patient should have a firm and complete understanding of the medical decision rather than half-truths or emotion-driven and limited knowledge often gained by cursory reading or the Internet. But some patients still demand immediate satisfaction or search for another doctor who will render inferior care. It takes a strong willed and self-confident doctor to refuse improper care at the expense of losing a patient.

Lastly, there's also the very important indication for primary and secondary prevention of SCD in those with normal EFs but with conditions that predispose to ventricular tachycardia and ventricular fibrillation. They include, but are not limited to, Long QT syndrome, Idiopathic Hypertrophic Cardiomyopathy (IHSS), and Brugada's Syndrome.

CONTRAINDICATIONS FOR AN ICD IMPLANT; WHEN NOT TO IMPLANT

There are multiple conditions that make an ICD not a choice for primary or secondary prevention. Certainly, there are patients who benefit from the placements of ICDs, but it's important to know the type of patients who won't. The studies of the ICD looked at medium and long-term benefit over a 2-5 year period. The conditions that preclude survival of greater than one year wouldn't be expected to benefit from an ICD implant such as terminal or advanced cancer.

First, for patients with reversible causes of a SCD episode, there's an absolute contraindication to receiving an ICD. This is a subject injected by much emotion and inappropriate ICD implants by physicians. The simple question is how one defines reversible. There are some obvious signs of temporary conditions that lead to SCD but eliminate the need for an ICD once corrected. These conditions are mainly associated with electrolyte abnormalities. The dialysis patient who misses a session might present with SCD or a fatal arrhythmia because of a high potassium or calcium blood level. These patients can have it reversed with acute dialysis, so an ICD implant for secondary prevention is not indicated.

Additionally, an athlete running a marathon may collapse with SCD due to an acute low potassium or magnesium with dehydration. If the athlete survives, it also wouldn't be an indication of an ICD for secondary prevention. The real difficulty is the patient with some form of structural heart disease who collapses during heavy exercise. The electrolyte abnormality might simply uncover this previously unknown condition that predisposes to SCD. Obviously, this individual with a minimal amount of long QT on the EKG that gets worse with exercise can simply refrain from heavy exercise. However, if the patient doesn't wish to curtail their lifestyle or fears a second episode of SCD, then an ICD implant may be indicated.

Many of these situations are unique and require frank discussions by all the parties involved to make educated and informed decisions. It must be understood that these decisions place an onerous responsibility on the electrophysiologist as it's life and death in the balance. The majority of these judgments aren't like that of King Solomon but rather conform to the ethical standards of the Hippocratic Oath. The responsibility of the doctor to do no harm results in the patient's best interest.

The use of drugs or intoxication is one such indication of a reversible cause of SCD. Acute toxicity of alcohol or high blood levels of cocaine is often associated with SCD and a fatal cardiac event. In the case of cocaine, the cause of an episode can be from a heart attack that causes the SCD episode or from the direct effects of the cocaine on the conduction system of the heart that causes a fatal cardiac rhythm. In the case of alcohol, the long-term damage to the heart by chronic alcoholism associated with the acute toxic effects of a high blood alcohol level can lead to a cardiac arrest. If the patient survives, then the question is whether or not they receive an ICD implant for secondary prevention. However, what if the person refuses to stop their addiction. This situation can lead to much struggle, but in general, the use of an ICD is simply contraindicated if the addiction continues; again, this can be a very contentious issue.

This leads to the next contraindication of severe psychiatric conditions. It must be understood that the decision to place an ICD must be based on the patient being able to independently take care of themselves and guide their future lifelong follow-up. I imagine that addiction can be considered a severe and irreversible psychiatric condition. But we're talking about the psychotic or schizophrenic individuals who often live in a group home and are dependent on others for their daily care. This also includes severely mentally challenged individuals who are incapable of comprehending the consequences and challenges of an ICD implant.

It's obvious that these decisions for an ICD implant are often challenging, and there's a social component to these decisions. In the case of a mentally challenged individual such as a patient with Down's Syndrome who often have heart abnormalities that predispose to SCD, the decision of an ICD implant can lead to conflict within the family as well as with the doctor. The decision must be based on the assurance of the ability to afford lifelong care to the patient, which is often simply impossible.

The same dilemma arises in consideration for a patient with severe or advanced dementia. The question arises as to how one defines "severe" and "advanced" to the satisfaction of the family who wants the best done for their loved one. It can cause a tremendous amount of strain in the doctor-patient relationship. I guess the best guideline is to see if the patient is self-sufficient rather than dependent on outside care for activities of daily living (ADL). This can be an issue of culture too. As I have said, there are cultures and medical systems in the world that simply don't implant an ICD in someone over the age of 60-70 years, except in very specific circumstances. Thus, these decisions must be based on more than emotion but rather on the blunt realities of the patient's condition and prospects for any meaningful and productive survival.

Similarly, a contraindication for an ICD implant is if the patient has an expected lifespan of less than one year. This can often be a very subjective decision by the doctor and is difficult to assess the probability of survival. In the case of patient who survives SCD and has metastatic cancer refractory to further therapy, the ICD wouldn't be placed. I must stress that the studies with the ICD demonstrated its efficacy in prolonging life for 2-5 year. Therefore, if the patient's lifespan is severely shortened, then the benefit of ICD implant won't be realized. There's no doubt that the emotions of the family and the patient play a large role in these decisions. I fear that the "entitlement" mentality and family-directed care will only make these decisions more confrontational as the family irrationally demands an ICD. I imagine its only God who truly knows who will survive less than one year, but nevertheless the physician must arrive at these difficult decisions for proper withholding of an ICD implant.

A far more difficult and often contentious issue of keeping all these contraindications in mind is the decision when to replace an ICD when the battery depletes in 5-8 years or if the leads fail to work and need replacement. The battery is fairly easy to remove or replace, and the ICD can certainly be turned off with the programmer. The ICD leads are more difficult to replace, but the problem is in the broken lead. It can lead to multiple spurious shocks due the misinterpretation by the ICD of electrical interference caused by the lead are not working properly and giving the patient many repetitive shocks. A basic question to be asked is whether or not the EF is still less than 35% to justify the ICD in the first place.

It's an everyday occurrence in this country where an ICD reaches battery depletion and the electrophysiologist finds the ejection fraction has improved better that 35%. In many of these cases, the ICD was inappropriately placed before the patient was given 3-9 months of adequate medical therapy. Then eight years later, one finds that the heart has actually healed and is working appropriately. Most electrophysiologists loathe the prospect of not replacing the ICD out of the fear of medical liability for when the decision for ICD implant was initially made.

If the heart has healed and the patient is not using or appropriately shocking with the ICD, it shouldn't be replaced and the rationale to be accurately documented in the medical records. In reality, there is essentially nothing to be gained by replacing the ICD if the EF has recovered and is greater than 35%, especially with the risk of the new ICD becoming infected and having life threatening sepsis being greater than the benefit to be gained by inappropriate replacement.

This dictum that is even more pertinent that is that if in the interim of the initial ICD placement the patient develops an incurable disease or becomes intellectually challenged with advanced dementia. In this, again, the physician may be loath to the idea of not replacing the ICD for the reasons I have discussed. It's essential that the family and the patient both have a firm understanding that the replacement would be ill advised.

Before ending this section, I'd like to add a very important discussion that must be breached. In much of this book, it seems that I've maligned many of the practices of physicians in the often difficult decisions that must be made. Without a doubt, there's a major problem in America with the cardiologist and electrophysiologists making inappropriate medical choices. However, it has to be understood from much of my previous discussions that the practice of medicine in the recent few years has become almost 100% adversarial in nature. The increasing patient attitudes of entitlement have only markedly increased under Obamacare, and the concept of "patient directed care" has forced the doctor to make decisions that he simply knows is wrong.

The legal reality in this country and the lack of any meaningful tort reform have forced that majority of "nice" guys to do "not nice" things as they're compromised by the fear of suits and the pressures of the patients that have no real knowledge of the situations. Additionally, for many of these physicians, their licenses are at stake, and there's absolutely no relief or solutions from organized medicine or Obamacare. At the end, physicians are all "brothers and sisters" and must continually strive to correct the dysfunctional system and to save modern medicine from the inexorable brink of becoming a third-world system. Unfortunately, I feel that it'll take the patients armed with the knowledge of this book to afford themselves the proper level of cardiological care as these reforms will probably take longer than the coming of the Messiah.

The issue of SCD remains a large public health problem, but the pioneering work of Michel Mirowski and his foresight has had a giant impact on minimizing this problem. Still, the prevalence of SCD is increasing daily with newer treatments of heart diseases that is prolonging life to the point of needing the ICD.

INVASIVE ELECTROPHYSIOLOGICAL TESTING AND SYNDROMES OF SCD

At this juncture, I'd like to cover the common syndromes leading to SCD and the evolution of electrophysiological testing in the understanding of these maladies. It's extremely important to follow this topic as it heralds the beginning of the analysis of common cardiac diseases and how one can understand the consequences and management of these disease states.

The modern era of invasive electrophysiological studies was started by the demonstration in 1969 by Scherlag with the recording of the bundle in the human heart. This was followed by Hein Wellens in Netherlands, who described the phenomenon of electrical reentry that was responsible for common arrhythmias of paroxysmal supraventricular tachycardia (PSVT) seen in Wolff Parkinson's White Syndrome and reentry involving the AV node called AV nodal reentry (ANNRT).

The electrophysiological testing became more than an intellectual tool in that it guided the efficacy of the pharmacological treatment of these reentrant arrhythmias. It was further advanced by Wellens's demonstration that life-threatening arrhythmias such as ventricular tachycardia that could lead to SCD were based on reentry and be treated with various medicines that were actively being developed at the time. One such medicine was amiodarone, initially developed and used in Europe, this drug was remarkably effective in the prevention of many reentrant arrhythmias.

It was fascinating to go to the yearly NASPE meetings as the ranks of electrophysiologist increased and to see the discovery of these new medicines and how effective they were against these common rhythm disturbances. Around this time, one discovered the remarkable efficacy of amiodarone in the treatment of atrial fibrillation and atrial flutter, which are the most common arrhythmias in man and was initially felt to be a form of "micro reentry." It was at this time that the electrophysiological testing was melded with the ICD in the treatment of a host of conditions that could lead to SCD.

LONG QT SYNDROME

We start out with the long QT Syndrome, which I've previously mentioned. This condition is seen on the EKG where the interval after depolarization on the EKG is prolonged to the end of repolarization and the T wave (Fig 69, Fig 70, and Fig.71). There are two forms. The congenital form of long QT present at birth that can either be a mutation in the genes that suddenly arises in that it is the first case in a family or can be familial in that other members of the family have the EKG abnormality. The other form of the syndrome is acquired and is seen in a host of electrolyte disorders and with various medications such as some antidepressants that can increase the risk of SCD and is always seen on the label and instructions.

Soon, two principal forms of the congenital syndrome were defined: the Jervell and Lange-Nielsen syndrome, which is associated with deafness, and the Romano-Ward syndrome that's associated with normal hearing. Both of these syndromes were initially described in the pediatric population and were associated with spells of passing out and premature death. Soon to follow were descriptions of the syndrome in sibling and with other relatives such as a great grandparent, who died suddenly with no explanation that probably was SCD in retrospect.

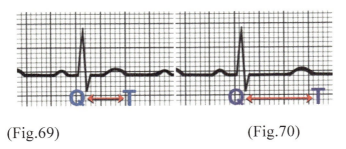

(Fig.69)   (Fig.70)

These are EKGs of a normal and a long QT interval. The degree of prolongation of the QT interval does have some prognostic implications, and an ICD is indicated for treatment the longer the interval over normal. Actually, drugs such a beta blockers have the ability to shorten the QT interval and can be the first line of therapy with borderline QT prolongation over 450 milliseconds in duration.

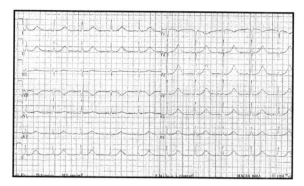

(Fig.71) Here is the EKG of a patient with a prolonged QT interval greater than 600 milliseconds. Note that the prolongation is mainly due to a wide and somewhat peaked T wave. In fact, the configuration of the T wave on the EKG can give a hint as to what gene type is the Long QT syndrome and act as a guide to therapy.

In 1957, a case was published of a Norwegian family with four out of six children were deaf mutes. All four children demonstrated marked prolongation of the QT interval and suffered recurrent syncopal spell. Four children died suddenly. Note that both of the parents of these children were healthy, but on their EKG was mild QT prolongation. Nevertheless, this family aided in identifying that the gene was recessive and not all family members demonstrated the full blown disease although they carried one of the two genes in their chromosomes.

Only recently, the science of gene mapping and characterization of the various cardiac conduction channels responsible for electrolytes movements in the conduction cells has led to an explosion of more than 10 gene abnormalities leading to 10 conduction channel or long QT diseases.

In 1961, Dr. Cesarino Romano from Italy described a 3-month-old baby with a very prolonged QT interval on the EKG. The baby had normal hearing but had two brothers who died suddenly. Later, he described a brother and sister who both had the long QT syndrome with many relatives who died suddenly and demonstrated classical recessive gene heredity on a mapped family tree. To this day, it's a challenge to identify the "normal" gene carriers without long QT on the EKG but may have a borderline long QT under the correct clinical circumstances, which can inappropriately prolong the QT due to various medicines or electrolyte abnormalities. In their cases, investigation of the relatives and unexplained deaths has lead to gene testing and proper counseling for the risk of having a child with the long QT Syndrome. One must ask whether the patient themselves should be treated with an ICD or medications like beta blockers.

The identification of the acquired long QT Syndrome was recognized when it was found that certain circumstances could prolong the QT interval when these patients initially come to the ER with a syncopal (passing out) spell. It must be understood that there may be the presentation as a presumed "seizure" in a patient who collapses but is actually an aborted episode of SCD and an associated arrhythmia. Plus, the patient may present as a drowning victim when it was an arrhythmia brought on the by the prolongation of the QT interval by exercise in the cold water. This is especially common in the pediatric population where a swimming child just stops breathing or appears to be having a seizure.

In actuality, there are many people with the hereditary or acquired long QT, who have no symptoms and live normal lives. Again, these are usually carriers of the recessive gene, but there are also some with the full blown syndrome who can go through life without incident. However, if there is a past history of SCD in the family tree, it's probably essential that one seek treatment from an electrophysiologist. This treatment may just be a beta blocking agent if the patient has had no syncope or dizziness.

However, in many cases with a very long QT, there is no other option than a lifelong ICD implant. The ICD is a miracle for these patients and allows a normal healthy lifestyle, which even includes contact sports or marathons. As the units get smaller, aesthetically, there's little change in one's appearance, allowing a woman to wear a low-cut dress.

The real difficult decision in the long QT syndrome is in whom to place the ICD. There is little doubt when one has the long QT and survives an episode of SCD, the ICD is indicated as a secondary prevention. In this case, the ICD becomes a lifelong therapy for the long QT syndrome until it's discovered how to change the gene itself or the expression of the gene leading to reversal of the long QT on the EKG. This also might take the form of a new medication that can change the ion channels in the heart to cure the long QT and reverse it back to normal.

The real challenge is when to place the ICD as primary prevention in a patient with the long QT syndrome who didn't have a near fatal arrhythmia. First, the patient must have a prolonged QT on the EKG and undergo genetic testing to ascertain if they carry the long QT gene and further determine what gene locus is the abnormality and to thus identify what type of long QT syndrome is present. So, it's helpful to do an accurate family tree to see what the gene expression is in the family based on those relatives who have the long QT or unexpectedly died with no explanation.

Based on these variables, the ICD implant is placed as primary prevention based on the probability the individual will have an episode on SCD. This becomes even more difficult with the very young patient who will possibly be committed to the ICD for the rest of their lives. Again, this decision should take at least two physicians' opinions and should be based on the recommendation of a primary specialty center for the treatment of long QT, probably in a pediatric hospital if the patient is less than 21 years old.

TORSADES DE POINTES

This arrhythmia is the most common form of ventricular tachycardia that leads to SCD in the patient with the Long QT Syndrome. It translates to "twisting or ballet of the points" that represents the RV and LV, beating with an EKG that looks like twisting. No matter how beautiful the name, Torsades is a life threatening arrhythmia that if gone untreated leads to ventricular fibrillation and death. If Torsades lasts a short time and corrects itself as we see in (Fig.72), the patient may feel nothing, a little dizziness, or pass out and regain consciousness. But again, if it persists and is not shocked back to normal rhythm, it deteriorates to ventricular fibrillation and SCD.

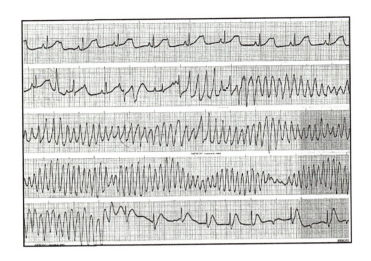

(Fig.72) (www.nms.ac.jp)

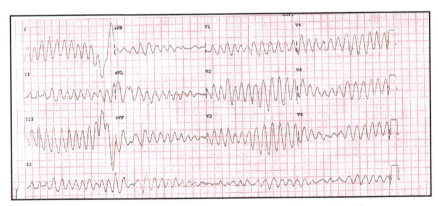

(Fig.72 and Fig.73) (www.heartpearls.com) Here are two beautiful EKGs of a few normal beats and the onset and deterioration to Torsades de Points. Although it's a life-threatening arrhythmia, one can appreciate the "dancing or ballet of the points" as the EKG shows a twisting configuration. As a young cardiologist, I first saw this in a patient who was given an overdose of a medicine that was known to cause this, and I was immediately fearful in seeing this recording. I also appreciated the symmetry of the EKG and made me all the more interested in becoming an electrophysiologist.

What was even more amazing was when a patient who came out of their room to chat with me and stood next to me suddenly collapsed. The nurse ran out with the rhythm strip of Torsades, and I immediately got a defibrillator and shocked the patient back to normal rhythm. Boy, that experience certainly woke me up and took a few years off my life. I'll never forget my utter terror and subsequent satisfaction in saving a life. Such is the life of a cardiologist. One second the patient was there and talking, and the next second he was near death. It was only my training that resulted in my immediate reflex to shock the patient and saved his life. Not to shock the readers, but I've seen doctors panic and simply run out of the room because they didn't know what to do. That is the reality of the young doctors' eight-hour shifts and lack of experience or training.

There are a variety of causes of Torsades de Pointes. Those include various medications that are known to prolong the QT interval and lead to the heart being vulnerable to SCD and Torsades. These medications can be taken at the same time for other conditions but if predisposed to Torsades, the combination can be deadly. These principal conditions are diarrhea, exercise, low magnesium, and low potassium. It's common to see a patient with chronic and explosive diarrhea develop marked depletion in their potassium and SCD.

If the patient is eating high amounts of grapefruit and is on an antibiotic like erythromycin, the combination can also exacerbate the prolonging of the QT interval. Other such medications include Biaxin, Tagamet, Celexa, Haldol, amphetamines, cocaine, and various antidepressants. It's wise, specifically in those who know that their QT intervals are borderline long or that they know they're carriers of the long QT gene, to read the literature or ask the doctor if any medication they're taking can increase their risk of Torsades.

The last common cause of Torsades is a very slow heart rate or a block in the conduction system such as AV block that causes a very slow heart rate, which may suggest the need for a pacemaker. As the heart slows, the QT interval increases. This is very pronounced when there's a long pause in the heartbeat above five seconds, especially in the elderly, where the beats following the pause have a very long QT interval and make the patient prone to Torsades. This is seen a lot in syncope patients while they're wearing a long-term heart monitor.

Interestingly, the first description of Torsades was in 1966 by the French doctor Dessertenne when it was documented in an 80-year-old survivor of SCD with heart block and a heart rate in the 20s. The word Torsades was coined by his wife from a French dictionary, which meant twisting of the threads in a helix for a sweater. Nevertheless, its not uncommon in patients getting a pacemaker for a slow heart, that the cause of syncope may be not only the slow heart rate and block but concomitant Torsades.

ARRYTHMOGENIC RIGHT VENTRICLAR DYSPLASIA

Arrhythmogenic right ventricular dysplasia (ARVD) or arrhythmogenic right ventricular cardiomyopathy is an inherited form of a non-ischemic cardiomyopathy. ARVD is caused by a genetic defect of the right ventricle in the connection of the cells and is characterized by fatty infiltration of the RV and thickening of the muscle in an autopsy of the heart. It's associated with life-threatening arrhythmias of the right ventricle, which is a rapid form of ventricular tachycardia and SCD.

In 1986, Dr. Nikos Protonotarios examined a group of families on the island of Naxos in Greece with the syndrome of ARDS and sudden cardiac death. He found that all had thickening of the skin on their palms and had very "woolly" hair. ARVD without these characteristics is found in North America, and this is because the genes lie close together. It's seen in 1/10,000 people and thus is fairly common.

In children and young adults, it presents itself like the long QT Syndrome with seizures, drowning, syncope, palpitations, and death. It's inherited as an autosomal dominant syndrome; therefore, it's very common in families and can be deduced from the family tree. In a group of young people genetically tested, up to 1/2000 may be the carrier of the autosomal recessive form of the gene, making it one of the more common forms of genetic disease and death in the pediatric population. ARVD has been traced to up to 12 different gene loci, and some of the forms tend to become evident at ages 40-50.

In actuality, ARVD is very common in the electrophysiologists' practices as it presents initially in 80% of ARVD patients as a syncopal spell and can be easily recognized by a peculiar EKG characteristic called an "epsilon" wave. I distinctly remember the first time I saw this EKG abnormality in an adolescent patient who had a syncopal spell and subsequently lived a normal life with an ICD. The young patient had no more syncopal spells but with frequent shocks by the ICD. Plus, it's a rather regular cause of syncope and death in the athletic population but can easily be screened by a simple EKG-again the need for athlete screening.

The ventricular tachycardia of ARVD arises from the right ventricle and has a typical LBBB configuration and a very characteristic appearance that immediately raises the suspicion for ARVD (Fig.74). The disease can be confirmed by an echocardiogram and more definitively by a cardiac MRI. It can be seen during a cardiac catheterization with contrast visualization of the right ventricle, but the gold standard for diagnosis is the cardiac MRI that shows a much thickened right ventricle that has mostly fatty infiltration in replacement of the normal right ventricular cells.

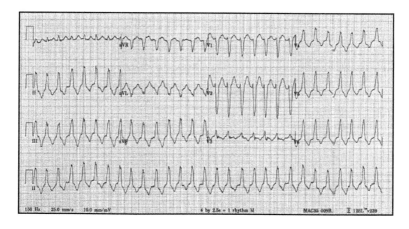

(Fig.74) (lifeinthefastlane.com) This is the EKG of ventricular tachycardia of ARVD. Note that the arrhythmia is very regular each beat is the same which is unlike the EKG of Torsaces. This looks like a LBBB and is easily recognized as possible ARVD. In the early presentation of the disease, this arrhythmia stops itself and may cause palpitations or syncope, but in the later stages continues and deteriorates to ventricular fibrillation and SCD.

Unfortunately, the first sign of ARVD may be SCD. It's interesting that in some individuals in the family who test positive for the disease may not have any manifestation until they're older. Nevertheless, they still have the disease, and the first sign of ARVD may be fatal. As the disease progresses, the right ventricle enlarges, and the patient develops congestive heart failure. At the end stages of the disease, the fat spreads to the left ventricle, and heart failure becomes critical.

The treatment of ARVD is very controversial and varies significantly from doctor to doctor. The problem lies in the fact that this is an actual progressive physical changes in the heart, not just an arrhythmia, so there can be drawbacks and limitations to whatever is done. The only real treatment and cure for this disease is cardiac transplantation. It's reserved for those that have survived to the stage of congestive heart failure as it may be the only viable option. There are multiple treatments available for early ARVD. The drawback of any medicine is that they may be effective for a period of time but fail later. As the physical changes of the right ventricle progress, the drug may fail and cause SCD.

Sotalol, a class III antiarrhythmic agent, is very effective in prevention of the episodes of ventricular tachycardia in ARVD as well as other diseases. The use of electrophysiological testing may be utilized to test if the electrophysiologist can stimulate the heart to go into the characteristic ventricular tachycardia. Then the doctor can treat the patient with Sotalol and do a second study to show that the drug prevents the doctor from initiating the tachycardia. If Sotalol works, the doctor does a cardiac MRI every two years to document to check for a progression of the disease. As the disease progresses, it may prove to be ineffective as the right ventricle is replaced with fat cells.

Thus, the ICD becomes the essential element in the treatment of ARVD. The complex decision becomes when one resorts to this treatment. The problem in ARVD is that when the muscle becomes completely infiltrated with fat, the ICD itself may not work as the electrodes of the ICD cannot make appropriate electrical contact with the healthy muscle tissue. This is described as a conduction block at the site of lead contact to the RV muscle. Nevertheless, the

ICD is placed, which may last a lifetime if the muscle infiltration remains stable over many years. As we saw in the long QT Syndrome, the challenge is when to place the ICD as primary prevention to anticipate an episode of ventricular tachycardia.

LEFT VENTRICULAR HYPERTROPHY; HYPERTROPHIC CARDIOMYOPATHY

Left ventricular hypertrophy is the thickening of the heart muscle as a secondary response to severe hypertension or seen as a primary hereditary disease process collectively known as the hypertrophic cardiomyopathies. As the heart muscle becomes more muscular, no different than in a weight lifter, there's the resultant thickening of the LV muscle as a response to pumping the blood at a very elevated blood pressure. This can also be seen in the reverse situation in a much-dilated heart with heart failure and thin muscle, but QT prolongation is most pronounced in the hypertrophic cardiomyopathies. In the patients with the many forms of hypertrophic cardiomyopathies, the heart muscle simply thickens with no known predisposing cause. This syndrome is very common and is felt to be responsible for up to 10% of pediatric and adult sports deaths. This can be significantly exacerbated by the use of illicit steroid ingestion.

The most common cause of significant left ventricular hypertrophy (LVH) is in uncontrolled hypertension. It's seen in a much higher proportion of the black population because hypertension is more common in the black population. Another cause is because that population doesn't seek medical treatment for the hypertension even those on dialysis who have a much higher incidence of the uncontrolled hypertension. In addition to being responsible for the majority of strokes with hypertension, over the years of high blood pressure, the heart muscle thickens and may fail with eventual dilation of the hypertrophied muscle losing its effectiveness and causing sever congestive heart failure.

Before this occurs, the hypertrophied muscle can lead to SCD and Torsades. It also causes a form of obstruction to the heart outflow in the aortic valve called obstructive cardiomyopathy where the enlarged muscle causes a blockage of the blood outflow out of the aortic valve. Interestingly enough, if the high blood pressure is treated, then the hypertrophy can resolve and reverse the propensity to CHF and SCD. Plus, the severe hypertrophy of the heart muscle can actually cause the coronaries to constrict. In certain instances of the LAD artery, there can be intermittent closure of the artery and a heart attack with the risk of heart damage and SCD due to ventricular arrhythmias such as VT and VF.

The other most common form of LVH is hypertrophic cardiomyopathy (HCM) or obstructive hypertrophic cardiomyopathy (HOCM). This condition is present in 0.5% of the population and often goes unrecognized until a SCD or collapse. These are forms of hereditary LVH that principally can cause heart failure: SCD due to an arrhythmia, severed CHF, and what is called a cardiomyopathy that produces a low ejection fraction and the high risk of SCD just from the low EF. The degree of hypertrophy may differ in various parts of the heart, and HOCM exhibits particular thickening of the septum between the LV and RV, specifically near the aortic valve. It's responsible for 40% of SCD in athletes and often unrecognized until the athlete collapses on the field but can easily be identified by a screening echocardiogram.

Like the long QT Syndrome, HOCM and HCM are hereditary. It's important to trace your family tree for a history of SCD if you have this condition. As with the long QT Syndrome, the ICD can be used for primary and secondary prevention of SCD. There are also guidelines for the primary use of an ICD based on the degree of septal hypertrophy measured with a simple echocardiogram. For that matter, an echocardiogram is the primary means of diagnosis of LVH and can be supplemented by heart catheterization and a heart MRI. There are various findings on the physical exam that can complement what is found on the echocardiogram when the doctor has you bear down in the Valsalva Maneuver to listen for a murmur and measure your blood pressure. These simple tests can offer hints for treatment as well as prognosis.

The use of genetic testing has added much to our knowledge of HCM and HOCM in that it can be caused by up to 12 known gene mutations. It can run in families or occur as a first time gene mutation. The form of genetic HCM and HOCM is important as one form called beta myosin heavy chain mutation can cause 50% of these patient having SCD before the age of 40. Recently, sarcomeric (structures in the cell) protein mutations have also been found to be associated with early death.

There a multiple forms of treatment for HCM, especially HOCM. The primary goal of medications is to relieve chest pains that may be caused by the heart muscle closing off the coronaries during the exercise. The main drugs that are use include beta blockers like Inderal or Atenolol as well as calcium channel inhibitors like verapamil or Nifedipine. These agents act to lessen the vigor of the heart contraction and the symptoms but have no proven efficacy in reducing the incidence of SCD. In the face of heart failure, one can be placed on a diuretic such as Lasix. These agents must be taken with caution and closely followed by your physician as they can actually cause a worsening of the outflow tract obstruction seen in HOCM.

More invasive treatments include surgical septal myectomy and alcohol septal ablation. A surgical myectomy involves an open-heart surgery where the septal hypertrophy is relieved by excising part of the hypertrophied septum in HOCM and in HCM to relieve the outflow obstruction as well as many of the symptoms of the hypertrophy. Complications from an open-heart surgery can include infection, bleeding, stroke, and heart perforation with death. Thus, a surgical myectomy is a very serious decision, and the fact that it doesn't lessen the incidence of SCD makes it useful only in the most symptomatic patients.

The technique of alcohol ablation involves the injection of alcohol through an LAD branch via a catheter to kill off some of the septal muscle. This can be a very effective treatment in terms of symptom and heart failure relief but is limited to a very small amount of specialists who are trained in such technique. Nevertheless, alcohol ablation remains a very effective technique, and frankly, should be considered before open heart surgery even if it involves traveling to a different city for an appropriately skilled specialist.

Lastly, we come to the issue of an ICD implant. This can be a very difficult issue and is mostly based on the family tree and the results of genetic testing. There are some forms of HCM that has a much higher incidences of SCD, and an ICD implant is absolutely indicated. However, the problem lies when the genetic tests come back positive for hereditary HCM, and the family tree indicates a history of SCD. In this instance, the degree of hypertrophy of the septum is assessed. With this information at hand, a decision for ICD implant can be made. As far as I'm concerned, if an aunt or uncle, a first cousin, or grandparent has a SCD episode irrespective of the degree of septal hypertrophy, then the ICD implant is absolutely indicated.

BRUGADA AND EARLY REPOLARIZATION SYNDROMES

There are a variety of abnormalities of repolarization that have been seen on the EKG such as the long QT syndrome. These repolarization abnormalities can be fairly common, and the problem is to ascertain if these abnormalities have any clinical relevance to a true disease state. It's only by meticulous observation and documentation that these associations can be made.

Brugada Syndrome is a hereditary condition characterized by specific EKG markers during repolarization that lead to SCD. Although the EKG findings of the Brugada Syndrome were described in 1989, it took the cardiologist Pedro Brugada and his brother Josep Brugada to recognize the association of the EKG variant to SCD as a distinct clinical entity (Fig.77). The incidence of Brugada Syndrome is estimated to be 5 in 10,000 individuals worldwide and usually becomes clinically evident in adulthood starting approximately at the age of 40. Estimates are that the Brugada Syndrome is responsible for 4-12% of all SCD, and it's the second most common cause of death following accidents in Southeast Asia. So, it's critical for individuals with Southeast Asian origin to have a screening EKG.

The apparent EKG evidence for Brugada's syndrome is seen in many individuals as a normal variant of the EKG, so it takes some analysis to determine if it's truly Brugada. The electrophysiologist may do a special EP study with the introduction of various intravenous medicines during the study to see if they further expose the EKG evidence for the syndrome and supported or negated the correct diagnosis. Plus, the EP study can be used to see if Torsades or ventricular tachycardia can be induced, which identifies those patients at a high risk for subsequent SCD.

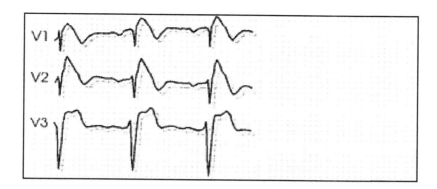

(Fig.77) This is an EKG of Brugada's syndrome. Note the repolarization wave after the QRS complex has a very high takeoff in the leads V1, V2, and V3. This is the characteristic EKG picture, but can also be present in a small percentage of normal individuals. It's important for a person with this EKG to look into his or her family tree and have a genetic testing if there's some unexplained deaths.

Similar to the Long QT syndrome, there are lots of pharmacological agents and conditions that can unmask the EKG of Brugada's and bring on SCD. These include febrile states that often are misinterpreted as febrile seizures, antihistamines, antidepressants, pregnancy, and most importantly, it's a very common cause of death with even minimal cocaine use. Brugada Syndrome may actually be the most common unidentified abnormality that is associated with cocaine and SCD. It's an unfortunate consequence of our society that recurrences of SCD are seen in up to 90% in cocaine abusers. These patients who cannot or will not abstain from the drug results in an incredible burden on humanity, family members, and the physician.

Clinical presentation may also take on the form of sudden infant death syndrome (SIDS). Another very common form is the sudden unexpected nocturnal death syndrome (SUNDS), or the "screaming death" in Southeast Asia where the individual screams loudly at night and has SCD; syndromes include bangungut (Philippines), non-lai-tai (Laos), lai-tai (Thailand), and pokkuri (Japan). Pathological variants in 16 genes have been associated with Brugada Syndrome, and every patient who is identified by the EKG or the EP study identification should be sent for a gene analysis and specific type identification. This is augmented by the family tree analysis of SCD.

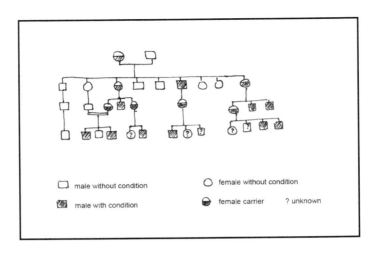

(Fig.78) (brusselsgenetics.be) This is a simple genetic tree of any disease that starts out at the top with the original parents and traces four generations of relatives, who may have or not have a condition as well as being a carrier of the gene without the full expression of the disease such as Brugada or Long QT. It's essential for the families with these diseases to create such a family tree to aid the doctor in making decisions for an ICD in conjunction with genetic testing.

The Brugada Syndrome can present as an EKG abnormality, unexplained syncope, or SCD. A unique variant of this syndrome presents with a "storm" of incessant syncopal spells or Torsades. This syndrome must be identified as the use of a specific drug, IV Isoproterenol, is unique for controlling the arrhythmia storm in Brugada patients.

The use of the ICD is critical in Brugada syndrome because the first clinical manifestation can be SCD. If the patient has a positive EP study and/or a positive family history, then an ICD implant is the recommended treatment of choice. The real dilemma comes when doing genetic counseling for a patient's immediate relative including the parents of the proband (patient who has the disease). This includes prenatal testing of a woman and man who may be carriers and with a strong possibility of a child born with Brugada's or, for that matter, any genetic disease with SCD as a clinical manifestation. With the development of genetic testing, these decisions have become much easier to make, but nevertheless, they should be subjected to multiple opinions before a relative has a primary prevention ICD implant or a pregnancy should be avoided.

The early repolarization syndrome is a recently observed syndrome where the prevalence of early repolarization changes in the EKG lead V4-V6 and III with AVF is more common than in the general population and is seen in survivors of SCD with no structural heart disease (Fig.79). There have been various studies looking at this EKG variant that occurs in 2-5% of the population. Also, sudden cardiac death is rare but more common than in the general population. This EKG abnormality is seen in athletes, young men, and African Americans and can be a very complex issue in terms of possible ICD implantation.

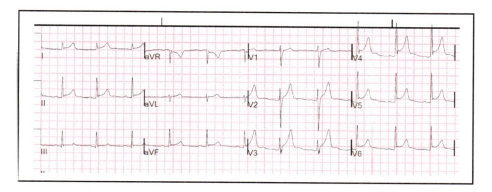

(Fig.79) This is an EKG of an Afro-American male with the early repolarization syndrome. Note that the ST segment is elevated right after the QRS, most pronounced in lead V54-V5 and lead II.

It's been found that the degree of the repolarization height over the QRS has important prognostic significance. In those with marked EKG abnormalities and with syncope, the implant of an ICD can be advised since there's no genetic testing or EP study evidence to aid in this decision. This syndrome is a recent addition to the repolarization abnormalities, and the difficulty in this particular syndrome is that there's no genetic testing for its presence as well as a specific therapy other than ICD if the family tree is suggestive of unexpected sudden deaths.

Catecholiminergic Ventricular Tachycardia

This is another rhythm disorder of the heart in genetically predisposed patients that affects one in ten thousand people but is responsible for 15% of unexplained SCD in the pediatric population.

Early signs and symptoms are syncope or dizziness brought on by exercise or acute emotional stress. Obviously, this syndrome can be mistaken for a simple fainting spell. But it accentuates the importance of not ignoring these symptoms especially with repeated episodes during competitive sports. This syndrome is very difficult to diagnose. It's usually picked up during a treadmill with heavy exertion and the patient starts to develop serious ventricular arrhythmias during peak stress. The patient should examine their family tree and be sent for genetic testing since it's been found in five gene abnormalities that control the movement of ions—specifically calcium—during the depolarization and repolarization process.

Beta blockers are used to treat this syndrome, but if the genetic testing is positive, the use of an ICD implant is the primary alternative when the beta blockers don't alleviate the symptoms. Of course, the next event after the initiation of beta blocker could be fatal SCD, so in my opinion, the ICD should be the first line of treatment with the addition of beta blockers to alleviate the palpitation or dizzy spells as backup.

Sick Sinus Syndrome, Tachycardia-Bradycardia Syndrome, Paroxysmal Supraventricular Tachycardia (PSVT), and Atrial Fibrillation.

At this juncture, we leave the genetic disease causing SCD and enter those acquired medical conditions that are common afflictions. Sick sinus syndrome (SSS) is a group of arrhythmias that are related at one level to the sinus node but has come to include multiple situations that cause both a fast and slow heart rate. I include the tachycardia-bradycardia (tachy-brady) syndrome in this context as the electrophysiologist often utilizes these terms interchangeably as a reason to place a pacemaker for the slow heart rate or to help control the fast heart rate. Realistically, it's not appropriate to bundle these two syndromes together as a justification for a pacemaker, but it has come to be such a standard of care that I feel it is appropriate to bundle this discussion.

These syndromes are often related to aging of the heart, ischemic heart disease, cardiomyopathy, hereditary, or valvular disorders. These syndromes include sinus bradycardia, sinus tachycardia, PSVT, and SSS (sick sinus syndrome).

Sinus bradycardia occurs when the primary natural pacemaker of the heart starts to slow down and doesn't send out the appropriate signals to meet the rate demands of the body. The heart beats slowly. A variant of this condition is chronotropic incompetency, which means that the heart rate is not too slow at rest but doesn't increase appropriately with exercise and limits one's exercise capacity. We have touched upon chronotropic incompetency already, but it is appropriate to reiterate at this point.

Sinus bradycardia is the most common cause for the placement of a permanent pacemaker and can also be the most abused indication. First, significant sinus bradycardia is a result of the natural aging process, and the real question is when the situation is true pathological (disease) versus physiological (natural result of aging). There is no doubt that in the trained athlete that sinus bradycardia is physiological and can be fairly pronounced with heart rates in the 30s to 40s at rest. Certainly, these athletes don't require a pacemaker. Plus, they aren't passing out (syncope) because of this bradycardia.

In the patient who is older and the untrained athlete in the age group of 40-70, the presence of sinus bradycardia and heart rate range can pose a very difficult clinical dilemma. What if these patients are passing out or experiencing significant fatigue presumably due to the slow heart rate and not meeting the oxygen requirements of the body?

There is really no good way of coming to the conclusion of a pathological situation in patients in the age range of 40-70. There are some who have had these slow heart rates since early childhood and are part of hereditary sinus node dysfunction. If these children demonstrate fatigue or difficulty with school, then a pacemaker may be a solution. However, the question of a pacemaker implant is much more difficult in the intermediate age group.

As a first step in almost any patient where the doctor suspects pathological sinus bradycardia, the primary test is a holter monitor or event monitor. These are short-term or long-term recorders that are affixed to the chest with leads and record or transmit the EKG over the airways or the Internet in the form of a single lead rhythm strip. Then the doctor analyzes the strips for any significant arrhythmia, heart block, or bradycardia to check if these episodes correlate with the patient's symptoms. This is how the doctor can actually come to a conclusion if an episode of bradycardia is truly pathological that caused such as dizziness or just the normal range for this patient.

It has been estimated that over 50% of pacemakers, especially in the elderly, are placed for bradycardia that isn't pathological. The pacemakers have the ability to store data and record how often they pace the heart upon interrogation that the doctor does regularly. In many of these studies, a majority of these implanted pacemakers in patients over the age of 70 paces less than 10% of the time. In the older age group of over 80, there're more cases of the pacemakers for bradycardia being placed for physiological bradycardia that's been improperly and incompletely evaluated. On the other hand, there are many circumstances that the bradycardia or heart block is transient and short lived but is significant enough to warrant a pacemaker implant.

It's all too common for an elderly patient to be admitted to the hospital for a completely unrelated reason and found to be bradycardic with a possible need for a surgical procedure. In this instance, the surgeon may ask for an electrophysiology consult for the pacemaker placement. The long term holter is not available, and the patient might have a component of dementia, which makes evaluation of associated symptoms and the decision regarding pacemaker implant difficult. Often, the electrophysiologist will appropriately want to do an electrophysiological study. This procedure is when temporary electrodes are placed in the heart and the doctor does a "programmed stimulation" of the heart to evaluate the components of the conduction system. There are established parameters to measure the function of the sinus node, AV node, His Bundle, and the bundle branches.

In terms of the sinus node, Dr. William Mandel, at Cedars Sinai Medical Center in Los Angeles, developed a series of parameters and guidelines regarding the need for a permanent pacemaker implant. In my opinion, the electrophysiological study is often underutilized, and the untrained electrophysiologist unfamiliar with sinus node disease may not know whether a pacemaker implant should be indicated. The decision for a pacemaker implant must be fully discussed with the family to understand the doctor's reasoning behind it while taking into account the mental and physical reality of the patient's clinical condition. If the patient has advanced dementia, the pacemaker implant just to facilitate a surgery can be excessive. Also, the surgery may take some appropriate consent from the family, who are willing to take the chance of having the surgery without the prior pacemaker implant.

One interesting statistic is that upon testing of patients with advanced dementia in a nursing home, 50% of the patients with holter monitoring had significant bradycardia. It's intriguing to contemplate whether this bradycardia, specifically at night during sleep, deprived the brain of sufficient oxygen and contributed to their dementia.

Lastly, in the evaluation of sinus bradycardia and many other incidental or symptomatic arrhythmias, the physician has the option of placing a long term "loop" event monitor under the chest skin near the heart. This device is the size of a stick of gum and is like a solid state miniature hard disk with the ability to record and store the heart rhythm in the patient with a diary to note the times and occurrence of any symptoms. It doesn't entail leads and is a simple but invaluable aid to the physician, evaluating whether an episode of bradycardia is symptomatic and requires a pacemaker implant.

Sinus tachycardia is when the heart goes fast due to speeding up of the natural pacemaker, which occurs normal while one exercises but pathological at rest or asleep, is called inappropriate sinus tachycardia (IST). This is a very complex syndrome and condition that often occurs in women with the common denominator of concurrent emotional disorders. Note the two scenarios: an emotional disorder coming about because the heart is always going fast and causing the emotional problem, or the emotional problem occurring first and is somehow linked to the ultimate development of their fast heartbeat.

Nevertheless, the treatment of this condition remains a significant challenge. The use of beta blockers to treat the fast heartbeat is usually ineffective, and all treatment modalities are doomed to failure if the baseline emotional disorder isn't addressed. Also, the patient will often go from doctor to doctor seeking some type of treatment.

Radiofrequency ablation is the treatment regularly utilized with the radiofrequency ablation (RFA) is a technique whereby the catheter is utilized to vaporize the specific tissue. In IST, an attempt is made to ablate the sinus node so that a new pacemaker down the chain of the conduction system takes over at a slower rate. In my experience, this treatment is almost always a failure and exposes the usually young patient with false hope, resulting often the ultimate need of a lifelong pacemaker. And going from doctor to doctor may result in three or four ablations that often culminate in failure, which gives the patient a life threatening complication or a pacemaker and a further becomes pretense to seek lifelong disability and a wasting of a life.

Sick sinus syndrome occurs most often in patients over 50. Its variant chronotropic incompetency can occur at a much younger age and may cause SSS as one grows older and the heart's conduction system becomes scarred and fibrotic. Sick sinus syndrome (SSS) is one of the most common arrhythmias encountered in the older age group. It is a complex interplay of rapid and slow heart rates while SSS and tachy-brady syndrome are often used in exchange although they're not exactly the same. It's difficult to treat SSS. The heart, because of aging or scarring of the conduction system, has periods of rapid heart rates with short bursts of atrial fibrillation, alternating with bouts of bradycardia when the atrial fibrillation converts into a significant sinus bradycardia while SSS often includes atrial fibrillation.

When a rhythmic mechanism malfunction naturally often go too fast and too slow; it can be compare to a car engine that whine too fast and suddenly going too slow. In nature, the diseased conduction cells speeds up and slows down on their own. The difficulty in treatment of SSS is that the modality for tachycardia that slows the heart down also makes the bradycardic episodes more severe and symptomatic. Thus, the rapid heart rates can be treated with beta blockers, and often, a pacemaker is placed to counteract the bradycardia.

In fact, SSS is one of the most common uses of a pacemaker, which should be reserved after exhaustive trials with medications. Sometimes, as the last resort, ablation is used to treat the tachycardia and sometimes with a pacemaker implant in the case of atrial fibrillation where the ablation basically cuts the AVN connection to the bottom of the heart so that the top can beat fast and not affect the pulse. The pacemaker is then placed to treat the resultant heart block and bradycardia. In this scenario, as of 2014, the doctor will use a more advance pacemaker called a biventricular pacemaker (BiV) or a cardiac resynchronization device (CRT).

As we have previously discussed, the CRT device paces the LV as well as the RV. A CRT device is pacemaker where a third lead is actually placed over the LV, utilizing the coronary sinus to access to the outside of the left ventricle for pacing of the left ventricle as well as the right atrial and right ventricular leads. Both can take the forms of a biventricular (BiV) pacemaker or a BiV defibrillator. In a standard dual-lead pacemaker, the leads are in the right atrium and the RV. In this arrangement, the RV may pace before the LV, which is opposite from the natural scenario where the LV and the RV almost beat simultaneously. Some people with a dual-chamber pacemaker develop fatigue as a symptom of this "dysyncrony" called the "pacemaker syndrome" where the CRT device can be a solution.

Paroxysmal Supraventricular Tachycardia (PSVT):

Often, these syndromes are associated with rapid heart rates that originate in the left or right atria and are composed of a multitude of specific syndromes. These include atrial fibrillation (AF), atrial tachycardia (AT), atrial flutter (AFL), AV nodal reentrant tachycardia (AVNRT), and tachycardia associated with the Wolff Parkinson White Syndrome (WPW).

This group of arrhythmias is very important to understand as they are very common in the general population. There are an estimated 2.2 million people in the United States with atrial fibrillation at an average age of 75. First, atrial fibrillation is the most common arrhythmia in man and accounts for a major portion of arrhythmia hospitalizations in America. It is basically a very rapid and irregular beating of the atrium up to 300 times/minute, which enter the AV node where it's slowed but can lead the ventricles pumping ineffectually and irregularly at rates up to 200 beats/minute.

The prevalence of atrial fibrillation is related to age. Anticoagulation with Coumadin or some newer novel blood thinning agents are highly effective in the prevention of strokes in patients with an AF. In the older population, 80 years and older, there's a high incidence of bleeding especially when the patient is having difficulty managing the drug and checking the INR (blood test measurement of blood thinning). The newer novel drugs such as dabigatran and rivaroxaban don't require the regular checking of the INR but can be remarkably expensive. These newer drugs have on major drawback which is not the case with Coumadin- the subsequent lack of an antidote in the prevalence of unexpected bleeding.

The prevalence of AF in the population of patients 40-50 years of age is only 2.5% while up to 15%-20% of all individuals aged 70 and older may suffer bouts of AF. It's a truly astounding number, and the causes of AF are multiple. The increase of incidence of AF in the elderly population obviously suggests that one of the most common causes is simply the changes in the heart conduction system. It's a result of the natural aging process, the inevitable fibrosis of the conduction system, and the resultant malfunction with deterioration to AF.

However, there are many associated triggers to atrial fibrillation that can be a chronic basis and lead to the atrial fibrillation becoming the permanent heart rhythm. The atrial fibrillation leads to a multitude of symptoms such as palpitations, fatigue, shortness of breath, and even the development of congestive heart failure (CHF). These triggering conditions included high blood pressure, coronary artery disease, valvular heart disease, smoking, cocaine usage, acute and chronic alcohol ingestion, obesity, electrolyte abnormalities lung disease, certain prescription drugs, hereditary forms, pericarditis (inflammation of the cardiac sac), hyperthyroidism, and viruses that infect the heart causing chronic weakness of the heart called a cardiomyopathy. Sometimes, AF seems to occur without a trigger and is short lived. This is called lone AF that's seen in the younger population and seems to just go away, but it's possibly associated with later recurrence with aging and some risk factors.

I mentioned obesity as a possible cause of atrial fibrillation. This association has been known for a long period of time, but the exact cause and effect has only recently been ascertained. It's my opinion that obstructive sleep apnea (OSA) is possibly one of the most common causes of atrial fibrillation, which frequently goes unrecognized and untreated. It appears that with the nighttime lack of oxygen to the body when one stops breathing, the apnea and low oxygen can lead to fibrosis and damage to the conduction system of the atrium. Also, the atrium can become stretched from the pressures that develop in the heart when one stops breathing. Because obesity is an epidemic in America, OSA is increasing and seen in a younger and younger population. It may be the primary cause of "lone" atrial fibrillation in the younger population or after alcohol ingestion.

The key here is that this can be cured by weight loss or the use of continuous positive airway pressure machines (CPAP) at night. Sadly, most doctors ignore obesity and proceed with complex medications, and at the worst, profit making radiofrequency ablation. It's my strong feeling that if one is obese, especially morbidly obese over 300 pounds, then it's dangerous to suggest surgical procedures that can be associated with multiple life-threatening complications. Of course, when the patient expects immediate results, it would be too much to demand that the patient just loses weight. So, the doctor would choose more rapid and dangerous treatments, which may have short-term effects but do absolutely nothing for the long-term health or survival of the patient.

These types of patients will persist in their habits of eating that will shorten their lives, place an amazing burden of their finances, and add the costs to the medical system. If the doctor insists on the patient doing the right thing, the patient often will find another doctor who will do what he wants. It's only the strong input from the knowledgeable family and possibly from a good psychiatric evaluation that one can take correct care in diseases and addictions that lead to atrial fibrillation. Overeating, aversion to exercise, alcohol, smoking, and drugs must be avoided.

The surest way to detect atrial fibrillation is with and EKG (Fig.80). If the EKG shows atrial fibrillation, your doctor may order further tests such as an echocardiogram to look for valvular heart disease or evidence of a weakening of the ventricles with enlargement of the atrium. If your nuclear treadmill is abnormal, he may recommend a diagnostic catheterization of your heart to look for significant coronary artery disease. Additionally, the doctor may recommend that he attempts to shock the atrium back to normal with electrical cardioversion, which is a simple procedure done at the hospital as an outpatient and takes only a few hours. If the atrial fibrillation returns or becomes persistent, he may recommend certain antiarrhythmic medication to either slow the ventricular rate (rate control) or keep your hear in sinus rhythm (rhythm control).

There is significant debate in the literature about which modality of these two to employ in the patient as there's a definite shortening of life if one remains in atrial fibrillation with simple control of the rate. The drugs that are used for rate control include beta blockers and can includes digoxin; however, recent studies have shown that digoxin used for rate control in AF can actually lead to an increase in cardiovascular causes of death. As of 2014, its use should be discouraged for AF rate control although it had been utilized as an herbal remedy since almost the beginning of medicine.

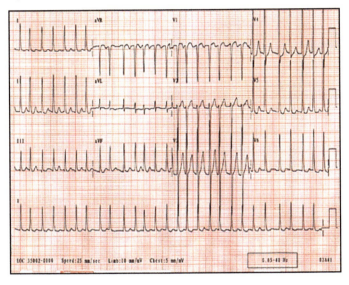

(Fig.80) (www.emedicinehealth.com) This is a 12-lead EKG of rapid atrial fibrillation. Note that the QRS complexes are close together, signifying a very rapid heart rate, which in this EKG approached 200 beats/minute. Note the spacing between the complexes is irregular, and there's absolutely no organization in the chaotic rhythm of the heart. There are some physicians who have used the analogy that atrial fibrillation is actually mathematically chaotic and signifies marked dysfunction of the atrial conduction system. Lastly, note that there's no P wave as the atrium is fibrillating like a bag flopping in wind and just undulating with minimal contractions.

Other medications that can be utilized for rate control include verapamil (Calan) or diltiazem (Cardizem). If you visit the ER with atrial fibrillation, your doctor or the ER physician will most likely start you on an intravenous (IV) drip of Cardizem. If this is your first episode, the Cardizem can help in the conversion back to normal rhythm. If unsuccessful, the doctor may start you on a new medicine for rhythm conversion or suggest electrical cardioversion. The important things to know is there are multiple options and to have your doctor communicate to you and your family his contemplated options for your treatment.

The biggest problem at this time is there are various new procedures for the possible "cure" of atrial fibrillation and further possible need for anticoagulation agents. As it's your first episode, the doctor may or may not admit you to the hospital to evaluate the status of your heart with an echocardiogram or treadmill and to establish a precise history of your lifestyle that can contribute to avoiding atrial fibrillation. If the primary disease or habit that is causing the atrial fibrillation is found, then hopefully, the atrial fibrillation can be cured. If not, the adage is that "atrial fibrillation begets atrial fibrillation." Should the atrial fibrillation recur and become permanent, then one's lifestyle and survival is permanently and negatively affected.

Some patients with atrial fibrillation have their arrhythmia discovered by the doctor on a routine physical exam without any previous symptoms except maybe some minor palpitations. There are a large amount of patients with AF who have unbearable symptoms such as palpitation, fatigue, malaise, and often the inability to sleep with the oppressive sensation of an irregular heartbeat. No one knows why there's this large range of symptomatic spectrum, but there's no doubt that many patients simply need an aggressive attempt at rhythm control rather than rate control as they're intolerant to the AF.

Before elaborating on blood thinners for atrial fibrillation, I'd like to mention depression briefly. When I listed off the symptoms of atrial fibrillation, I added malaise with fatigue and the inability to sleep or concentrate, which are very prominent in atrial fibrillation and significant symptoms of and depression. The patient is literally "heart sick." I strongly feel that these symptoms, as has been demonstrated in various studies, are also the signs of profound depression. Depression is often unrecognized by the doctor in those cardiac diseases, which are relentless in their symptoms and can lead to severe depression with a further worsening of the disease. This has been shown to be factual in patients with congestive heart failure, constant shortness of breath, and those who survived a heart attack or have undergone coronary bypass surgery.

There are visionary cardiologists who have suggested placing these patients on an SSRI or newer atypical antidepressant drug, which can actually help in the healing process. Some heart surgeons in this country who will do a psychological profile in patients before coronary bypass. If the patient is profoundly depressed, they don't undergo surgery. The real problem is that if the disease cannot be reversed and the depression only increases, the quality of life diminishes. This will eventually require psychopharmacology and psychotherapy as the patient sinks into profound depression and loses any joy in life. It can be tragic for the patient and family and requires intense treatment for the primary cardiac disease as well as well as facing the inevitable emotional toll leading to depression or even suicide. It's critical for the patient and family to understand these complex psychodynamics in severely symptomatic atrial fibrillation and not to forego the psychological aspects in the medical management.

The next critical step in the care for the patient with atrial fibrillation is using blood thinners to prevent a blood clot that can form in the atrium while not beating but quivering with a blood clot forming and breaking off and with a blood clot (embolism) going up the carotids to the brain and causing a stroke. This has been a very controversial issue and a very complicated decision for many years. The mainstay of anticoagulation for atrial fibrillation has been warfarin (Coumadin) that affects the clotting factors produced by the liver. The degree of blood thinning by Coumadin is measured by a test call an INR and should be between 1.8 and 2.3. This test requires a quick visit to a local laboratory or to your doctor's office must done on a regular basis. Test results can be expedited as fast as within minutes.

In actuality, Coumadin can be a relatively safe drug, but the reported side effects are inevitably related to the INR getting too high and causing bleeding. These can be minimized by regular testing of the INR, but the problem is the patient not complying with the tests or inadvertently taking too much Coumadin, resulting in overly thin blood and bleeding that can be in the brain. It's often the elderly who inadvertently takes inappropriate dose of the drug. This is a major cause of ER admission for over anticoagulation and minor or major bleeding and requires the need for Vitamin K as an antidote to counter the Coumadin effects on the liver.

There are several newer alternative agents that can substitute for Coumadin in atrial fibrillation that is not related to valvular disease. These include dabigatran or rivaroxaban, which can be taken and don't require the regular checking of the INR. Additionally, these agents take only 3-4 hours to take effect versus up to 2-3 days needed for INR to be therapeutic with Coumadin. Because there's no antidote for drugs' side effects, and in the case of spontaneous bleeding, one must wait up to 12 hours for much of the blood thinning to lose effect. However, the fast speed of the onset of blood thinning, especially if you're in the hospital, can lead to expedited discharge versus waiting for the effects of Coumadin. It can then lead to Medicare having the potential to deem it as a delay in service because alternative quicker agents are available.

In this scenario, the patient is placed at financial liability by Medicare converting a possible IP service to as OP even though you were in the hospital for more than two midnights. Furthermore, most of the large cardiology organized groups have published guidelines that the possible one week delay in full anticoagulation with Coumadin is a statistically safe option in atrial fibrillation. Most electrophysiologists and cardiologists don't of this or ignore these new guidelines, so it's up to the patient or the family to demand outpatient out of the hospital establishment of Coumadin therapy.

Even though you have atrial fibrillation, it doesn't always mean the doctor will place you on a blood thinner. If this was the first episode of atrial fibrillation with no structural damage to the heart on echocardiography, the cardiologist may not elect anticoagulation. Over the past few years, numerous formulas such as the CHADS score (Fig.81) have been developed. Based on your age, structural disease, hypertension, vascular disease, and congestive heart failure, there's a derived probability of a stroke and the concomitant need for prophylactic anticoagulation. If you're a male less than 65 with no heart failure or hypertension and remain in atrial fibrillation, the CHADS score would be 0-1, and the probability of a stroke would be low. However, if you are a female over 75 with heart failure and hypertension, then your CHADS score would be 4, and there would be the need for anticoagulation.

	Condition	Points
C	Congestive heart failure	1
H	Hypertension (or treated hypertension)	1
A	Age >75 years	1
D	Diabetes	1
S	Prior stroke or transient ischaemic attack	2

(Fig.81) (bjcardio.co.uk) This is a table of the conditions that compromise the CHADS score and the associated points. A number of 0 or 1 suggests that there is no need for anticoagulation if you have atrial fibrillation; a number of 2 or above confers the need for the use of anticoagulants as part of your care.

Anyone with atrial fibrillation must know their CHADS score. The CHADS score can change as conditions change, and this may convert you to a higher or lower number, changing the need for anticoagulation. If you move, change doctors, or end up in the hospital, it would be very helpful if you were able to relay your CHADS score along with your past medical history that was used to create the CHADS score. Over the past few years, there have been attempts to add to the CHADS score to make a prediction of stroke risk, but at this time, the basic CHADS score and the concept behind its creation are sufficient for your information.

Next, there are several types of medications that can be utilized for rhythm control of atrial fibrillation. These are fairly complicated as the usage and the dosage have a lot of variability. Their overall efficacy in maintaining sinus rhythm varies. If you have early or new atrial fibrillation and are controlled and maintained in sinus rhythm on one of the drugs, there's a chance that there will be no recurrence of atrial fibrillation. This is especially true when there's no structural heart disease, and you never develop significant coronary artery disease. As you reach age of 75 or older, the heart and the atrium go through a natural stage of aging, and the occurrence (prevalence) of atrial fibrillation in the age group of 75-85 can reach actually 20%.

Others can be tried as well as cardioversion when the medication stops working, but some patients may be left with rate control and anticoagulation.

The older of the drugs utilized included Quinidine and Procainamide. They were used for many years with limited efficacy, but they were all that were available. In recent years, Quinidine has been show to actually have negative effects on your lifespan and is no longer utilized. On the other hand, Procainamide does have some use and can be an excellent first line drug tried for rhythm control. In same light, Digoxin had efficacy in rate control and in rhythm control especially in combination with other drugs. But Digoxin has been shown to have a negative effect on survival and was recommended against being used in most cases as of 2014.

The advent of amiodarone (Cordarone) was simply a revolution in the rhythm control of atrial fibrillation. At first, it was a very controversial drug and was only available in Europe. American electrophysiologists had to get import licenses to obtain the drug as it was not approved by the FDA. Amiodarone was simply a miracle drug in maintaining normal sinus rhythm in atrial fibrillation and atrial flutter. When I was in practice, I obtained the license for amiodarone to use it in most of my patients with atrial fibrillation. In almost 80% of the patients with atrial fibrillation at all stages of the disease, amiodarone was able to maintain them in normal sinus rhythm. This is a truly remarkable number for a drug, and as I've said, electrophysiologists who read the literature were aware of its miracle properties.

Alas, there were also very unusual side effects of the medicine including sun sensitivity that could turn a face into a blue like mask. This could be minimized with the use of sun screen, but at that time, most people didn't even know about the presence of sunscreen. Another complication was the development of corneal deposits that didn't interfere with vision but could be of a surprise to an ophthalmologist looking into your eyes. Nevertheless, amiodarone became widely utilized and is still employed in much lower doses than previously prescribed as it has alleviated many of the untoward side effects. There are some who have forsaken amiodarone for newer agents, but this a mistake since there's no question that amiodarone remains a mainstay treatment for atrial fibrillation.

Amiodarone still remains a primary therapy, but there's another drug called dronederone (Multaq) with similar efficacy when used correctly and is without the side effects of amiodarone.

I was involved in the early FDA controlled studies with this drug, and over 20 years, it's been shown be effective in the control of many arrhythmias when used correctly in specific circumstances. Interestingly, when taking this drug, one should not eat grapefruit or grapefruit juice as it interferes with the drug metabolism and can lead to overdose.

Additionally, as with most of the drugs in this group, therapy should not be contemplated if there is the presence of severe heart failure. This doesn't apply to amiodarone but does in the case of dronederone. The difficulty lies in the definition of "severe" heart failure and the ejection fraction cutoff. In this scenario, the decision to use dronederone as well as other drugs with the same precaution must be left up to the cardiologist. As far as I'm concerned, every patient should have an electrophysiologist who will add to these critical decisions; it's prudent and wise to consult and rely on the opinion of a board certified electrophysiologist in the management of the arrhythmia.

The newer drugs to have shown efficacy in the control of atrial fibrillation include Sotalol (Betapace), flecainide (Tambacor), dofetilide (Tikosyn), and propafenone (Rhythmol). There are some newer agents that specifically target atrial fibrillation on the horizon, but these drugs are the mainstay of modern therapy. Betapace and Tikosyn must be initiated in an inpatient admission of more than 2 midnights as they take at least 48 hours to take full effect and initially can immediately cause life-threatening arrhythmias (proarrhythmia). If it doesn't occur, they're very effective in up to 60% of atrial fibrillation especially when the atrial fibrillation is new or in a young individual with no structural heart disease and normal left atrial size on an echocardiogram.

Before we end this discussion I would like to comment on a recent development in the care of patients with atrial fibrillation. It's the initiation of the "multidisciplinary approach" to atrial fibrillation care. One recent study called the "SAFETY" study (Lancet 12/01/2014) was designed to measure the short-term survival in patients having had atrial fibrillation but now converted to sinus rhythm and living out of the hospital. I feel that many studies initiated to support Obamacare and the switch to corporate medicine have good intentions, but they're basically a bunch of unscientifically designed malarkey. They promote the "multidisciplinary" approaches to atrial fibrillation care, which means that your care is by nurses and paramedical personnel. It frees up the doctor to work in the office with new patients and spend time in the catheterization laboratory doing expensive and profitable procedure to increase the financial bottom line at the expense of the patient. Furthermore, this lets all the paramedical personnel to bill for patient care and profit for the institution, whereas before, the patient was only billed for doctor to patient interaction.

RADIOFREQUENCY ABLATION

In any discussion of atrial fibrillation as well as many arrhythmias such as supraventricular tachycardia, PVCs, and ventricular tachycardia, radiofrequency ablation (RFA), it's of essential importance having become an indispensable therapeutic modality in the treatment of these arrhythmias over the past 20 years. This is the subject most close to my heart as this was the primary part of my practice of electrophysiology.

The first catheter ablation was performed by Dr. Melvin Scheinman in 1981 to case AV block in rapid atrial fibrillation. He did this by using a shock from a form of a defibrillator through a catheter placed next to the AV node and the His bundle.

Radiofrequency (RF) energy, a low voltage form of electrical energy utilized by surgeons for bleeding, quickly supplanted the method of intracardiac shock as the energy source for AV nodal ablation and all forms of arrhythmias until this time. The relative safety of this energy source contributed to the widespread adoption of RF ablation for many arrhythmias. This method of treatment was all based on the initial demonstration of Scherlag in identifying structures in the heart by their specific recording in the age where RF ablation was the basis for many of the techniques of selective ablation of structures within the heart.

A major advance and one of the milestones of electrophysiology was that of Dr. Warren "Sonny" Jackman, who worked with Dr. Ben

Scherlag at the University of Oklahoma. At first, the work of Jackman was met with much skepticism because it was very tedious and complex that required a great amount of teaching and study. This is a frequent situation in medicine as the physician often wants the quick and easier way out when it comes to newer and challenging techniques. Nevertheless, many electrophysiologists in this country chose to study with Jackman, and it became obvious that these techniques led to the highest success rates with less complications.

He first developed a technique for ablation of AV nodal reentry and the Wolff Parkinson White, syndrome which was effective in up to 98% of the patients when utilized by electrophysiologist with proper training. In addition, his technique led to a significantly lower occurrence of heart block that required a pacemaker as a complication of the procedure and also allowed for much lower energy levels with less tissue damage. This was called the "slow pathway (SP)" ablation and " action potential (AP) ablation". If you're a patient who has AV nodal reentry or the Wolff Parkinson White syndrome (WPW), RF ablation is the treatment of choice after failure of one or two drugs to control the arrhythmia. Plus, you must make sure that you have an electrophysiologist who is trained in the SP or AP ablation technique and has a good track record for success without complications.

The hospitals are not obligated to be transparent in your care regarding the track record of the doctor for ablation, or for that matter, any medical procedure except perhaps bypass surgery. It's your right to obtain these records to know the complication rate tracked by most institutions at the least. If the institution refuses this information, it may be wise to seek a second opinion at a major hospital or university that assure some measure of transparency and success rates for your procedure. For that matter, if I were to have an ablation, I'd try the Internet to find the institution with the highest volume of cases, the qualifications, and patient ratings for the electrophysiologist. If you're to use an electrophysiologist, all of the websites list whether they are board certified, which is absolutely essential.

Again, if your procedure isn't urgent as most ablations aren't, then do your research before you chose the right electrophysiologist and hospital or university for you procedure. There's absolutely no reason you can't seek the care of a local cardiologist or electrophysiologist after you have had an ablation or a cardiac catheterization at a specialized institution and subsequently return to the local physician for your ongoing care. A lot of patients feels uncomfortable with this situation, but I assure you, it will guarantee you the highest success with the fewest complications with the possibly reluctant but inevitable acceptance by your local physician.

INDICATIONS FOR RADIOFREQUENCY ABLATION

There are many indications for radiofrequency ablation for various cardiac arrhythmias. The important idea is that usually ablation is a secondary indication for treatment. It's to be utilized after there's an attempt to control the arrhythmia with a primary means, which is usually medications. I'll go through each of these indications and when they should be utilized.

In general, ablation is a complex procedure, and in most cases, it can qualify for an inpatient stay in the hospital. Most of the procedures can qualify for Medicare Part A reimbursement at a far lower cost to the patient than if the procedure were admitted as an outpatient or Part B procedure. As of 2014, most electrophysiologists are aware of this fact but fail to "certify" a two-midnight stay for some reason. The patient and the family must discuss with the interventional electrophysiologist and demand that he properly admits you as an inpatient according to the Medicare rules. In his chart, he must declare that there's a compelling reason based on the complexity of the procedure that could result in your staying for two midnights.

This "certification" doesn't obligate the doctor to keep you over two days; it's just stating this is a distinct possibility. There are Medicare sites (just google Medicare Inpatient procedures) that list all the Medicare procedures that they consider an inpatient. Furthermore, if you google (inpatient ablations) you'll find discussions of the qualifications for most of the ablations to be done as inpatient services. There is no doubt that a major portion of the physician population of this country fails to document this "certification," but it's absolutely essential that the patient and the family do their due diligence to be admitted under correct status as inpatient instead of outpatient. Although the Medicare sites take a PhD to decipher, all this information can be derived on the Internet or from this book.

After your ablation, it's not inappropriate that the doctor discharges you after a one overnight stay as this doesn't negate his initial certification for an expected inpatient two-midnight status. Medicare in its Internet sites calls this "early recovery," and it's unequivocally appropriate that your status remains inpatient. For some unknown reason to me, some electrophysiologist and cardiologist find it some kind of perverse "red badge of courage" to discharge you after an ablation for atrial fibrillation without even an overnight hospitalization.

As far as I'm concerned, this is simply malpractice and based on the narcissism of the doctor, which clouds his best judgment and opens the patient up to a multitude of risks. Thus, I strongly advise that the patient insists on at least one overnight stay for ablations, and any complex cardiological procedure that may be contrary to the intent of the doctor but should be firmly insisted.

I've consistently mentioned radiofrequency as the energy source of choice for the ablation. There are also newer energy modalities that have been developed such as the use of extreme cold (cryoablation) or laser energy for the destruction of the target tissue. In my mind, the use of radiofrequency energy is the tried and true way to have your ablation, and although cryoablation is advertised to have fewer complications, it's probably not as effective and has a lower success rate. Thus, I'd strongly advise you to avoid cryoablation or laser ablation.

There are many indications for ablation as an attempt to actually cure your arrhythmia. Contrary to medication that only controls the heart rhythm abnormality, ablation is an attempt to actually cure the arrhythmia so that you no longer have symptoms and the need to be on medications. Of course, like all procedures that involve placing a catheter in the body or using energy to actually burn the culprit area, the procedure in not without complications and a chance of death. In almost all circumstances with an arrhythmia, ablation should only be used as the second line treatment. There are exceptions, which I will mention later, but this guideline will serve you well as a general rule.

I will now list the basic clinical conditions for ablation and try to go through each individually. Keep in mind that there may be more indications as the technique evolves, but I will try to be complete and give you some hints to the future:

1. Atrial fibrillation
2. Atrial flutter
3. AV nodal ablation for atrial fibrillation
4. Paroxysmal supraventricular tachycardia
a. AV nodal reentry
b. Left and right atrial tachycardia
c. Wolff Parkinson White syndrome-in all its forms including Long Ganong Levine syndrome
d. Sick Sinus syndrome with multiple areas of atrial tachycardia-multifocal atrial tachycardia
e. Junctional tachycardia
f. Symptomatic sinus tachycardia
g. Symptomatic extra beats (ectopic) in the atrium of the AV junction area
5. Ventricular tachycardia-many of these ablations are utilized in association or an adjunct (addition) to an ICD implant
a. RV and LV outflow tract ventricular tachycardia
b. RV dysplasia with ventricular tachycardia
c. Idiopathic catecholiminergic ventricular tachycardia
d. Substrate based ventricular tachycardia associated with a previous myocardial infarction and a scar
e. Mitral and aortic valve idiopathic ventricular tachycardia
6. Ventricular Fibrillation (Trigger ablations)

COMPLICATIONS OF ABLATION

There are many complications of ablation, but overall the rate is less than 1%. This may vary from one electrophysiologist to another and based on the experience of the physician. It's okay to ask the doctor how long he has been doing ablations, how many he has done, and his complication rate with. In general, you'd want an electrophysiologist who has done more than 100 cases and has at least two years' experience with a low complication rate. One resource for the complication rate may be the hospital; however, this may be hard to obtain due to the reluctance of the hospital even though they do keep these records by law. There are some websites that attempt to list the doctor by the procedures he does (Heathgrades.com) without the list of the complication rate. Again, you may simply ask the doctor and get an answer.

Those that involve the left atrium such as atrial fibrillation ablation or the LV such as a ventricular tachycardia that originates in the left ventricle are the most complex ablation procedures. One important complication if the procedure involves the left side of the heart has a blood clot that can form in the chamber or on the ablation catheter itself and travel up the carotids to the brain with a resulting stroke. The risk of a clinical stroke may be less than 1% in atrial fibrillation ablations, but in studies that look at the incidence of a small subclinical (not obvious) strokes utilizing MRI, it may be up to 41%. (Journal of Cardiovascular Electrophysiology 2013 Jan; 24 (1) 14-21 Haeuslerj et al.) This is a very concerning number and may result in lessening of one's mental acuity in the long run. It should be taken into consideration if such an ablation is contemplated in an already mentally compromised patient.

Another important complication of atrial fibrillation includes bleeding into the sack around the heart, which is called a pericardial effusion. This can occur at multiple stages of the ablation, especially at the step that involves crossing of the atrium from the right to the left atrium in a procedure called a transeptal puncture. This can be a fairly dangerous part of the ablation procedure and demands an experienced doctor without question. It took me many months to learn this technique, and frankly, I was uncomfortable every time I did a transeptal puncture.

Needless to say, I'd specifically have your electrophysiologist spell out the possible consequences of this complication and how he would handle it. As well as a possible stroke, this would qualify the procedure as an inpatient hospitalization and incur Medicare A payment. If you have a pericardial effusion or stroke as a complication of the atrial fibrillation ablation, the doctor must be compelled to switch your order to inpatient especially if he hasn't signed the two-midnight certification.

The last serious complication of the procedure that I wish to discuss is the creation of a fistula or a communication between the esophagus and the left atrium. This is a longer-term side effect and usually wouldn't occur on your initial admission for the procedure. It's not a common complication but is often a fatal. When one starts out with bleeding from the mouth, then it requires immediate hospitalization and open heart surgery. The reason for this complication is that the esophagus lies right behind the left atrium and can possibly heat up during the procedure leading to its damage and late rupture. If not a rupture, a minor esophageal damage can result in chest pain post procedure and can be investigated by the electrophysiologist. This is a reason to convert the procedure to an inpatient hospitalization. In this circumstance, it's completely within your rights to query the physician and make sure that he converts the order to inpatient.

I'd like to end this section by reemphasizing this concept of inpatient versus outpatient for any of the ablations. If you google to find radiofrequency ablation and outpatient versus inpatient, you'll get a bunch of sites associated with the government (CMS-Center for Medicare and Medicaid) that approach this subject in usually an unintelligible way. As I've said, it's only with the knowledge of this book that you can make some headway into understanding these discussions. The bottom line is that Medicare does have a list of inpatient only list of procedure that is easily retrieved on the Internet, but ablation is not on the list. Most ablations, especially for atrial fibrillation and ventricular tachycardia, should be classified as an inpatient admission upon your hospitalization with the proper order of two-midnight certification—even if released as "early recovery."

ATRIAL FIBRILLATION ABLATION.

The most common indication use of radiofrequency ablation is in the cure of atrial fibrillation because atrial fibrillation is the most common of the arrhythmias. The technique of radiofrequency ablation for atrial fibrillation is rather new, and the indications and technique are still going through their outcome-based studies, which document its safety and efficacy. The basic, and often skirted, guideline is that the ablation be reserved for atrial fibrillation that has failed at least therapy with two rhythm-control medications. This isn't an absolute rule but should be followed in general. As of late and as the technique of ablation has improved, there are some patients with atrial fibrillation who are extremely symptomatic with the arrhythmia and a marked decline in their lifestyle. In these patients, the ablation can actually considered as a first line therapy.

Since the ablation works the best as a cure for atrial fibrillation, the use of atrial fibrillation ablation can be considered if the patient is less than 50 years old and has failed at least one drug trial. I must stress, although this is not adhered to by many electrophysiologist, atrial fibrillation ablation should never by utilized in a patient over the age of 80. This incidence of side effects in these patients approaches 20%, and the risk of stroke or cardiac perforation with a pericardial effusion is simply too high and can be immediately life threatening. Plus, the complication of small strokes in these patients threatens their cognitive abilities.

The history of ablation for atrial fibrillation is rather fascinating. The real breakthrough came in 1998 at a meeting of HRS when Michelle Haissaguerre, an electrophysiologist in Bordeaux, France, first described the use of catheter ablation for patients with atrial fibrillation. Believe me this caused a great stir from the electrophysiologists at that meeting as it was well known that atrial fibrillation was remarkably common and very difficult to treat with medications. Basically, he put catheters in the left and right atrium and mapped the "triggers" that he felt started atrial fibrillation and ultimately found that the triggers perpetuated the persistence of the arrhythmia. He found that in 96% of the time these triggers originated in the pulmonary veins as they led into the left atrium draining the blood from the lungs leading into the left ventricle and to the body (Fig.77).

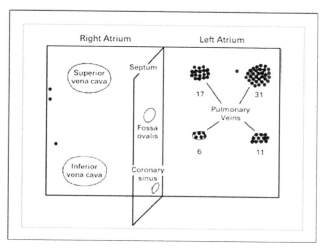

(Fig.77) This is a picture from the first article from Haissaguerre et al. (New England Journal of Medicine 1998). It shows that 96% of the triggers for atrial fibrillation come from the sleeves of the four pulmonary veins that enter the left atrium: left upper, left lower, right upper, and right lower pulmonary veins. This was an absolutely landmark finding and remains one of the great discoveries of modern medicine.

Haissaguerre had his catheter in the left atrium from the right atrium by perforating the septum that separates the two in a transeptal puncture. This technique was very precise and difficult, so it led to many of the electrophysiologist learning the technique while causing many of the early complications during the ablation procedure. The interventional cardiologists had been using the technique for years as they studied the mitral valve and complex congenital heart disease. These interventionalists were enlisted to teach the electrophysiologists in their hospital or in classes at the HRS meetings.

These pioneers utilized fluoroscopy guidance to place the transeptal puncture catheters, and this technique was very effective in experienced hands. Luckily, this technique has been refined in recent years by the introduction of intracardiac echocardiogram instruments that allows the visualization of the atrial septum and makes the procedure far easier and safer. I had a beautiful model of the heart made out of clear plexiglass that allowed me to visualize the position of the catheters for transeptal puncture in three dimensions and correlate them to the x-ray visualization. I spent countless hours at classes on the classical technique, and by the time intracardiac echo became available, I was an expert at the initial radiological guidance procedure as the echo just made it a little easier. Nevertheless, the experience at the original technique served me well over the years, and I had very little complications from transeptal puncture.

By mapping of these pulmonary vein triggers, they're subsequently ablated and eradicated so not to initiate atrial fibrillation. As a result, the heart would remain in normal sinus rhythm as the triggers were no longer available to jump-start the atrial fibrillation. Special catheters that were rounded like a Lasso, with multiple electrodes, were placed into the pulmonary veins and facilitated the tedious chore or multiple simultaneous recordings of these often fleeting pulmonary vein triggers.

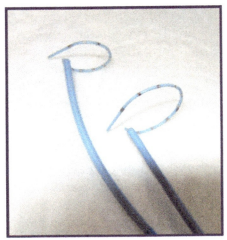

(Fig.78) This is a picture of a circular catheter that is introduced through a sheath in the atrial septum in the four pulmonary veins in the hopes of recording trigger. A drug is given intravenously to try to stimulate these triggers, and once the patient goes into atrial fibrillation and is subsequently cardioverted back no normal rhythm, these triggers are ablated and validated by repeat drug testing that they were gone. Obviously, this painstaking and long process would often take 8-12 hours and had quite a bit of radiation exposure from the x-ray machine.

Thus, ablation of atrial fibrillation initially was aimed at eradicating these triggers and sending the patient home in normal sinus rhythm. The problem was that a good percent of the patients would either go back into atrial fibrillation that night in the hospital with up to 1/3 of the patients within 12 months. Only 13% would remain free of atrial fibrillation, and most of these remained on drugs and blood thinners. This procedure was minimally effective and exposed the patient to very high amounts of x-ray radiation. At this juncture, the amount of indications for overall ablation suddenly took on a large leap forward with atrial fibrillation ablations and were very lucrative for the electrophysiologists. So many of them dove into this procedure head first although it had limited efficacy; however, it did herald much more effective procedures to come for atrial fibrillation.

I'd like to add more discussions of the technique for atrial fibrillation ablation. The Medicare coverage for atrial fibrillation ablation is rather nebulous as is almost everything with Medicare. It's associated with transeptal puncture for access to the left atrium, and if one takes liberties with Medicare's list of inpatient only procedures on their website, this procedure with its complication rate and complexity with time for the procedure can easily be interpreted as inpatient only. That means that the physician must certify in the beginning of your hospitalization that he has a "reasonable expectation" that your hospitalization will span 2 midnights even with "early recovery."

Under this ideal scenario, the remainder of the bill, which would usually be 20%, will be paid by your coinsurance or out of your pocket or if you don't have a coinsurance of "gap" policy. When you sign the consent, remind your doctor of his responsibility of cerification before you're admitted to the hospital as I have repeatedly reiterated in this book. You can also ask the case manager who is assigned to you case. I have found that these nurse case managers are simply angels in disguise, and they're the most useful for understanding and facilitating your proper classification during your hospitalization.

If you have a complication and have to stay in the hospital for 2 nights or more, then all the doctor has to do is make sure the inpatient order is in the chart to assure your inpatient status. The Medicare rules are very specific that the doctor must write and sign the order. Also, the Medicare guidelines are remarkably stringent in elucidating the exact documentation requirements, and as of 2014, Medicare has the right to request the doctor's office medical records to assure proper documentation of the need for inpatient as well as if the procedure is indicated in the first place!

Every doctor group known to mankind has protested what they consider draconian rules and regulations. However, Medicare has taken on a very proactive stance regarding these stringent rules, and for once, Medicare is exactly right and is basically protecting the patients' rights to a proper procedure that is actually indicated and is further appropriately documented to pass Medicare scrutiny. These doctor groups simply have their members' rights and best interests placed before that of the patients'. In that aspect, they're acting contrary to their Hippocratic Oath, the basis of their physician responsibilities.

They make obtuse and undiscernible arguments in the favor of the doctor and try to justify their behavior as in the patients' best interests. In my opinion, if one reads their reasoning, it becomes all too evident that it's a bunch of nonsense and has everything to do with the doctors' rights to do inappropriate care and documentation, exposing the doctors lack of professionalism. These groups may further justify their behavior as forced upon them by the unreal expectations. As I've said, the doctor makes most of his money by patient volume at the expense of patient care.

There are excellent physicians in the community who are competent and do the due diligence in the care of their patients. I have honestly found these are those that have gone to the proper classes on documentation for procedure indications and applicable admission status. University hospitals are usually very compulsive to assure that all the doctors attend and understand these new rules. It's the small private hospital or a corporate-run facility that constantly wants to put profit ahead of patient care with the lack of doctor education principally at fault. If I needed a complex procedure such as an atrial fibrillation ablation, I'd do my homework and go to a possible independent university hospital or a private physician that demonstrates competence and puts in my best interests first.

It's time to go back to the complexities of atrial fibrillation ablation. I'm spending so much time on this specific example as it's a basic outline of the techniques and vagaries of all ablations as well as many of the complex cardiology procedures and the rules that assure your proper care and procedure documentation.

In 1991, Haissaguerre described a new approach called Pulmonary Vein (PV) isolation. Instead of mapping the multitude of individual pulmonary vein triggers, this procedure attempted to isolate these triggers from entering the atrium from the pulmonary vein sleeve and initiating and perpetuating atrial fibrillation. It was at this time that Dr. Jackman and Scherlag proposed ablation of left atrial autonomic ganglion for the cure of atrial fibrillation. Until then, the ganglion approach had never taken on the acceptance although it's distinctly possible that pulmonary vein ablation through the ganglion approach was probably the correct procedure.

In actuality, the PV isolation procedure is most likely ablating the ganglion and may account for its apparent efficacy. Similar to the PV trigger ablation, the ganglion ablation is time consuming and highly complex, so this technique takes expertise and patience. Additionally, the PV isolation approach has more defined, although partially arbitrary, end points whereas the end result of the ganglion ablation is usually less burns in the heart and complications with possible better efficacy. There have even been newer approaches called "complex fractionated electrogram" ablations that involve making charcoal of the complete atrium, preventing the atrial fibrillation but rendering the atrium as useless sack with far less contractile efficacy and probable long-term higher incidence of atrial fibrillation or even more complex left atrial flutter arrhythmias. Unfortunately this may also be the fate of many patients with the PV isolation technique if the doctor is too vigorous in his attempts to achieve what he sees as complete isolation.

The technique of PV isolation has taken on a highly computerized aspect that is like a burn and connect multiple dots technique (Fig.78). In this technique, a computerized rendering of the atrium is generated and burns that go around each pulmonary vein are documented. This individual pulmonary vein technique was found to be associated with a complication of long term PV vein stenosis that can be difficult to impossible to treat with severe consequences. Thus, a technique called "left atrial antrum isolation" or wide area circumferential ablation (WACA) was pursued. This is the technique of choice as of 2014, but it has introduced another dire complication of severe damage to the esophagus and life-threatening esophageal rupture.

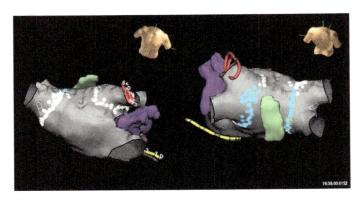

(Fig.78) This is a picture of two views of a computerized rendering of the left atrium and in yellow the ablation catheter. The white and blue dots are the areas of ablation for the electrical isolation of the pulmonary veins in the WACA technique. There is also a way to validate the complete isolation that is done with intracardiac recordings and is an essential part of the technique. This electrical validation can also be used in a second procedure if the isolation is incomplete and has "gaps" in the blocking line of ablations. The green is rendering of the position of the esophagus, and as you can see, the dots try to avoid any burn over the esophagus. Lastly, the red is a rendering of the round helical or Lasso catheter we discussed in the PV vein ablation.

The PV atrial isolation technique has been accepted as the standard approach in the patient with atrial fibrillation. It has been modified to include extra burns in a patient where the atrial fibrillation is permanently present. Also, the technique has been facilitated by the development of catheters with water running through them to the catheter electrode that irrigates the tip and cools the area of ablation (Fig.80). The real problem of all these techniques is that the long-term efficacy over about 5 years has come into question. The short to medium term efficacy of over 70% is not within question, and the improved medium term lack of complications and increased efficacy over just rhythm control medications are not questioned.

However, the initial effects of the procedure may actually prove to be detrimental to left atrial function and possibly recurrent strokes in the long term. Over the years, the atrium naturally dilates, scars, and develops structural abnormalities that facilitate atrial fibrillation. In the long term (>10 years), efficacy of these procedure may not improve survival or grant freedom from atrial fibrillation. It may actually be shown to be detrimental in that it promotes not only atrial fibrillation but more complex and difficult to control left atrial arrhythmias as a result of the atrial scarring from the ablations. Only time will tell with the appropriately designed longer term follow-up clinical studies.

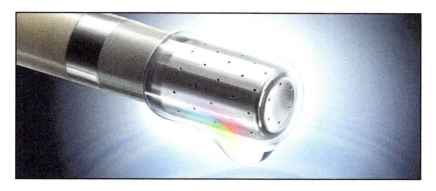

(Fig.80) (biosensewebster.com) This is a rendering of an irrigated tip ablation catheter that has small holes in electrode where water comes out and irrigates and cools the area of the ablation and has significantly improved the efficacy and safety all ablation procedures.

ABLATION FOR ATRIAL FLUTTER

The arrhythmia of atrial flutter can be very symptomatic and difficult to control with drugs. Also, a variant left atrial form of atrial flutter is a very common complication as a result ablation and can be extremely challenging to cure. This left atrial flutter technique is beyond the capability of many electrophysiologists. An additional problem is that variant and normal atrial flutter can be a trigger to the development of recurrence and production of atrial fibrillation as it leads to structural disease in the right and left atrium as well as an electrical trigger for the initiation of atrial fibrillation. The heart often goes very fast, causing severe palpitations and even heart failure. We will mainly cover the most common classical right atrial flutter.

In actuality, if the arrhythmia is not easily controlled with one medication, a right atrial flutter ablation should be considered as a quick second line or even first line primary treatment since it nearly cures 100%. The ablation technique was first demonstrated in the laboratories of Dr. Warren Jackman at the University of Oklahoma by a remarkably intelligent and talented electrophysiologist from China, Dr. Xunshang Wang. He is now at Cedars Sinai Medical Center in Los Angeles, California. Frankly, I consider him probably one of the best electrophysiologists in the world. If I needed an ablation, I most likely would travel from my home in Philadelphia to Beverly Hills for my ablation by Dr. Wang.

He was the first to actually show me the intracardiac electrograms (recordings) of what is called cavotricuspid isthmus (CTI) ablation for the common form of right atrial flutter before publication. He shared with me that this would be the ablation of choice for atrial flutter and be a 100% cure; he was right. This ablation, when properly done and verified with electrical block at the CTI, is nearly a 100% cure. Plus, it's free of most complications and doesn't require medications any longer. The real art in this ablation is doing it early enough in the disease that it doesn't eventually lead to atrial fibrillation and its concomitant consequences. In my opinion, ablation of atrial flutter can be done as an outpatient procedure with one overnight stay and does not warrant inpatient status.

ABLATION FOR VENTRICULAR TACHYCARDIA (VT)

In general, it can be said for ablation of many forms of ventricular tachycardia, that the ablation can be nearly 100% effective and verifiable by electrophysiological techniques. The techniques of ablation of idiopathic, and many hereditary forms of ventricular tachycardia can be performed with few complications and a very high rate of complete cure. In the case of ventricular tachycardia caused by a heart attack and scarring with severe weakness of the heart, ablation is done in addition to an ICD implant for safety.

These ablations can be used as a primary therapy or in addition to an ICD implant because the ventricular tachycardia is too frequent and causes a lot of ICD shocks. This is a situation called "arrhythmia storm" and consists of a lot of repetitive tachycardias with repetitive ICD shocks that can often be life threatening. Much of the work on ablation of scar associated ventricular tachycardia was pioneered by Dr. William Stevenson at the Brigham and Woman's Hospital in

Boston. He's an absolutely brilliant electrophysiologist whose work has improved the lifestyle of many patients with recurrent ventricular tachycardia and has saved countless lives.

Recurrent ventricular tachycardia develops in up to 40-60% of patients with an ICD. The incidence of VT starting from the first implant of the ICD is seen in 20% of patients within the first five years of the implantation. In many of these patients, after five years a good percent of the patients have VT episodes that are terminated by the ICD but can become frequent and interfere significantly with life style. More importantly, there is suggestion that the overall lifespan is reduced more than ten years on average in patients with frequent shocks.

Thus, the techniques of VT ablation can be important not only in the idiopathic and heredity form of VT, but most importantly, in the large population of heart attack survivors with a large scar and reduced ejection fraction with recurrent episodes of VT.

There are various technical considerations in the ablation of VT. First is whether the tachycardia can be reproducibly induced during an electrophysiological study and whether or not the VT is tolerated by the patient during the procedure without significant hypotension (low blood pressure) or deteriorating to a cardiac arrest. Most of the idiopathic forms of VT such as RV and LV outflow VT, bundle branch reentry, RV dysplasia, and Mitral annular VT can be accomplished with the patient remaining stable. This group of sustained inducible VTs with tolerable blood pressures remains the subgroup of greatest success rates and possible cure. Every one of these ablations is highly complex and can be very time consuming. Therefore, all of these VT ablations can unequivocally meet the criteria for an inpatient admission to the hospital.

These ablations involve the need to map the tachycardia for the ablation to be successful. By this, contrary to the ablation of AF and atrial flutter at a specific anatomic site, these arrhythmias can arise at various ill-defined parts of the LV or the RV. It uses the same technique as in atrial fibrillation ablations where a virtual computer map is generated of the atrium. In a similar fashion with VT ablations, the electrophysiologist generates a computer image of the LV and the RV, depending on which ventricle is the focus of the VT. This way, the area of the arrhythmia can be isolated and successfully ablated. These computer generated images have tremendously facilitated the safe and rapid ablation of many forms of VT with up to 100% success rates.

In the past, the electrophysiologist had to rely principally on the x-ray to get an idea of the arrhythmia focus. Obviously, this exposed the patient to a large amount of radiation. The problem with all these techniques is that the VT must be initiated and sustained without hemodynamic deterioration and hypotension leading to a cardiac arrest in many cases. The computerized techniques have greatly improved the safety of the technique by quickly allowing the mapping of the principal arrhythmia focus before the patient deteriorates.

The techniques of Dr. Stevenson advanced the ablation of VT associated with an old myocardial infarction and scar acting as the focus for the ventricular tachycardia. He developed a technique based on the older work of Dr. Albert Waldo in atrial flutter of "entrainment mapping" of the VT focus. This method allowed a relatively quicker and more accurate identification of the proper area to ablate in the ventricular scar and lead to a high rate of cure. Before this work, the EKG would often identify multiple areas of ventricular tachycardia and the need for multiple ablations in different locations in the ventricle. However, the work of Stevenson demonstrated that many different EKG forms of VT could all be coming from one area of the scar. With the aid of the computerized images and proper use of this technique, the VT ablation became a relatively useful and frequently used technique (Fig.81).

Furthermore, as this technique matured, it became obvious that many forms of the VTs that originated in the scar originated both from the inside of the heart or endocardium and the outside of the heart or epicardium. This led to some very novel approaches to ablation of the epicardium, which should be done only at very specialized university centers that can do these complex procedures. The use of the epicardium as well as the endocardium for ablation is a fairly new procedure, but in many of these tachycardias that are associated with a scar as a result of an old heart attack, they can only be approached for ablation with catheters in the epicardium, which is within the pericardial sack and surrounds the heart (Fig.81 and 82).

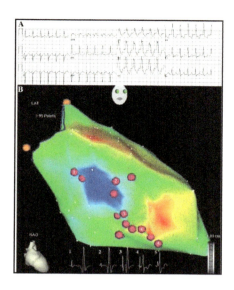

(Fig.81) (by permission of Dr. William Stevenson) This is a computer-generated image of the left ventricle and the mapping of the ventricular tachycardia. The EKG on top is that of the stable ventricular tachycardia. The red and blue representing areas of scar and tachycardia focus with the red dots representing the areas of ablation to terminate the tachycardia and hopefully afford a cure.

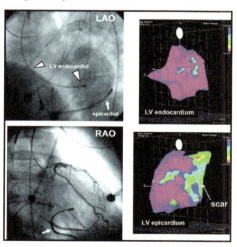

(Fig.82) This is picture (By permission of Dr. William Stevenson) is of the left catheters in the LV endocardium and epicardium. On the right is the computerized rendering of the LV endocardium and epicardium with the green scar seen on the epicardium and only minimally in the endocardium. The scarred area is the area of the ablation on the epicardium.

Before we proceed with more tachycardias, I should mention some additional complications and situations specifically with ablation within the left ventricle. First, your doctor will do a special echocardiogram called a transesophogeal echocardiogram (TEE) before the procedure, which will look for any old clots in the LV. IF these are found, then you will be placed on blood thinners before the procedure and may become a candidate for an epicardial procedure. Also, many doctors will want to admit you to the hospital the day before the ablation to do the TEE with the ablation to be done on the second day.

This extra day admission for a TEE is to be absolutely avoided as Medicare and private insurance companies will not pay for a simple procedure that could've been done either on the same day or some days before the ablation as an ambulatory outpatient procedure. If your doctor insists, then find another institution if your procedure is not emergent. The new rules of Medicare could deny the payment for the TEE and delay, or even withhold, payment to the hospital for the whole ablation procedure, which could mean immense financial liability to the patient.

Other complications and situations with any procedure done in the left ventricle is the possibility of a blood clot or emboli forming at the ablation site or on the catheter and traveling to the brain with a subsequent stroke. To avoid this, the doctor will place you on the intravenous blood thinner, heparin, to prevent these emboli during the procedure. Still, there's a small but less than 1% chance of a stroke. Other major complication, especially in scar ablation, is that there is actual perforation of the myocardium and some bleeding around the heart in the pericardial space called a pericardial effusion and possible tamponade.

ABLATION OF NON SCAR RELATED VENTRICULAR TACHCARDIAS

This category is an important subject as these ablations can have a high cure rate and are approached from the RV with basically no risk of a stroke since the outflow of the RV is into the lung and not the brain. A group of VTs in patients with a dilated cardiomyopathy but with no coronary disease is seen mainly in patients with a previous ICD implant, who have many ICD shocks for VT or even ventricular fibrillation. These idiopathic cardiomyopathies can have an area of scar, but in most instances, there's a discrete common focus without scar that can be approached accurately with the aid of computerized mapping. With the newer mapping systems, the tachycardia doesn't have to be sustained as the systems rapidly map with only a few beats of the VT, promoting a higher degree of procedure safety.

There are many of these tachycardias that can be approached in this manner for a high rate of cure. RV outflow and LV outflow tachycardia are fairly common cases of VT, and specifically in RV outflow, VT the success rate for cure is high (>95%) with fairly low complication rates. These are idiopathic tachycardias, which means that they have no known cause and occur spontaneously. They can be associated with some weakness of the heart, and they can actually lead to some additional loss of heart strength if they become very frequent.

There is a fairly common VT called bundle branch reentry, which has as a characteristic EKG appearance and a very high success ablation rate with no need for a subsequent ICD or pacemaker. It's common after a heart attack or can be idiopathic and is fairly simple to recognize and cure. There is a group of tachycardias that themselves arise in the bundle branches or in their outcropping of the bundle fascicles or the purkinje fibers themselves. Again, these can be idiopathic or associated with an old heart attack, but all are associated with a common intracardiac marker called pre-potentials that facilitate a good success rate with a relatively rapid and safe procedure.

ABLATION FOR POLYMORPHIC VT AND VENTRICULAR TACHYCARDIA

These two circumstances are relatively uncommon but present a very difficult therapeutic challenge. Most of the patients already or will soon have an ICD implant. The most common presentation is an arrhythmia "storm" where the ICD is firing repetitively and the patient is in an extremely dangerous clinical situation. This can also be a consequence of some of the hereditary forms of sudden death such as the long QT syndrome. In these syndromes, the tachycardias are unstable and immediately lead to a cardiac arrest, so mapping of the tachycardia is impossible. These ablations involve identification of a trigger area, which actually initiates the rhythm. This is a very difficult and specialized procedure that can only be done in specialized centers with electrophysiologists who have experience and are trained in these ablations.

These trigger procedures can have a high risk of failure and even death. Thus, initiation of these procedures must be associated with a full understanding of what is involved when they are contemplated. If you have arrhythmia storms often, they can be temporarily controlled with drugs as you're transported by ambulance or a helicopter to a specialized center in your state.

INSURANCE COVERAGE

Before we end this discussion of ablations, I'd like to review some of the options you have in regard to ablations as a proactive consumer of medical care. Most of these ablation procedures would qualify you for inpatient care. There may be some exception such as AV nodal ablation, atrial flutter ablations, and even some of the VT ablations such as bundle branch reentry, RV outflow VT, and fascicular tachycardia that involves the RV but not the LV. Again, it's extremely important that you discuss your options with the attending physician, who is responsible for your admission orders.

This should be an electrophysiologist although some hospitals may assign a hospitalist as your primary doctor. In this circumstance, you must firmly reject such notion of the hospitalist as your primary doctor and demand that your admitting doctor be the cardiologist or the consulting electrophysiologist. Having a hospitalist take care of this responsibility and your care is simply irresponsible and is often done as expediency for the hospital, which is not in your best interests. After your procedure, they may attempt to assign a hospitalist for your post procedure and discharge care. Again, you must reject the hospitalist simply has no expertise in recognizing complications and their subsequent management. They may even inappropriately facilitate an early discharge to lower their patient load.

For some reason, this is becoming all too common. In most of these complex procedures, two midnights in the hospital or the expectation of two midnights is completely appropriate and correct approach. The omnipotent corporate heads of many of the hospitals with their hospitalist employees and the case managers, have adopted the dictum to quickly discharge the patients to save money. Of course, these corporate hospital CEOs put their hospitals' best interests before the proper medical care. If for an untoward complication that you must remain in the hospital for more than two days, it's essential that your admission status be changed to inpatient. The hospital will be saddled with an added financial burden and bureaucracy, but armed with the knowledge of this book, you must insist on your status changed to inpatient.

Unfortunately, there is a very unfortunate cohort of electrophysiologists and cardiologists, who promote premature early discharge to the point of even considering an ablation for VT to be a same-day discharge. This behavior is simple incompetency and overtly dangerous. Somehow, it's promoted by doctors under the misdirected notion that this is a sign of his unique expertise and "manhood and prowess" but has nothing do with the patient's safety and proper care. In many of these procedures, there can be late or delayed complications such as bleeding from the groin site that cannot be properly managed if you're at home. Plus, if this complication occurs at home within the first 48 hours of discharge, your readmission to the hospital would result in additional and unnecessary billing for two related admissions.

More importantly, if the readmission is within 48 hour, it may trigger close Medicare scrutiny because of a 48-hour readmission. This could delay payment and cause very negative financial considerations to the hospital's bottom line under new Medicare rules. If improperly billed, the whole reimbursement can be delayed or potentially not reimbursed. In my experience, the hospital would rather bill improperly with the hope of not being caught than do the billing properly. This is a sad comment on the American system, but it has nothing to do with the patient's best interests.

If you consider your ablation or procedure to be complex enough to warrant a 2-midnight consideration, any notion of same day discharge must simply be rejected. If there's a suspicion of inappropriate discharge or level of service, this deserves mention to the doctor and often the case manager, who will listen more intently. In summary, it is not my aim to scare you about such procedures; I simply want to instill in you the power of knowledge that can facilitate your proper care when it is necessary.

There are some very excellent companies available to all hospitals that can determine your appropriate admission status and to deal with issues such as readmission reviews. Although these review companies are hired by the hospital, recommending the proper management of admission status and documentation ultimately is in the patient's best interests. However, Medicare in the last few years has stopped audits of hospital charts probably based on pressure from Medical lobby groups. And as usual, this lack of appropriate audit has allowed many hospitals, especially corporate hospitals, to act with impunity from any reasonable oversight. For this reason, many hospitals continue to manage admission status to their own benefit and act directly in conflict with the recent Medicare rules. This behavior only improves the bottom line on the CEO's spreadsheet for his hospital.

For many hospitals, because Medicare obviously can't audit or review the millions of patients' charts just from a monetary basis, it's simply better to do the more profitable admission status with a chance of only a few being audited. These audits can and should result in large sanctions and punitive damages for these hospitals and require them to establish oversight and utilization services many aforementioned companies offer. Luckily, as I write this book, up to 50% of the hospitals in this county use some form of this compliance review, but the doctor must cooperate for this to work, which sadly is a rare occurrence.

Before we continue I must add to what was just discussed. As of now, 50% of the specialist in this country have been bought out by the corporate medical businesses, the hospitalists have become salaried employees with benefits and performance bonuses. Bonuses are based on productivity and the money they make for the corporations. Although I'm a firm believer in free enterprise, such arrangements have no business in medicine. There are private medical specialists who are fighting the trend, but they have no ally in our present administration.

If I were to have an ablation, I'd absolutely avoid a specialist who was a corporate employee. Unlike the hospitalist, he would not be under the same edict to early hospital discharge and forced hospitalist attending admissions. Corporate-owned hospitals can charge more for almost any service under the auspices of hospital reimbursement for services versus the services done by a private independent institution or doctor. Thus, I'd avoid these corporate hospitals if at all possible unless it's the only type of institution in my area. Although the university hospitals may be corporate owned, these institutions have some assemblance of morality and the proper safeguards and admission practices in place to protect the patient. A majority of hospitals that pay for outside utilization review, must still implement the compliance recommendations, but at least, they're attempting to demonstrate the proper behavior.

CARDIAC CATHETERIZATION, HEART ATTACKS, AND BYPASS SURGERY

Now, we will do some review but with a few additional points to highlight important management issues. Like some ablations, cardiac catheterization can be a very complex procedure. There are some instances where the procedure is unequivocally an inpatient procedure in the eyes of Medicare and most private insurance companies. We have gone over the anatomy of the coronary system and placement of a stent in the left main coronary artery or high up in the left anterior descending coronary artery. Many of these complex procedures require the placement of something called an Impella devise to augment your heart if it's weak or if there is left main disease. Again, this qualifies the procedure as highly complex and dictates that the doctor certify a reasonable expectation of a two-midnight hospital stay.

As of January 1, 2015, the certification rule has been somewhat changed keeping with Medicare and CMS history of political motivation with rules that are nearly uninterruptable. Now, the doctor must certify someplace in his notes that you required inpatient care rather than directly in the initial order. Unless absolutely requested by the proactive patient, such chart documentation will rarely be provided by the doctor, and the admission level of care will be even more difficult to ascertain accurately and subject to CMS interpretation. I believe this change is definitely purposeful and designed to give CMS the ability to lower the admission status to outpatient as much as they can for them to save them money.

In this manner, they switch more financial burden to the patient although it may be contrary to the reality of the needed inpatient complexity. A change like this is utterly ridiculous and just makes it harder for the patient and the doctor to validate the proper level of care. As before, this is keeping with the precedent of deteriorating care set up by Obamacare, which is unequivocally to the detriment of the patient. Thus, the key here is for the patient to breach the discussion with the cardiologist as to your proper admission status and to utilize the knowledge learned from this book to get the proper documentation or certification accomplished in the medical record or the records in the doctor's office documentation.

With any of the catheterization procedures, you would warrant inpatient status if there is major complication. If a complication arises out of an outpatient procedure and the doctor doesn't change you to an inpatient with proper certification, and if you're discharged with only one midnight stay, you'll never be covered by Medicare A as an inpatient. Medicare guidelines that are easily accessible on the Internet under googling the two-midnight rule specifically address the presence of a major complication to convert to a more complex inpatient qualifying situation.

However, most cardiac catheterization with a cardiac intervention or stent is considered an outpatient service and does not warrant a two-midnight certification. It's interesting and unfortunate to note that the cardiologist will improperly document for inpatient when there should've only been an outpatient order. It takes a specialized case manager nurse to reverse this mistaken classification to an outpatient procedure. Unfortunately, unless there is a supportable and defensive recommendation from an outside or hospital utilization watchdog, the case manager may be operating under some ridiculous and oppressive corporate edicts and guidelines, which prevent her or him from classifying the proper service level.

The next issue I want to revisit what is called chronic total occlusion of a coronary artery. As we have discussed, a patient may have a heart attack that is "silent" and has no idea of any cardiac damage. Often, when you have a doctor screening EKG for a physical or an insurance exam, the EKG may abnormal and have a Q wave indicative of an old heart attack. In the same regard, when you are a having a cardiac catheterization for a heart attack or for a positive stress test, the doctor may find that one of your coronary arteries is totally closed or occluded by plaque. Frequently, there's significant calcium in the occlusion as it has been present for a prolonged period of time. Chronic total occlusion (CTO) of a coronary artery is defined as occlusion of the coronary artery that is total or near total (99%) that has been present for at least three months. It can be difficult to identify that the artery has been closed for more than three months, but clues are significant calcification of the lesion, which is a gauge of its chronicity as well as the development of what are called collaterals.

If the artery is totally closed, there are parts of the heart muscle that are completely deprived of blood flow. For this reason, a good part of that muscle will die and form a scar, but some of the outlying muscle will still get some blood supply from small braches of other arteries of the heart and remain in a form of hibernation where they are alive but functioning at a lesser degree. If the RCA occludes in its middle, then some of the muscle in the RV and lateral LV may die, but some of the blood from the circumflex and its obtuse marginal branches may also feed part of the lateral wall of the LV and the distal RV, offering some blood supply to these parts of the RCA occlusion. This hibernation or ischemia of the distal muscle produces abnormal byproducts of metabolism with less oxygen and may stimulate the circumflex branches to grow extra blood supply to these areas over time.

Now, the key point in this arrangement of collaterals is that they may become so extensive as to actually return blood flow to the hibernating muscle and prevent ischemia with exertion or at rest and not be a source of angina pectoris. Those who followed the previous section on coronary artery disease will know that a nuclear treadmill will expose abnormal areas of perfusion and ischemia if you're a patient with angina. The size and area of this ischemia on the nuclear treadmill can correlate to the area that is found to have a CTO or not. If it does, then the size of the ischemia on the nuclear treadmill can be a gauge of the extent of ischemia called the ischemic "burden."

The reason I go into such detail regarding CTO is that the cardiologist or interventionalist may see a CTO when he's visualizing the coronaries for target or culprit lesion in an elective or emergent left heart catheterization with placement of a stent. I've talked about the oculostenotic reflex. After the target lesion is fixed, the doctor may reflexively want to approach the CTO just because it's there. He may do it at the same time or have you stay in the hospital one or two extra days to further in a second procedure intervention and try to fix the CTO.

This scenario can thus occur whenever the doctor sees an additional occlusion aside from the culprit lesion. These are called bystander lesions that have no proven significance for survival or angina symptoms. If this bystander lesion is felt to be life threatening such as a lesion far up (proximal) in one or more of the three major coronary arteries, this approach may be warranted. This is solely up to the interventionalist, and his motives may be correct in the notion that the other bystander lesions are life threatening or may have a high risk for further angina.

However, this's the more uncommon situation, and the usual circumstance is actually that the lesion isn't life threatening and the doctor has absolutely no clue as the ischemic burden of these additional lesions or a CTO without a repeat nuclear study after the first intervention. The prudent approach with these bystander lesions and CTO is to do the first procedure and then discharge you. I assure you that after the culprit intervention, the cardiologist or interventionalist will discuss what he found and try to appeal to your gut reaction that since it occluded, it should be fixed and try to compel you to stay in the hospital for the second procedure.

Well, as of January 2015, Medicare won't pay separately for this second outpatient procedure, which isn't considered complex enough for inpatient status. They'll only pay a comprehensive payment for the first procedure, which is less that the cost of both procedures. In all likelihood, the doctor will be oblivious of this reality or just want to ignore it. The most prudent course of action in these situations is to be discharged and to see how you do at home. If you still suffer from angina pectoris and the doctor is aware of your bystander CTO or extra bystander occlusions from the previous catheterization, he should do a treadmill first to see if it is still abnormal and to gauge the ischemic burden. Plus, he should gauge the area of the heart if it truly matches the area of the CTO or bystander lesion and consider a second procedure to open up the CTO or bystander occlusion with an angioplasty or a stent.

Furthermore, there are some critical technical issues when it comes to intervention on a CTO. Because it's totally occluded, the interventionalist can't advance a wire through the occlusion. If it's a fresh and soft occlusion as in an acute heart attack with a new occlusion or "thrombus," it's possible to pass a wire and afford a pathway and guide through the artery for a stent of angioplasty. With a CTO and its heavy calcium, the approach is like a roto-rooter to use rotational atherectomy, which actually bores through the occlusion. There's also a newer technique of using a laser angioplasty that burns through the obstruction. Just as a house pipe could burst, so can a coronary artery.

The rotational atherectomy can not only perforate the artery, but it can cause the whole artery to split or "dissect" with the total loss of blood supply to the tissue resulting in a new heart attack. Furthermore, the success rate of opening the CTO is only 50-70% with the complication rate of myocardial infarction or dissection and perforation approaching 5% with many resulting in emergency bypass surgery. So, this CTO procedure is not to be taken lightly and must be thoroughly thought out before consenting to the procedure.

In addition to having a very skilled and experienced operator of the procedure, it is imperative that the centers doing the CTO interventions have the correct resources. Not only is the newer equipment such as computerized tomography of the vessels with the newer visualization and guide wire techniques required, but the institution must have surgical backup when minutes and is of the essence. This often is not the case.

Lastly, with CTO and other significant occlusions, the most prudent course of action at the start would be coronary bypass surgery. There have been various studies that have shown that when the angiogram shows a culprit lesion and other CTO areas, CABG is indicated rather than a staged procedure with multiple stents or angioplasties. So, the medium and long-term survival is better with bypass, but there's a marked decrease in the need for further cardiac catheterizations and the concomitant risks with the interventionalist having additional profit.

Before we leave this discussion of CTO, I would like to add the use of CTO after bypass surgery, including the intervention on bystander interventions both post CABG or as a separate procedure after culprit lesion PCI. First, a newer phenomenon is if the patient develops angina after bypass, which was done on arteries initially felt to be better managed by bypass, then with PCI, they're subsequently intervened upon with a stent of angioplasty. There have been virtually no studies on this practice, and especially with CTO, a nuclear treadmill must first be done to demonstrate the exact area of the presumed ischemia and the ischemic burden. If this isn't done and the operator simply acts on his oculostenotic reflex on the bypassed vessel, then the results are questionable and the risk of serious dissection of the arteries and failure of the CABG are very real.

The more prudent approach to this situation would be a vigorous medical management and lifestyle changes such as diet manipulation, blood pressure control, stopping smoking, diabetic control, and lowering of cholesterol. Unfortunately, many patients simply can't or won't take this course of action but want immediate results. This practice can have unfortunate results. As I've said before, there is no doubt that the vegan diet can reverse cholesterol buildup in especially these minor arteries and should be considered for those subjected to these very questionable PCI procedures.

CORONARY ARTERY BYPASS SURGERY

Coronary artery bypass surgery (CABG) is a surgical procedure like PCI and is performed to relieve angina pectoris and reduce the risk of death from coronary artery disease. In this procedure, usually veins from the leg and the intact internal mammary artery in the chest are grafted to the coronary arteries after or distal to the obstruction to restore blood flow to the heart muscle. At first, the surgery was performed with the heart stopped on a coronary bypass pump to substitute for the heart pumping. However, more recently, CABG is performed on the beating heart called "off pump" bypass surgery.

Cardiac surgery itself was done in the 1940s with just a handful of surgeries that could be done on a beating heart without a bypass pump. These procedures were done on congenital heart disease with the Blalock-Taussig shunt, atrial septal defect repair, and closure of a patent ductus arteriosus in children. As a side note, there's a movie called "Something the Lord Made" about the two remarkable individuals. Vivian Thomas was a black cardiac pioneer, and he had a complex relationship with the southern white surgeon, Dr. Alfred Blalock. It captures the high drama of the first open heart surgery on a beating child's heart as well as the incredible bravery of two exemplary individuals. One risked his license for having a black man in surgery, and the black man saw the fruition of his dreams amidst the prejudice of the 1940s.

However, it became obvious due to the complexity and dangers of these surgeries that there was a necessity for the development of a heart lung machine to allow one to stop the heart for surgery and proper suturing to critical structures such as the coronary arteries for cardiac bypass surgery. The first attempts at cardiopulmonary bypass occurred between 1951 and 1955. The machines had three requirements: 1. To anti-coagulate the blood so it did not clot in the machine. 2. To prevent the machine from destroying the red blood cells due to trauma as they passed through the machine. 3. To oxygenate the blood while the same time remove the CO_2 buildup as a waste product of metabolism both of which are normally done by the lungs.

These proved to be daunting tasks, and during these early years, the death rate was more than 50% during attempts at coronary bypass surgery. The part of the problem was that each surgeon was self-taught, and many crucial details of successful open heart surgery had to be learned the hard way, which was by trial and error. Because of this mortality rate, only the sickest of patients had open heart surgery so that the grim statistics could be justified. It wasn't until the late 1950s that Dr. C. Walton Lillehei and Dr. Richard DeWall at the University of Minnesota developed the bubble oxygenator that allowed the safe exchange of oxygen and CO_2. Doctors would come to the university in droves to observe these surgeries and take back the technology to their respective centers.

During the next ten years, the operative death rate from open heart surgery dramatically decreased to less than one in one hundred. No one at that time would've predicted the incredible efficacy of coronary bypass as a lifesaving procedure that could be done with such good results.

It's a great testament to the tenacity and expertise of these early innovators, to whom we owe a great deal for the saving of pediatric and adult lives.

The first modern coronary bypass surgery was done in America on May 2, 1960, at the Albert Einstein College of Medicine-Bronx Municipal Hospital Center by a team led by Dr. Robert H. Goetz and Dr. Michael Rohman. At first, just the intact internal mammary artery was used to bypass an occluded proximal LAD (at the origin of the vessel) as this was such a dangerous lesion often called the "widow maker." (Fig.83 and 84).

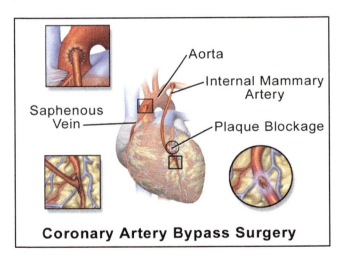

Coronary Artery Bypass Surgery

(Fig.83) This truly remarkable picture comes from Blausen.com "Blausen gallery 2014" Wikiversity Journal of Medicine, 10.15347. Here, you see the way the saphenous veins and internal mammary artery are sutured (sewed) into the LAD and the RCA from the aorta into the coronary past the obstruction. One can imagine the amazing skill of the surgeon doing these complex small sutures that are leak proof and precise. In this picture, you can see that the blockage is on the top or proximal part of the LAD, and the LAD provides blood to the whole front of the heart muscle that if becomes completely closed could cause a fatal heart attack and thus called the "widow maker" lesion.

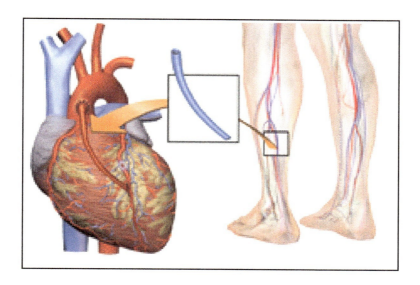

(Fig.84) This picture depicts the harvesting of a saphenous vein (SVG) from the leg for the coronary bypass surgery. In this picture, the SVG used to bypass the LAD. A second bypass surgery is often not able to be done as proper veins cannot be found by what is called vein mapping by a special Doppler echo machine.

CABG is one of the most common procedures performed during U.S hospital stays; it accounts for more than 10.5% of operating room time. From 2001 to 2011, CABG frequency decreased by 46% due mainly to the use of complex multi-vessel PCI but increased again in 2011 due to the PCI predictably late failures, many of which were done inappropriately in the first place. Moreover, the rise of safe off bypass procedures and hybrid procedures that involve PCI and LIMA (left internal artery) bypass of the LAD have become more prevalent.

There have been reports in literatures of patients who had up to 20-30 stents. This is more than irresponsible that it borders on neglect as there's never 20 culprit lesions and the use of CABG should've been considered far earlier in patients with multi-vessel disease and presumably angina. Obviously, there are never 20 life-threatening scenarios with only three major coronary arteries. Almost assuredly, these were stents placed in minor branches, which are almost never life threatening, and angina is more amenable to medical diet and drug therapy; this is usually frank malpractice.

According to the United States Centers for Disease Control, the average cost for just the hospitalization for CABG in the United States in 2013 was $38,707 (www.cdc.gov). However, adding the doctor costs to the total changes it to an astounding $75,343. Compare that to the total costs in Netherlands, which is $15,742 (www.static.squarespace.com). This discrepancy in costs can be explained in part by the fact that Netherlands has proper control of CABG that is reviewed and performed only when it's indicated in patients felt to have a reasonable prognosis without predictable serious complications and limited to patients under the age of 80. This is an excellent example for the United States to follow, but there would be uninformed and indignant protests against restrictions in care irrespective of the fact that elderly patients have significant complications and cognitive deterioration post CABG.

In 2004, the guidelines of the American Heart Association and the American College of Cardiology (AHA/ACC) (Eagle et al: Circulation 110(14): e340-437) covered situations where CABG was indicated specifically as the preferred treatment over PCI and the adequate trials that have demonstrated the superiority of CABG. These include:

1. Disease of the left main coronary artery. This includes the relative contraindication against attempts at left main PCI unless there are significant reasons and another disease (co-morbidities) that preclude CABG.

2. Disease of all three major coronary arteries (LAD, Circumflex, and RCA)

3. Diffuse disease not amenable to PCI. This can certainly be controversial and dependent on the observations and the opinions of the interventionalist; there would be much variability in the opinions from operator to operator and when to properly proceed with CABG versus attempts at PCI.

4. Patient with severe left ventricular dysfunction (low ejection fraction less than 30% or weakening of the heart). This is certainly a guideline that is widely ignored. The amount of PCI done in patients with low ejection fractions may account for 30% of all PCI procedures and are most simply unwarranted.

5. Lastly, patients with diabetes mellitus. This is a recommendation most commonly based on the elderly with insulin-dependent diabetes or a patient with diabetes, who has demonstrated end organ disease caused by the diabetes including but not limited to strokes, kidney disease, or peripheral vascular disease. This is also a guideline that is often overlooked or ignored.

As of 2015, many cases with advancement in PCI technology and numerous cases of this guideline for multi-vessel PCI can be less stringent, and the data is fairly compelling that the incidence of closure (restenosis) of the stent is higher in diabetics, and the medium to long term survival is better with CABG and multi-vessel disease.

In terms of PCI to patients with low EFs, a PCI may be warranted under some circumstances such as an emergent PCI. However, the amount of cardiac catheterizations, in what is so often the case of a catheterization is done in a patient with a low EF in the hopes of finding a coronary lesion that the doctor feels can be causing the low EF. This usually has no scientific or medical basis. More often than not, these PCIs are just cosmetic improvements in the coronaries without any real benefits to the patients, and many of these patients just have shortness of breath and no angina. When the time comes to cover congestive heart failure (CHF), I'll provide details of cardiac catheterization under these circumstances.

Prognosis following CABG is based on the typically successful coronary bypass graft lasting 8-15 years. In terms of grafts using the LIMA, these grafts can have a longer longevity. It appears that at 10 years, the survival of CABG patients can approach medical therapy, specifically in patients with stable angina. In patients with multi-vessel disease, the survival continues to be better for those with multi-vessel

PCI. Interestingly, the younger patients seem to do much better in long term than the older patient, and the stenosis rate of the bypass grafts approaches 50% in patients over the age of 75. CABG in patients over the age of 75 must be balanced with their other disease states (comorbidity) as well as the cognitive and mental capacity before a decision is made for CABG. Loss of mental function after the bypass is a very frequent complication in CABG and must be factored into any decision for CABG, especially in the elderly with a component of vascular or Alzheimer's dementia.

Like the native coronaries, these saphenous veins bypass grafts (SVG) can collect cholesterol plaque no different than what is seen in the natural (native) coronary vessels. Specifically, the saphenous veins undergo fibrosis and deteriorate with slow closure that promotes the growth of collateral vessels. In recent years, the use of PCI to the LIMA and the SVGs has markedly increased. This has been a very successful development as PCI may extend the longevity of grafts. In the grafts to the three major arteries, revascularization with PCI extends lifespan and can restore quality of life. There is no question that PCI for failing bypass grafts can be successfully performed with relative safety and significantly extent the longevity and the functioning of these grafts. There appears to be both short term and long term efficacy in vein graft patency with PCI and graft stents, which may avoid a second redo CABG. But the interventionalist must have adequate experience with PCI of the SVGs as there are additional complications that include, but are not limited to, actual perforation of the graft with the stent or angioplasty that can have dire consequences.

As a closing note, one of the most depressing scenarios in medicine is when a patient is recovering in the hospital from CABG and asks to leave for a "smoke break." This is sheer insanity. In more advanced countries, due to the remarkable cost of CABG, the national health system denies CABG in patients who continue to smoke or they'll have the patient actually sign a contract, acknowledging the consequences of losing health coverage if they continue to smoke after the CABG! In America, the lobbyists and action groups will firmly accuse the health system of withholding medical care against the patient's rights. I have no doubt that such actions are based on greed and sheer ignorance of the cost of smoking to human life and medical resources. As far as I am concerned Medicare and insurance companies should simply never approve or pay for any human being who insists on continuation of smoking after a bypass. These patients should be required to sign a contact which specifies they would reimburse the payer if they are found to continue smoking or further a punitive fine.

PERIPHERAL VASCULAR DISEASE AND VASCULAR BYPASS SURGERY

Peripheral vascular disease (PVD) or peripheral artery disease (PAD) refers to the obstruction of large arteries of the extremities and aorta, the carotids, or the vasculature of the brain. PVD usually results from atherosclerosis and cholesterol buildup in the large arteries similar to the situation in the coronaries. In this book, I'll mainly cover diseases in the lower extremities. The use of the techniques and treatments can be utilized in virtually any artery of the body including the aorta itself, renal arteries, celiac (intestinal) arteries, and arteries of the upper extremities. However, I'll primarily discuss PVD in legs although similar PTA (percutaneous transluminal angioplasty) and stents can be done in all of these arteries as well as arteries of the brain recently in select hospitals.

About 20-30% of patients may be asymptomatic, and the blockage is discovered during a screening exam with the lack leg pulses. A Doppler echo exam of the legs is often done as routine screening in asymptomatic individuals as part of a physical examination. The other symptoms and signs may include (Fig.86 and Fig.87):

1. Claudication-severe cramping at rest or exertional pain with numbness in the legs due to decreased blood flow in the legs.

2. Sores or ulcers on the legs, feet, and toes that can be similar to that seen in diabetes that do not heal properly.

3. Coolness in the legs often associated with a blue color change (cyanosis) and either both or one of the legs or feet being colder than normal.

4. Diminished and often abnormal nail growth in the foot and associated with distinct and well-demarcated hair loss of the lower leg.

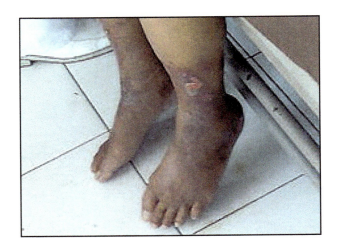

(Fig.86) (Wikipedia) In this picture, one can see many of the signs of PVD. First, it's obvious that the lower leg and foot are blue, and there is a well-demarcated area in the lower leg where the leg is whitish and then suddenly is blue (cyanotic). The lower leg can be seen to be free of hair with unhealed ulcers on the lower leg.

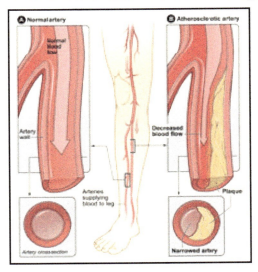

(Fig.87) (Wikipedia) This is a picture of a normal and a disease artery in the lower leg. On the right is an artery with a cholesterol deposit in the arterial wall that limits the blood flow to the leg and causes claudication. Eventually, this deposit can grow and cause complete occlusion of the artery that can cause severe claudication even at rest, jeopardizing the viability and survivability of the leg, which can lead to the amputation of the affected leg.

The risk factors for PVD are basically the same as with coronary artery disease, but with these striking differences:

1. Smoking in any form is the single most common risk factor for PVD. It's an undeniable fact that 80-90% of all PVD across the word is seen in current or past smokers with a high correlation to the years and amount of cigarettes smoked. Smokers are three times more likely to have PVD than coronary disease, and second hand smoke has also been implicated in changes in the peripheral arteries that promote cholesterol deposits. It appears that the mechanism for this is that the carbon monoxide in the smoke blocks the red blood cells from picking up oxygen and deprives the legs as well as the whole body of oxygen with the resultant long-terms effects on the body's arteries and damage to the vessels lining the arteries- (endothelium). Obviously, this is major health problem that has remarkable cost in medical resources, but more importantly, the quality and longevity of life. In our society, it's not uncommon to see an individual in a wheelchair, hobbling around with one or both legs amputated due to severe PVD and smoking cigarettes with tar stained and overgrown fingernails from PVD in the arms. Believe it or not, as an intern at a large county hospital in Torrance, California, I saw a family hold a cigarette to a patient's tracheostomy from lung disease due to smoking who also had a leg and arm amputation due to severe PVD. Such is the power of the habit where smoking may be the patient's only pleasure in life.

2. Diabetes mellitus results in between two to four times the risk of PVD and is proportional to the severity and closeness of glucose control as well as the overall duration of the diabetes. Basically, if the diabetes has been present since adolescence, the development of PVD in adulthood is almost inevitable.

3. Hyperlipidemia (high cholesterol) is the principal culprit as a risk factor in the low density lipoprotein. Basically, when you have your lipids checked as part of a physical exam, the report gives you the total cholesterol and breaks it up into the low density lipoprotein (LDL) and the high density lipoprotein (HDL). The LDL is a bad risk factor, and the HDL is a good risk factor. Correction of the LDL to less than 100 is associated with a major improvement in the rates of heart attack and stroke, and to a lesser degree with PVD.

4. Hypertension with elevated blood pressure is correlated with an increased risk of PVD, heart attacks, stroke, and kidney failure. The risk is correlated to the degree of high blood pressure, and you're relatively protected if you can keep your upper blood pressure reading (systolic BP) less than 120 mm. of mercury. The risk of claudication and PVD is 4 times higher than normal if the systolic is greater than 150 mm. of mercury.

5. Chronic inflammation where there are certain markers in the blood that are a measure of the amount of inflammation in your body. Chronic inflammation can be seen in such diseases as rheumatoid arthritis, lupus erythematosus, and ulcerative colitis.

6. Obesity. especially in the sedentary individual, who does no exercise and weighs more than 250 pounds. The effects of obesity are multifold and have a component just because of the extra burden on the arteries in the standing individual and the probable disruption of the blood flow and simple damage to the arteries.

The diagnosis of PVD can be relatively easy with office outpatient tests. The first test is called an ABI index that's basically comparing the blood pressures in parts of the leg and seeing if there is an area of relatively low blood pressure, which means that the artery is partially or totally closed.

If the ABI is normal and the patient has significant signs and symptoms of PVD, the next test is a form of echo of the leg called a duplex scan that can actually visualize the obstruction in the leg (Fig.88). Once these two test are done, the doctor can then have the option of doing an angiogram of the lower extremity with catheters, or ordering even further sophisticated non- invasive (outpatient tests in the hospital not involving catheters) such as computerized tomography (CT) or magnetic resonance angiography (MRA) both of which can visualize all the blood vessels in your leg and pelvis as well as the aorta.

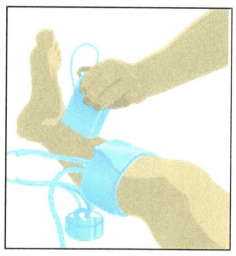

(Fig.89) (Society of Interventional Radiology) This is a picture of the ABI index and a Doppler duplex ultrasound. A blood pressure cuff is placed around the leg, and the pressure and waveform of the blood flowing through the artery are measured by the Doppler probe placed down the leg after the blood pressure cuff. In this way, it can be shown how the blood pressure differential relates to an occlusion in the artery at the level of the blood pressure cuff. Also, the presence of the arterial occlusion can be detected solely by the Doppler machine, which can take a picture using painless echo waves of the occlusion and make an estimate as to the percent occlusion of the vessel at the specific arterial level.

Once the presence of PVD is confirmed by mainly using these non-invasive tests, the doctor will easily classify the severity of the disease to determine the treatment and further diagnostic strategy. There are many staging systems, but stage I and II are the asymptomatic presence of PVD on a screening test or mild claudication with exertion in a limb. Furthermore, severity in stage III and IV with rapid claudication over minimal walking distance and rest claudication with no exertion or often awakening the patient from sleep when the oxygen in the blood stream is lower. The last findings in subgroup level V range from ulcers only on the toes of the foot, and to tissue loss or frank gangrene of the foot.

The final aspect of PVD is the treatment. Contrary to the situation in CAD and targeting the culprit lesion and ultimately the bystander lesions and the oculostenotic reflex, a similar situation doesn't exist when it comes to interventions such as angioplasty and stents to the arteries of the lower extremities (Fig.89, Fig.90, and Fig.91)

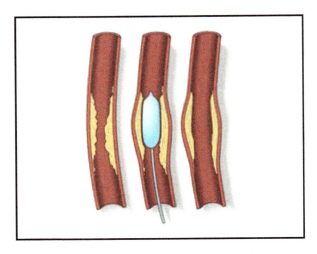

(Fig.89) (Society of Interventional Radiology)

This is a depiction of angioplasty with a catheter balloon of a large artery in the leg. The plaque or cholesterol deposit is compressed against the wall of the artery and opened. Without adequate diet, exercise, cessation of smoking, and lowering of cholesterol, ultimately, there can be a high rate of recurrence and regrowth of the cholesterol deposit. These arteries are much larger than the coronary arteries and take a greater diameter of balloon for the procedure.

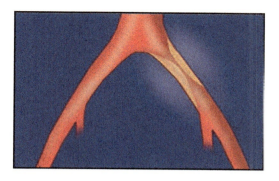

(Fig.90) (Society of Interventional Radiology).

This is a picture of the large descending aorta as it divides into the left and right iliac arteries leading into the legs. One can see an almost total occlusion of the left iliac, which would unequivocally cause the patient to have claudication and blue legs and non-healing ulcers if untreated.

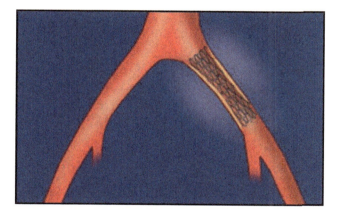

(Fig.91) (Society of Interventional Radiology)

This is a picture of the same left iliac artery as in (Fig.90) after placement of a stent. First, the artery is opened with angioplasty, then a stent is placed, which not only opens the artery more but also makes the opening last longer, and lifestyle changes prevent lifetime recurrence. Notice that because this is a very large artery, the stent is appropriately much larger than the stents utilized in the coronary arteries, and many are not coated like the coronary stents to prevent recurrent thrombosis (bare metal stents).

In the case of peripheral vascular disease, the arteries that are occluded and candidates for angioplasty and a stent are usually very obvious. The most common artery is the superficial femoral artery (SFA) that lies in the middle of the leg. There are multiple branches that reach into the feet, and any of these arteries can be subject to a stent. Unlike the situation in coronary artery disease, all the arteries of the leg lead down to the feet; thus, various levels can cause claudication and the demarcation of a blue leg and foot. As in the coronary arteries, you'll be obligated to take an antiplatelet drug such as a Plavix and aspirin for at least a year or the rest of your life after such a peripheral stent.

Likewise, if there is no alteration if lifestyle after the first intervention to your legs, it's inevitable that there'll be a recurrence of the closure. It seems that as it recurs, it goes farther and farther down the leg to smaller arteries in the feet. In the common, worst-case scenario, these patients develop non-healing ulcers and gangrene that lead to amputation of the foot or the whole leg. It seems unimaginable that someone would continue to smoke and eat freely after the development of sever PVD with amputation, but the power of a habit or addiction wins over as the nicotine or food is the only pleasure the patient has in his life and the patient is simply ignorant or wishes to ignore the disastrous consequences of their non-compliance. Inevitably, these habits can lead to the loss of their legs and destruction of their lifestyle. It's a sad reality of our country that many of these patients end up on lifelong disability and Medicare at age 45 rather than 65 and place a remarkable financial burden on the entitlement system until they die.

These patients most often feel unemployable due to their severe, self-caused diseases, and the government entitlement programs just perpetuates the habit and dependency with no negative monetary consequences. In this system, there's absolutely no incentive to quit or change lifestyle, not to mention the lack of proficient amount counseling and prevention education. This is the American way where the leaders have self-serving motives to not improve the system. The amputees aren't directed to any useful program, which could theoretically end their habits and improve their functions enough to get a job. Rather, these individuals are content with their government financial help while ignoring their well-being and supporting their various self-destructive habits as they go on to lose their second leg. They then remain a perpetual burden on the society and especially the family.

Ultimately, this type of medical system is destined under Obamacare to become a single payer system of totally socialized Medicine, which is the basic aim of Obamacare since its inception. It's difficult to imagine what form socialized medicine will take in the United States, but it most likely will take on aspects of the VA system, Medicaid, and federally qualified Health Centers (FQHC). In the case of the VA, there are some very obvious flaws to the system that have been exposed in 2014. It's run by bureaucrats who have really no concept of how to triage patient care for the sickest and properly delegate the patient in the correct avenues for their care. The system is broken, understaffed, and with overworked with undertrained doctors who work within a massive corporate mentality under a quota incentivized system where the patient ultimately pays the price.

In many of these scenarios, the patients often die waiting for appointments. This isn't due to computer error but due to the lack of available doctors or trained staffs for the ever increasing population. The exact situation exists in government mandated universal medical coverage and socialized medical care as they don't deliver the proper medical care with the time, expertise, and attention that are required. Furthermore, there is absolutely no incentive for the patient to seek cure but rather to perpetuate his entitled dependence of the system. Not only would the system be overwhelmed and overburdened by the sheer magnitude of patient coverage, but it isn't able to triage the patients with their new found power of entitlement, who abuse the system with non-emergent and often non-existent disease that don't need immediate attention. The extreme example is the homeless who simply have no other place than the hospital ER for their ever present mental and physical disease as well as for food and shelter (three hots and a cot). Such is the frank lie and catastrophe of Obamacare that simply results in frank extermination of the sick and elderly by sheer lack of proper management-cost containment at the expense of lives.

Well, let's go back to PVD. There are some very innovative methods of intervention in the leg arteries that can facilitate the opening of completely closed arteries, which aid the treatment of coronary artery disease. Multiple studies have shown that percutaneous interventional therapy has become the first line therapy of peripheral arterial occlusion and are as effective as a first line therapy over vascular bypass surgery. Aside from just the use of angioplasty and stents, new innovative techniques that facilitate and aid in intervention for PVD has evolved.

First of these innovations is the use of rotational atherectomy to open the arteries of the legs. Basically, this utilizes a catheter that is like a mini roto-rooter with rapidly spinning cutting blades that can open up a partially or a totally closed artery. This technique is especially useful when the occlusion has been present and symptomatic for a long time and has significant calcification. Other techniques open the arteries include the use of a laser catheter that is a relatively newer technique that can be utilized in very specialized study centers. When the clot is new and there is an acute "thrombus" that causes sudden severe leg pains, there's a catheter like mini vacuum cleaner that can suck out the thrombus or clot followed by giving the patient supplemental clot busting drugs to keep the area open for the next 24 hours.

In the last few years, there has been the development of cryotherapy catheters that freeze the occlusion and facilitate subsequent angioplasty. All of these techniques have special efficacy as a second procedure when a previous stent occludes and there's a need to intervene on "in stent restenosis." These repeat procedures can be very challenging and may require the use of some of these newer modalities.

The real controversy over the technique of interventions for PVD is that the patency rate of angioplasty is significantly better for the large arteries at the point of the iliac artery and the subsequent femoral and superficial femoral arteries as they come off the aorta. The success rate and long-term patency of these interventions may reach 90%. The problem arises when one tries to do an angioplasty or a stent in the small arteries of the lower leg and the foot itself. As one gets to the smaller arteries in the foot, the success and patency rate may only be 30-40%. It's important to stress to these patients the need for radical lifestyle changes and the use of various cholesterol and clot preventing drugs. If the situation progresses to non-healing foot ulcers or frank gangrene, especially those unable or unwilling to make the changes in the diet or stop smoking, amputation may be the only reasonable option.

Finally, the vascular bypass surgery in the treatment of PVD must be mentioned. The various non-surgical angioplasties and stents for PVD probably have better long-term results than the vascular bypass surgery. The vascular bypass surgery involves the use of a vein, an actual Dacron, or cloth graft to sew into the aorta and down to the leg past the closed artery such as the femoral artery in a procedure called an aortofemoral bypass surgery (Fig.92). The surgeon can also cut directly into the clot in the leg and try to cut it out in a procedure called endarterectomy.

Many of the readers may be familiar with carotid endarterectomy where the clot is surgically removed from the carotid artery leading to the brain. This endarterectomy procedure can be performed on the legs. These procedures have a long-term patency rate of up to 70% and depend primarily of the blood flow below the graft or endarterectomy and whether the patient decided to make a lifestyle change and take the appropriate medications to lower cholesterol and control diabetes. The disease can progress so severely in smokers that there's even a name coined called smoker's leg with advanced gangrene of the toes and feet (Fig.93).

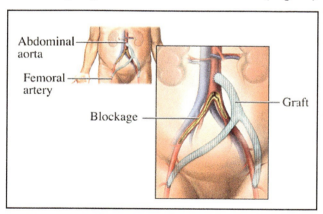

(Fig.92) (University of Nebraska Medical Center website) This picture is a depiction of a vascular bypass surgery where a Dacron graft is sewed into the aorta then in a Y fashion is sewn into the femoral arteries essentially bypassing the blockages in both of the large bilateral iliac arteries as they come off the aorta; thus, this is called an aortobifemoral bypass graft surgery. This procedure may not be the first line therapy, but in this example, if the iliac arteries cannot be opened with angioplasties or a stent, then there's no other option short of vascular bypass surgery. Also, in the face of imminent gangrene and possible amputation, vascular bypass may allow some salvage of the leg when endovascular intervention (stent and angioplasty) is not feasible.

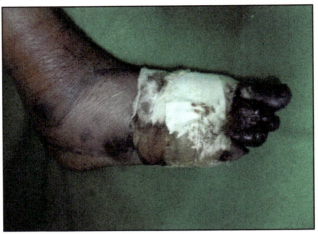

(Fig.95) (Internet doc website) This is a photograph of a foot with advanced dry gangrene of the toes. Notice the ankle with a sharp demarcation line where the skin is darker and reddish. This suggests the PVD is in the smaller arteries of the foot. At this advanced stage of PVD, there may be no other option but an immediate amputation of the toes. A vascular bypass may allow salvage of the rest of the foot, but this may be a last-ditch effort at saving the whole lower leg from amputation. However, amazingly, there are some patients who refuse amputation even at this advanced stage of gangrene. They're destined to die of infection with sepsis or a high rise in the potassium from the destruction of tissue in the foot and a cardiac arrest. This happens to be the foot of a smoker and is appropriately called "smoker's leg."

Within this discussion, it's appropriate to review these various procedures for PVD and the appropriate admission status. Unequivocally, most of the peripheral interventions like angioplasty and stent as well as the even more complex procedures like rotational atherectomy don't warrant inpatient status but will require at the most two days (one midnight) of hospital care as outpatient classification. Of course, if there are complications, this may warrant switching to inpatient services, but in general, some may only require an overnight hospital stay. Similar to coronary artery disease, a discharge on the same day as the procedure is strongly discouraged as it can be dangerous to the viability of a limb.

The more complex surgeries, such a vascular bypass, are definitely inpatient situations. When the patient is placed on 24-48 hours of blood thinners for an acute vascular clot, the inpatient services are also warranted. It is extremely important to ascertain the exact admission status from the doctor, to be proactive, and to review the appropriate documentation and certifications required for Medicare's approval for inpatient admission status. One can never assume that the doctor will do the appropriate paper work even though he's the only one who can tell you whether you're inpatient or outpatient status. Remember, the hospital is under no legal obligation to divulge your exact admission status.

In conclusion, the treatment of PVD has radically changed with the advent of various non-invasive techniques of angioplasty and stents. Unlike the treatment of CAD, the presence of this disease is much more obvious to the naked eye and has a much greater dependency for its development on the patient's cholesterol, glucose, hereditary, age, sex, and smoking patterns. Smokers, especially with concomitant diabetes, will develop a degree of PVD, and if gone untreated, it can ultimately result in multiple limb amputation. The ultimate financial and emotional toll on the family, patient, and system is immeasurable, but it's a lifelong, great burden to all those involved.

CONGESTIVE HEART FAILURE AND CARDIOMYOPATHY

Now it is time to discuss congestive heart failure, which is a remarkably common cardiac disease. Heart failure (HF) or congestive heart failure (CHF) are used interchangeably but aren't quite the same. HF occurs when the heart is unable to pump to maintain blood flow to meet the needs of the body. The signs and symptoms of the most common manifestation of HF, which is CHF, are shortness of breath, waking up at night with difficulty breathing that seems to improve with sitting up, excessive fatigue, difficulty catching one's breath with exercise, excessive nighttime urination, and swelling or edema of the legs. All of these symptoms are due to congestion with fluid in the lungs and with excessive water buildup in the body, hence the description of CHF.

However, heart failure can subsequently lead to the decrease in blood supply to all the organs of the body and cause damage and malfunction to these organs. It can also result in kidney failure with the kidneys stopping to excrete the appropriate amount of urine and byproducts of the body's metabolism. This situation is worsened by the low blood pressure that is so often seen with severe heart failure, which can even lead to shock. In terms of the liver, HF can cause the liver to fail and cause jaundice with the buildup of pressure in the liver, resulting in accumulation of fluid within the belly called ascites. In the lungs, the fluid builds up and causes pulmonary edema with wheezes and shortness of breath. The fluid can accumulate around the lungs, which called a pleural effusion. (Fig.95)

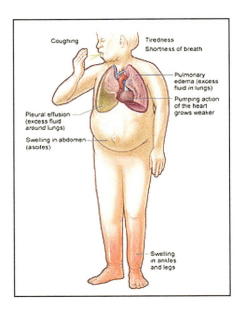

(Fig.95) (Wikipedia website) This picture is a depiction of the various signs and symptom of CHF. The cough is due to the fluid buildup in the lungs, especially if the cough is persistent and primarily occurs at night after lying flat. The legs often can swell and turn red due to the buildup of fluid, which is called pitting edema where by pressing down on the leg will leave an indentation. The swelling of the stomach is due to fluid in the peritoneum (empty space in your gut) and is called appropriately peritoneal fluid or ascites.

HF is a common and costly. If untreated, it can progress and potentially be a fatal condition. In the United States, heart failure is present in 2% of the population and in 10% of adults over the age of 65. HF can be a very insidious condition but overlooked as a common consequence of deconditioning or aging when many patients as old as in their 90s may never experience significant shortness of breath with exertion. Heart failure has been known since the times of the Egyptians in 1550 B.C.E with the Ebers papyrus commenting on shortness of breath and fluid in the lungs associated with premature death.

For that matter, in the year after the diagnosis of HF, the risk of death reaches 35%. In the case of severe heart failure that results in admission to the intensive care unit (ICU), the death rate in the first year approaches 75%. The yearly death rate after the first year of the development of HF is about 10%. This is truly an astounding number and just points out the fact that the treatments for heart failure primarily controls the symptoms but has a lesser impact on the incidence of death.

Common causes of HF include coronary artery disease with or without a previous myocardial infarction, high blood pressure for a prolonged period of time, valvular heart disease, atrial fibrillation, and a cardiomyopathy. Cardiomyopathy is a weakness of the heart muscle typically caused by a virus or of unknown cause (idiopathic) and is becoming a more recognized cause of HF. There are two basic form of HF: First is systolic heart failure, which is the weakness of the heart, and a low ejection fraction (EF-normal greater than 50%) or the ability to completely contract and expel the proper amount of blood with a low cardiac output. The other form is called diastolic HF, which is universally misunderstood and unrecognized by cardiologist, and is the inability of the heart to relax properly with a resultant rise in the pressures in the right left ventricle.

The symptoms of heart failure are the mainstay of diagnosis. The problem with the diagnosis is that under the newer paradigms of medical care, the doctor must rely upon screening computer questions and answers with a nurse interview for HF symptoms. This limits the time of a comprehensive history and physical with the doctor doing face to face examination and has led to the diagnosis primarily being made by computer rather than confirmed by various diagnostic tests and doctor input. This has led to multitudes of patients thinking they have heart failure when they are simply deconditioned. The symptoms lead to a staging of disease from stage I that is minor shortness of breath to stage IV that is the inability to get out of bed or lie flat without disabling symptoms. It's impossible for a computer question and answer spreadsheet to properly sort out the patient's symptoms for proper, tailor-made treatment modalities.

The various tools for diagnosis are primarily the timely history and physical. There is a blood test called the brain natriuretic peptide (BNP) that can detect the presence and severity of CHF as well as an elevated pressure in the heart. However, there are other disease and states that can give elevation of the BNP, and it takes a trained physician to interpret and make sense of an elevated result accurately. Echocardiography, which is done in the office and uses sound waves, can measure the EF for systolic HF and the parameters of heart relaxation for diastolic HF and is easily and readily done. The problem with the test, specifically for interpretation of the relaxation parameters, is that they take some time and training to interpret and correlate to the history and physical with the proper classification stage of heart failure.

The mainstay of HF diagnosis are the plain CXR (Fig.97) and a CT (CAT) scan of the lungs in some subtle cases. The CXR can demonstrate fluid in the lungs called pulmonary edema and the blood flow to the top of the lungs, showing a marked increase (cephalization of blood flow). Plus, the CXR can show fluid around the lung called a pleural effusion, which can persists even with therapy and lead to shortness of breath. The CT of the lungs can pick up very minor changes in the lungs at a very early heart failure but doesn't substitute for a good history and physical and is most often over interpreted as heart failure which is not substantiated by the gold standard of the plain and inexpensive CXR.

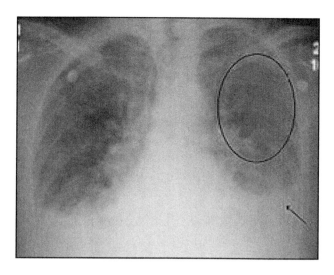

(Fig.97) (Wikipedia) This is a chest X-ray of a lung with CHF and pulmonary edema. First, note the circle at the top right, demonstrating the increased whitish lines that show increased blood flow to the top of lungs rather than the dependent bottom of the lungs (when you are standing for the x-ray). The heart itself is markedly enlarged, and the arrow points to pleural fluid or collection of fluid around the heart. Overall, the lungs are too white and represent increase blood and fluid within the lungs, which is called pulmonary edema. This condition leads to wheezing and rales or crackles on physical exam of the heart when one properly listens through a stethoscope.

Heart failure can present as an acute episode of CHF with rapid onset or chronic symptoms, commonly under outpatient treatment by the internist or cardiologist. Acute decompensated heart failure is the rapid change in symptoms that results in emergent hospitalization for immediate and often life-saving treatment. If a patient is hospitalized for a severe and acute decompensated heart failure situation, this will warrant inpatient classification of the admission that requires more than a two-day hospitalization and admission to the ICU or the coronary care unit. This is different than the situation with chronic or newly diagnosed heart failure where there can be a short-term hospitalization that never warrants inpatient services but is classified as observation, requiring at the most 2-3 days of hospitalization. There can be much overlap as to the severity of the heart failure and the inpatient status, so there should be a frank discussion with the physician at the onset of the hospitalization. There's a tremendous amount of ambiguity as to the appropriate hospital status for chronic congestive heart failure based on whether the doctor documents the episode as acute, acute decompensation, or chronic heart failure.

Chronic heart failure can easily decompensate. This situation generally results from a coexisting illness such as pneumonia, myocardial infarction, atrial fibrillation, acute cocaine or alcohol ingestion, and a patient's failure to maintain the fluid and salt restriction that comes with the prescribed medications.

Now back to the causes of HF. As I have said, HF is so common and is one of the five most frequent causes of acute hospitalization and ER visits. Some of the important risk factors include:

1. Ischemic heart disease
2. Cigarette smoking
3. Obesity
4. Diabetes Mellitus
5. Valvular heart disease
6. Hypertension

There are various causes of HF, and one of the more common is a cardiomyopathy that we will further discuss in the next section of this book:

1. Coronary artery disease angina or a previous myocardial infarction
2. Dilated cardiomyopathy
3. Valvular heart disease
4. Viral myocarditis (a viral infection of the heart muscle)
5. Infiltrations of the heart muscle, which is often idiopathic (unknown cause), or by a substance called amyloid that is seen in elderly patients

6. HIV cardiomyopathy

7. Connective tissue disease such as lupus erythematosus or rheumatoid arthritis.

8. Abuse of drugs such as cocaine, alcohol, and amphetamines.

9. Chemotherapeutic drugs used to treat cancer but can also cause an acute or chronic weakness of the heart

10. Pregnancy, which can lead to the weakening of the heart muscle and is seen in multiple pregnancies. Furthermore, for some reason, it's seen in the lower socio-economic status of patients and may be due to a virus infection of the heart in specific regions of the United States.

There are two basic types of heart failure: left and right failure with the associated dysfunction of the RV and LV. The differentiation of these two is somewhat artificial as LV failure or systolic dysfunction, which is the more common of the two, will ultimately lead to RV failure; however, RV failure or diastolic dysfunction can stand alone and doesn't perpetuate LV failure.

Left sided failure is primarily associated with a low ejection fraction (EF) of the heart and is easily picked up by echocardiography. Also, on physical examination, the heart is usually enlarged. The cardiologist can use his hand on the chest to feel the tip of the heart (apex) beating against the chest and detect displacement to the left indicating an enlarged heart. While listening to the heart, extra sounds called an S3 can be heard, and these signify significant heart failure. The problem is that most contemporary cardiologist doesn't know to listen for this sound and possibly only 1-2% documents an S3 when it's probably present in over 90% of patients with EFs less than 35%. It takes a very quiet room and time with a good stethoscope, which rarely is the condition in the ER. Various heart murmurs can be heard in the heart due to such valvular disease as aortic stenosis or mitral regurgitation, I'll cover next.

Left sided failure primarily leads to backup of the blood into the lungs and decreased perfusion of the organs and the body due to a low cardiac output with the low EF. To counteract this low output, the heart goes faster in what is called sinus tachycardia, and it's not unusual for a patient to present with a heart rate greater than 100/minute (normal 60/minute). The backup of blood into the lungs fills them with fluid and causes the lungs to ineffectively oxygenate the blood. This leads to low oxygen levels in the bloodstream and is why the first therapy you get in the ER is oxygen therapy through your nose with a nasal cannula. Compromise of the forward pumping of blood can lead to symptoms of low perfusion of the various critical organs. In the case of the brain, the patient often complains of dizziness or confusion.

A very common cause for the geriatric population to present to the ER with these very symptoms, and is screened for CHF with an echocardiogram which is ordered on an emergency basis. In many ERs, this can be done by a trained cardiologist with a machine made available in the ER. The physician looks for a low EF along with signs of scarring and death of heart muscle with areas of muscle abnormal movement (hypokinesia), no movement (akinesia), or backward movement (dyskinesia). The liver can malfunction and cease to produce clotting factors that may lead to types of bleeding. The kidneys can stop producing urine, and an easy blood test checks the creatinine that can build up rapidly if the kidneys are suffering from acute kidney injury. The low oxygen in the blood steam can lead to the blood lacking the rich red color and cause bluish tints to the lips called cyanosis.

Backward failure of RV failure doesn't lead to fluid in the lung but rather excess fluid in the venous system of the body and a high venous pressure. This can lead to fluid buildup in the legs called pitting edema and fluid in the stomach space called a peritoneal effusion (ascites). A peritoneal effusion can also been seen in patients with cirrhosis often due to alcoholism and is not uncommon for both of these simultaneous conditions to be operative in the production of ascites as alcoholism itself is a very common cause of heart failure as the alcohol "pickles" the heart muscle. Contrary to most contemporary health gurus, who perpetuate the idea of low amounts of alcohol for heart health, in terms of heart failure I feel that even a small amount of daily regular alcohol can perpetuate and lead to HF, not to mention alcohol addiction.

The treatment of left and right sided heart failure can be rather complex and may take up to 3-4 months to come up with an optimal and effective treatment plan. Thus, in chronic or minimally decompensated heart failure, observation or outpatient therapy is justified most of the time and doesn't require more than a two-day hospital stay. The mainstay of therapy remains diuretic treatment with drugs like Lasix or Bumex. The diuretics are utilized to rid the body of extra fluid, reduce some back pressure of the lungs, and clear up the pulmonary edema. In severe cases of "flash" or sudden pulmonary edema or acutely decompensated heart failure, the doctor may elect to place you on a constant IV drip of the diuretic. This is mostly seen when there's concomitant acute or chronic kidney injury, and there's no doubt that if one reaches this state of treatment and complexity, the inpatient treatment status is appropriate and most likely will entail a greater than two-midnight stay in the monitored (telemetry or constant EKG) unit.

In this same respect, the patient will be placed on a restricted salt and fluid intake. Secondly, the use of beta blockers to relax the heart and lower the heart pressures has become a mainstay of drug therapy. As an historical note, beta blockers used to be contraindicated (felt to be of negative effect) in heart failure. Later, there was some evidence that showed beneficial symptomatic relief, and numerous studies have demonstrated a marked improvement in short and long-term heart failure survival. Plus, drugs called ACE inhibitors affect the kidneys and are complex but improve kidney function and improve survival in heart failure patients. Drugs called aldosterone inhibitors have been shown to improve survival in only the severe class III-IV cases.

Ultimately, many of these cases of severe heart failure may not respond to drug therapy. The doctor may elect to do a right and left heart catheterization to determine if there's any coronary artery disease that can be fixed and measure the pressures in the heart. Many of these patients develop very severe kidney injury and severe shortness of breath that the doctor elects to start IV vasopressor agents such as Dopamine or Dobutamine in the hospital and continue daily IV therapy through an infusion catheter in the neck on a daily basis. If all else fails, there's another option, especially in the younger patients with class IV heart failure, to place a device in the body called an LVAD (left ventricular assist device) as a bridge to heart transplant.

These are very aggressive interventions and much thought and discussion go into their individualized use. As before, if one reaches this advanced stage, any hospitalization is extremely complex and unequivocally deserves inpatient status. Heart failure is one of the most common causes of death in America, and the use of LVADs and transplant in class V patients are extremely expensive. It also takes a very long-term commitment to compulsive lifestyle change, which are the lifelong dependency and the expense of multiple medications and the antirejection medication with concomitant intense medical care in transplant.

Recently, there has been development of a catheter that can be placed into the pulmonary artery of the patient to constantly monitor its pressures, which are a direct reflection of the amount of systolic heart failure and the buildup of fluid in the heart. This catheter has a built-in sensor and is connected to a device that uses telemetry to transmit the numbers to a central monitoring station. This way, if the pressure is building up and not yet resulting in the need for hospital treatment of the heart failure, the patient can be advised to increase or change his medications at home to avoid hospitalizations. This is obviously a wonderful technology theoretically that can save a great amount of money and improve a patient's overall lifestyle.

Yet, like so much technological improvement in medicine such as robotic surgery, advances like this inevitably lead to increased costs, which seems to be the opposite goal of all other advanced countries. The cause of this is complex, but it seems to inevitably revolve around the increased cost of the technology that is passed on the insurer with the lack of efficient outpatient intervention and lifestyle change, which could've translated into less medical expense. In other words, the dysfunctional system simply relies on technical advances irrespective of any overall changes in patient behavior or the medical system's inability to evolve to take advantage of possible cost saving measures.

Diastolic dysfunction is probably one of the most misunderstood and improperly identified conditions of the heart causing HF. The key physical finding is an S3, but only 1-2% of cardiologists are able to identify and document when it's presented greater than 90% of the time. On echocardiography, there's a very subtle abnormality of relaxation of the LV heart muscle after it pumps and subsequently refilling from the lungs for the next heart beat and pumping of the blood. This just cannot be identified in the ER by quick echo techniques.

The key to this diagnosis is realizing that the symptoms are very subtle and not as overt and obvious as with CHF. For that matter, the presence of mild pulmonary edema can only be made by a CT of the lungs that shows fluid buildup, which is too small to detect by CXR. Diastolic dysfunction doesn't lead to enlargement of the heart, and although diastolic heart failure is often used when there are symptoms of CHF, this isn't usually appropriate. The one good finding in diastolic HF is an elevated BNP level in face of normal left ventricular function on the echocardiogram (normal EF>50%).

Again, diastolic heart failure is certainly hard if not impossible to detect by cursory examination in the ER. Perhaps, the most common error in cardiology occurs when identifying and diagnosing diastolic heart failure as the reason for hospital admission. Although many cardiologists label diastolic dysfunction as a justification for inpatient admission, this is ridiculous and should be an observation status admission with only one overnight admission for treatment and proper diagnosis. When it's obvious that diastolic dysfunction is the erroneous diagnosis and the doctor orders a barrage of unrelated test that prolong observation admission, it's a red flag for Medicare to review the case for appropriateness of the admission. In my estimation, diastolic dysfunction is the erroneous diagnosis in up to 80% of the cases.

The treatment of diastolic dysfunction is rather complex too. One of the very basic tenets of therapy is to treat hypertension, which is one of the most common causes of the RV not relaxing properly. It's my experience that these patients often present with significant hypertension, which isn't properly attended to, and don't consider its significance as contributing factor to heart failure. Plus, it may take months of outpatient adjustment of medicines to control the blood pressure. This generally requires trial and error and the need for the patient to monitor and keep a log of their blood pressure throughout the day at home. The ultimate problem with contemporary hospital care and treatment of hypertension is that the attending is most frequently a hospitalist, who only treats you in the hospital and has no self-interest or personal gain as a paying client in treating the patient after they leave the hospital setting. For this very same reason, simple hypertension and diastolic dysfunction are rarely a justification for inpatient services classification as heart failure and blood pressure control can rarely be properly be attained during the short hospital stay.

Further treatment of the glucose level in diabetics is essential in therapy of diastolic HF. It seems that the elevated glucose in diabetics has an effect on the heart muscle to impede relaxation with hypertension and diabetes being the most common causes of diastolic dysfunction. A rapid heart rate such as seen in atrial fibrillation gives little time of the muscle to relax, and compulsive control of tachycardia is also a mainstay of treatment and can be the primary reason for acute decompensation. Drugs such as beta blockers, and Cardizem can be utilized to achieve this aim. Like everything else in diastolic heart failure, rate control can rarely be achieved adequately in the hospital setting but takes precise titration of the proper medications over an extended period of time.

Lastly, the use of Lasix or other diuretics are simply inappropriate and overused in the treatment of true diastolic dysfunction. Often, the patient actually has systolic dysfunction that goes unrecognized, and Lasix just causes the patient to be dehydrated with concomitant relative tachycardia and the detrimental effects of minor rises in the average heart rate over time. The improper limiting of salt or fluid intake can also result in this same detrimental dehydrating effect when the predisposing cause in not fluid overload.

Thus, heart failure can be a real challenge to diagnose and to treat. The real key to heart failure management is the compulsive attention to the physical exam and documentation of the various symptoms for proper treatment and classification of the heart failure stage. Most of these situations that require hospitalization can be managed as observation or outpatient status with the true control of symptoms done over months of individualized medical therapy primarily in the outpatient situation.

The future for the treatment of heart failure and even overall cardiology disease is taking on a marked revolution as I write this book. As individual genes are identified in patients with heart failure or coronary disease that runs in the families and control abnormal outputs such as an increased cellular propensity to collect cholesterol plaque or in detrimental effects in heart failure and cardiomyopathy. Abnormally functioning mitochondria can be seen as an overriding case of heart failure. In this respect, drugs can be specifically tailored to block specific abnormal gene output or supplement lack of gene expression and mitigate the disease progression with resultant prolongation of survival.

CARDIOMYOPATHY

Cardiomyopathy (heart muscle disease) is the deterioration in the heart muscle's ability to contract, which usually leads to heart failure. The most common form of a cardiomyopathy is a dilated cardiomyopathy with the heart enlarged and with a low EF. As the definition of cardiomyopathy expanded over the past 50 years, it was recognized that there was dilated cardiomyopathy, thickening of the heart called hypertrophic cardiomyopathy, and restrictive cardiomyopathy usually due to disease of the pericardium (sac surrounding the heart) or infiltration with amyloid or fibrosis that is seen in many connective tissue diseases such as Lupus Erythematosus. These groups can be further broken down into specific instances, which incorporate new genetic and molecular biology knowledge. For example, there's a specific gene mutation that causes arrhythmogenic RV cardiomyopathy.

In addition, to these three main forms of primary cardiomyopathies, there are a host secondary cardiomyopathies resulting from extrinsic condition or disease. The important ones include:

1. Peripartum cardiomyopathy associated with pregnancy, leading to a severe irreversible dilated cardiomyopathy considered possibly due to a virus in mothers with multiple previous births.

2. Takatsubo's cardiomyopathy, which is a recently described condition also called "stress cardiomyopathy," is seen in women under sudden stress and mimicking an acute heart attack but leading to a form of dilated cardiomyopathy.

3. Obesity-associated cardiomyopathy seen in the moderate to morbidly obese individuals, usually heavier than 250 pounds.

4. Ischemic cardiomyopathy is a dilated cardiomyopathy due to coronary artery disease resulting from the lack of blood flow and oxygen to the myocardium, which in most instances may not be reversed by any coronary intervention as the changes are due to permanent scarring of the heart muscle.

Unfortunately, many of these patients are subject to PCI procedures that are unwarranted and as result of the oculostenotic reflex with the interventionalist fixing whatever occlusion is seen irrespective of its physiological consequences (whether the PCI makes any medical difference at all). In actuality, this situation deserves precise evaluation with exercise echocardiography and nuclear tests called viability studies that can gauge the viability of the tissue supplied by these stenotic arteries and whether or not opening the artery will have any significant impact on the ventricular function with resultant improvement in the EF after the artery is opened. Again, this depends on whether the patient actually has angina or shortness of breath that's an angina equivalent in a patient with heart failure and the symptomatology having nothing to do with the coronary artery disease.

Many of these patients with a cardiomyopathy undergo cardiac catheterization to check for any significant CAD and a biopsy of RV using a special catheter that takes a small chunk of myocardium for pathological evaluation. This can be important in identification of any infectious or infiltrative etiology with specific microscopic changes that can be seen in acute viral or idiopathic cardiomyopathies.

Aside from the effects of cardiomyopathy on the overall left ventricular function, the low EF, and in some cases, the specific type of infection or infiltration can have profound effects on the conduction system of the heart and the electrophysiological consequences. EKG abnormalities are often present, and they may often mimic significant CAD associated with nonspecific, vague symptoms. Generally, the EKG is of a low voltage, and there may be blocks in the right or left bundle as well and in the sinus and AV node. In many of these cardiomyopathies, it's determined that a pacemaker implant is indicated.

As of 2014, many of these situations in cardiomyopathy are treated with a biventricular pacemaker or ICD that can actually augment the strength of the heart and lessen the symptoms of CHF. The biventricular device is a major technological breakthrough, and if you already have a previous standard pacemaker, the electrophysiologist may strongly suggest an upgrade to a biventricular device. These devices are most effective in the patient with a LBBB, which may actually occur in the majority of patient with a dilated and specific infiltrative cardiomyopathy.

The most important aspect of a cardiomyopathy is the need for the implant of an AICD. As discussed, the incidence of sudden death and ventricular tachycardia rises exponentially as the EF is less than 35%. Mostly, an ICD is warranted and should be a biventricular device if there are III-IV symptoms of CHF. However, it's surprising how some patients have a low EF with no symptoms or are just class I CHF with minimal fatigue and no symptoms with moderate physical exertion. If the patient with a cardiomyopathy has frequent PVCs or atrial fibrillation, then the electrophysiologist may suggest ablation for amelioration of symptoms and complete cure of the arrhythmia. An ablation of these arrhythmias may help slow the progression of the cardiomyopathy.

Lastly, there are some institutions in the world that are experimenting with the use of stem cell therapy to help replace the damaged myocardium in a cardiomyopathy or in a scar from a myocardial infarction. Interestingly, these studies have demonstrated some significant improvement in the LV function. This therapy entails replacement of damaged myocardial scar from a heart attack or cardiomyopathy and offers some great hope for the future of these patients. This is true, especially for those that are at the end stage of their disease and have very few other options. Such is the excitement in the study of cardiology and therapies of the future.

VALVULAR HEART DISEASE

Valvular heart disease is any pathological condition that involves one of the four valves of the heart: the left sided aortic a mitral valves and the right sided pulmonic and tricuspid valves. Although one can be born with some congenital valve abnormalities, valvular heart disease is primarily an acquired disease of aging and seen in the patient 50 years or older. Interestingly, over 10% of patients greater than 75 years old have a component of valvular heart disease. If the disease is picked up early, then surgical repair or replacement (insertion of an artificial heart valve) of the affected valve can result in a normal asymptomatic lifestyle.

We will review the following valve diseases: 1. Aortic stenosis, 2. Aortic regurgitation, 3. Mitral stenosis, 4. Mitral regurgitation, and 5. Tricuspid regurgitation.

Aortic stenosis is present in 3-4% of all people over the age of 75. It can be seen in younger patients born with a bicuspid instead of tricuspid valve and can be the cause of a heart murmur. This isn't to say that all heart murmurs are significant because most are normal, benign sounds of the blood flowing through a normal aortic valve and have no pathological significance. An incredible amount of people with benign murmurs are continually anxious about a normal finding on physical examination. These individuals feel compelled to have an expensive echocardiogram to confirm their benign nature when simple physical exam can differentiate a benign verses significant murmur. Even then, they remain under the impression that they have some sort of heart abnormality and may even remarkably seek disability for a heart murmur of absolutely no consequence to their lives other than undue mental anguish.

Rheumatic disease and inflammatory disease of the aortic valve at one time in history was the most common cause of all types of valvular disease, especially aortic stenosis. However, with early antibiotic treatment of streptococcal bacterial disease in the throat (strep throat), rheumatic fever has almost been eliminated as a cause of rheumatic heart disease. Many developing countries still carry a significant burden of rheumatic fever and subsequent heart disease; however, the World Health Organization and Doctors without Borders is helping eradicate this serious problem.

One very serious disease state leading to inflammation of the heart remains a very prevalent problem called bacterial endocarditis of the heart. Bacterial endocarditis is an infection mainly on the heart valves that is caused by bacteria in the blood stream leading to the infection of the aortic or mitral valve. The bacterial infection can come from sepsis in the elderly patient associated with a degree of abnormal degenerative disease of these valves, making them more prone to infection. It's a bigger medical problem in IV drug abusers, whose dirty needles and unsterile drugs leads to bacteria entering the blood steam and seeding an infection in the heart valves. Working in a major urban medical center, this is one of the most common problems seen in drug addicts and can be a cause of death or significant medical problems that require long term antibiotic treatment, which can be very difficult as many of these patient simply live outside of the norms of sociological behavior and become a monumental burden to the medical system.

Furthermore, the dramatic rise in IV heroin and opiate abuse, which is occurring in middle class America, threatens to create a whole new patient class with acute bacterial endocarditis. Gone untreated or partially treated, the only treatment option for endocarditis causes valvular disease can be an artificial heart valve. However, because of deviant behavior and psychological disease seen in these patients, this becomes a very difficult option with almost total lack of patient cooperation and compliance with proper medical care as well as a remarkable rate of recurrent infection as they continue with their IV drug habits.

Endocarditis on the heart is easily diagnosed by a standard echocardiography but needs to be confirmed with a special form of echocardiography called a transesophogeal echocardiogram employing a probe placed down the esophagus to be close to the heart (TEE). Using these techniques, one can actually see a growth on the valve that causes the valve to leak and not properly close. In the case of the mitral valve and aortic valve, it causes mitral or aortic stenosis (close) and mitral and aortic or mitral regurgitation (leak). In the worst case scenario, the valve can actually rupture and stops functioning, causing acute valvular regurgitation, which is most common with the mitral valve. In this situation, there's an acute heart failure and cardiovascular collapse, which requires emergent valve replacement. The growth on the valve can break off, in the case of the aortic valve, travel to the brain causing a stroke or to the leg as an embolism and close off all blood supply and an imminent threat to the leg viability.

Valvular heart disease in pregnancy can be a very difficult problem. If the mother has a tiniest component of valvular disease that would otherwise not be a problem, the 50% increases in blood volume during pregnancy, and the subsequent stresses on the heart can be a significant strain on the body, which can lead to actual heart failure. If there's any suspicion of old rheumatic fever or a heart murmur due to being born with a bicuspid aortic valve, serious discussion must be made regarding potential risks to the mother as well as the baby during pregnancy. Additionally, if the mother has a mechanical aortic valve replacement, there's an additional complex management of the blood thinning medicine to prevent maternal and fetal bleeding.

Aortic stenosis (Fig.80) in its mild form can be treated with simple control of blood pressure and basic attention to diet and salt intake. The symptoms of aortic stenosis can be fatigue, shortness of breath, and dizziness. As the valve becomes more stenotic, the heart muscle thickens and hypertrophies occur due to the high pressures in the LV necessary to push blood out through a smaller outlet. Also, there's a serious triad of symptoms that can develop in severe aortic stenosis, which foreshadows possible death. This triad includes syncope (loss of consciousness), heart failure, and angina. These three symptoms together predicts up to a 50% death rate within one year and require serious consideration of aortic heart valve replacement.

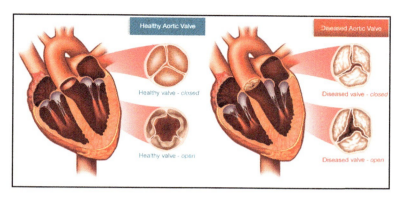

(Fig.80) (Wikipedia) This is a depiction of a normal and abnormal aortic valve. In the healthy heart, the valve closes completely during diastole and prevents blood from regurgitation from the aorta back into the left ventricle (aortic regurgitation). In systole, the LV contracts and the valve completely opens to allow uninhibited flow of the blood into the aorta. If diseased, the closed valve doesn't close completely and allows blood to regurgitate back into the LV and cause a heart murmur. This is a very difficult heart murmur to hear, so it requires an echocardiogram and a cardiac catheterization to recognize most of the times. The most common is the stenotic valve on the bottom right that doesn't open completely during LV systole, and the blood is blocked from flowing out freely, causing a loud heart murmur and requiring evaluation. If the stenosis is severe, it causes the pressures in the LV to build up and results in severe LV hypertrophy.

The use of valvular replacement itself is a complex subject. The most important aspect is the overall health and age of the patient, including whether they have any serious coexisting disease such as being on dialysis or severe COPD. The choices are basically four: mechanical prosthetic valve with open heart surgery, bioprosthetic heart valve replacement, aortic valvuloplasty, and TAVR (transcutaneous aortic valve replacement. In the case of mitral regurgitation and tricuspid regurgitation aside from surgical valve replacement, there is the option of surgical valve repair of the native valve.

There are two basic types of heart valves that can be implanted with open heart surgery: mechanical and tissue bioprosthetic valves. Modern mechanical valves that have been used for the past 50 years and been significantly improved upon have the significant advantage since they can last a lifetime and are made of various cloths and metals. However, all current mechanical heart valves require a lifelong use of the blood thinner Coumadin and a monthly close attention to the dose and degree of blood thinning to what are considered therapeutic levels. Coumadin is used to prevent clots forming on the valve with the mechanical heart valves. In contrast, tissue bioprosthetic heart valves don't need anticoagulation as they are biological tissue, typically made from pig tissue, and don't form clots. However, they have the significant disadvantage of lasting an average of 15 years before needing replacement, even shorter longevity in the younger active individual (Fig.81)

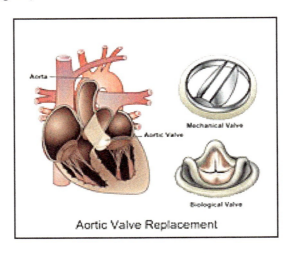

(Fig.81) (www.yalesurgery.org) On the top is a mechanical tilt valve that's made of metal and has an almost indefinite lifespan and requires the use of blood thinners (anticoagulation) to prevent blood clots. Most importantly, this blood thinning must be managed very closely with contemplated unrelated surgeries. The tendency for blood clots to form is immediate and may require hospitalization before the elective procedure to place the patient on IV heparin blood thinning as the patient is taken off the Coumadin in preparation for the surgical procedure. The second valve is a biological valve that can last up to 15 years before it becomes either stenotic or leaks and doesn't require any anticoagulation.

Tissue heart valves were traditionally made from pig connective tissue that's been treated by chemicals to not form clots or be rejected by the valve recipient. Over the past ten years, improvements in technology resulted in tissue valves made of horse or cow pericardial tissue that are less prone to human rejection with longevity and efficacy in improving the overall function of the heart. For that matter, if the patient has a valve replaced at the correct time before any permanent heart damage, there's essentially no shortening of the average lifespan. Thus, it's important to have follow-up yearly physical examinations and echocardiogram to evaluate the inevitable progression of the valvular disease and to if a valve replacement is ever necessary.

When it comes to mitral valve disease, if there's mitral stenosis, then the only real option is a valve replacement surgery. However, mitral regurgitation is much more complex as there are multiple causes of mitral valve leakage. First, in contradistinction to the thick and rigid tricuspid aortic valve, the mitral valve is a bicuspid valve, which is a much more delicate heat valve that's tethered to the LV by structures (tendinous cords) that are attached the anterior and posterior papillary muscles. Mitral regurgitation can occur for four reasons: 1. Damage to the valve itself that's usually due to rheumatic heart disease. 2. The aging process with degenerative valve disease or dilatation and functional enlargement of the valve orifice with a cardiomyopathy or heart failure. 3. Rupture of one or two of the tendinous chords (chordae tendinae) with a flail or loose mitral leaflet. 4. Rupture or scarring and dysfunction of the papillary muscles, which act to pull the mitral valve closed through the tendinous cords.

In actuality, the dilation of the valve orifice and the valve is probably the most common form of mitral regurgitation and is improved by treatment of the heart failure and reduction in the enlargement of the LV. Medication such as beta blockers and ACE inhibitors can act to reduce functional mitral regurgitation and possibly forestall the need for surgery. In this form of mitral regurgitation, the surgery may not necessarily require a new valve. It involves sewing the valve structure together to reduce the leakage or to place a ring in the mitral annulus (mitral support around the valve) and reduce the size of the overall mitral orifice. Amazingly, a recent technique called the percutaneous mitral clip has been developed whereby using catheters into the LV mitral valve clips are actually placed to bond together the two mitral leaflets and lead to less functional regurgitation.

This procedure had just been approved for use, and only very specialized interventionalists have the knowledge or skill to do this technically very difficult procedure. However, in the very sick patient with class III or IV heart failure and mitral regurgitation, this can an absolutely lifesaving percutaneous procedure without the prohibitive risk of surgery. Unequivocally, this same procedure will be perfected for clipping of the tricuspid valve in the RV, which shares the same functional and structural pathology of mitral valve regurgitation.

The second most common cause of mitral regurgitation is papillary muscle rupture or dysfunction. It's a very important subject because the papillary muscles can become damaged in a heart attack and can be rendered nonfunctional, or more importantly, imminently jeopardized by ischemia and lack of blood flow. In the case of complete death of the muscle, a surgical replacement of the valve was the only option before mitral valve clipping. However, in the case of papillary muscle dysfunction due to ischemia, the patient may not necessarily have angina pectoris but significant mitral regurgitation and heart failure resulted from the muscle not contracting properly to tether closed the mitral leaflets with LV contraction.

In this instance, it'd be very critical to identify the usual small branch coronary artery that's the culprit. Thus it's critical to identify the usual small branch coronary artery that's responsible for the lack of blood supply for the jeopardized papillary muscle. The use of echocardiography with exercise can visualize and quantify the degree of mitral regurgitation. If the regurgitation increases or shows up with exercise, it's a strong indication that a coronary occlusion is the culprit for this reversible papillary muscle dysfunction. Its rather straightforward diagnosis can lead to very effective PCI in minimizing this form of functional mitral regurgitation.

Lastly, I want to revisit aortic valve surgery because aortic stenosis is a major cause of disability and death (morbidity and mortality) in patients over the age of 70. Since the 1950s, the only real option for these patients was prosthetic valve surgery. These were open heart surgeries on the bypass pump that had a very high complication and death rate, specifically in the patient older than 80 and in those patients with other diseases like COPD, severe heart failure, or renal disease with chronic kidney injury. Furthermore, as in the coronary bypass surgery, there can be significant cognitive and mental deterioration after aortic valve surgery with the added risk of cerebral emboli and a stroke during or after the procedure. Recently, a percutaneous balloon valvuloplasty was developed to open up the valve area and lessen the stenosis with minimal effectiveness. Plus, it had the complications of a stroke and bleeding with short-lived results with no permanent solution.

In the past two years, transcutaneous aortic valve replacement (TAVR) has been widely approved, which meant a true lifesaving revolution in the treatment of aortic stenosis, specifically in the elderly and patient with multiple comorbidities that couldn't be expected to survive an open heart surgery (Fig.82), (Fig.83). TAVR is a percutaneous procedure that wedges an artificial valve into the patient's native (natural) stenotic valve done in the catheterization laboratory under sedation or anesthesia. The survival rates with this procedure are just now being evaluated, but it's simply a miracle for the patient who would've had up to 50% chance of death within one year due to the severe aortic stenosis. The complication rate with TAVR is relatively low, which is a testament of modern technology and medical expertise given the dire illness of these patients.

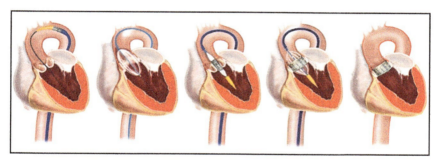

(Fig.82) (www.raneyzusman.com-Raney Zusman Medical Group) In this series of pictures, we follow a TAVR procedure. First, on the left two frames, a balloon catheter is threaded up through the aorta to the stenotic aortic valve, and the balloon is inflated in the valve in an aortic valvuloplasty to break open the valve. In the last three frames, the prosthetic aortic valve is placed and seated in the old aortic valve. This valve doesn't require anticoagulation. Since it's done mostly in the elderly, it will last their lifetime and can be lifesaving in these patients who would otherwise be dead within one year.

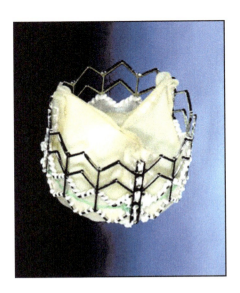

(Fig.83) (www.cathlabdigest.com) This is a picture of a TAVR aortic valve. Note, that it's a tissue valve with metal struts, which doesn't require anticoagulation to prevent clots and can usually last for the lifetime of the elderly patients who receive a TAVR.

Before we leave this discussion of valvular disease, it's important to review some of the concepts of admission status. Obviously, inpatient is always the admission status of a patient undergoing surgical valve replacement. Although obvious, it's not inconceivable that the doctor or the surgeon never writes or signs an order, which results in Medicare relegating the patient's surgery to outpatient Medicare B reimbursement and outpatient admission status. As of 2015, the consequence for the hospital payments can be very complex and put the patient or family at significant financial jeopardy. Basically, the hospital is being reimbursed as if were a simple outpatient one or two day surgery when the patient is on a ventilator in the ICU for up to 5-10 days with a bill surpassing 100,000 dollars in an aortic valve replacement! Medicare isn't designed for the patient's benefit but is to support the doctor and the hospital. It takes constant vigilance by the proactive patient and family to protect the patient rights and pocketbook. It speaks directly to the ignorance or arrogance of the attending physician or surgeon.

There's one more point to be made about the TAVR. It has become a very deleterious problem in American medicine that the patient is admitted the day before a TAVR or open heart surgery. This admission of one or two days before the surgery or procedure has been done for years and without significant consequence to the doctor, hospital, or patient. As of 2015, Medicare will be more draconian in its enforcement of new rules applying to this specific situation. Doctors will often use in their documentation that the patient is debilitated or lives too far away to come to the hospital on the day of the procedure. They will often order some cursory outpatient procedures such as a chest x-ray or echocardiogram to justify the pre-surgical hospitalization. This is considered by Medicare to be custodial care and does not warrant any admission of inpatient or observation service. Although the CMS rules are written and on the books, like any government legislation, it's always a crapshoot what Medicare rules they'll elect to enforce. It's my opinion that the TAVR justifies an inpatient admission status and the expectation of at least a two-midnight stay in the admission orders but no a one day admission before the procedure. Again, the constant vigilance by the patient and the family is in order.

PERICARDITIS AND PERICARDIAL EFFUSION

Pericarditis is an inflammation of the pericardium, the sac that surrounds the heart. The importance of the pericardium has been known since antiquity, but its exact function was not known. It's now known that the pericardium holds a small amount of fluid that actually lubricates the heart as it beats like an oil in a car's engine. The heart beats within the sac, and the outside of the heart is bathed in a thick protein fluid.

There are many causes for this structure and the fluid to become an irritant. The most important are infections of the pericardium by viruses or bacteria, uremic pericarditis in patient with kidney failure on or off dialysis, and Dressler's Syndrome that happens immediately or months after a heart attack. Further there are iatrogenic (doctor caused) forms of pericarditis after ablations or cardiac surgery.

Pericarditis can lead to increase fluid around the heart called a pericardial effusion because it's a form of irritation and inflammation. This fluid can be classified according to its composition such as water-like (serous), infections (purulent), fibrous (connective tissue), or hemorrhagic (blood). Depending on the type and the rapidity of the fluid developing, the inflammation can cause a sound in the heart called a "friction rub" that can be recognized by the cardiologist with auscultation of the heart as well as with placing his hand over the chest to find a sandpaper type of sensation on the skin. The importance of the findings is that they're a fast way of detecting pericarditis, which is one of the most frequent causes of chest pain in the ER after a heart attack or angina. If the cardiologist is unfamiliar or has lack the inexperience, they must resort to an echocardiogram for the definitive diagnosis. A quick echocardiogram in the ER or right after admission can detect the fluid to make the correct diagnosis.

The symptoms of pericarditis are principally substernal or left precordial "pleuritic" type chest pain. The pleuritic the pain is often described as a sharp scratchy pain compared to the pain of a heart attack or angina that's more of a pressure-like sensation. The pain of pericarditis classically is made worse by lying down or coughing and is significantly relieved by sitting up and leaning forward.

Most often, the pericarditis is caused by a virus and is associated with cold-like symptoms and a mild fever. Because of the similarity to the pain of a heart attack, the cardiologist must have a high suspicion for pericarditis based on his physical exam and the character of the pain before he orders an echocardiogram of the heart (Fig.85) to confirm the diagnosis and avoid the improper diagnosis of angina that may lead an emergent and unnecessary cardiac catheterization. This is compounded by the fact that there can be the immediate formation of pericardial fluid and the development of pericarditis in an acute heart attack, which makes the differential diagnosis of pericarditis even more complex and ambiguous. It's interesting to note that up to 22% of the patients who die of a heart attack will show a component of pericarditis around their hearts at autopsy as pericarditis often goes clinically unrecognized.

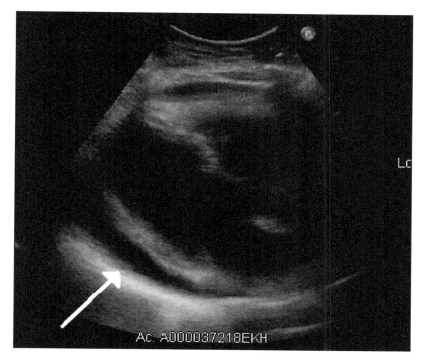

(Fig.85) (en.wikipedia.com) This is an echocardiogram of the heart with pericarditis and a pericardial effusion. I show this picture to make you all budding echocardiographers and to show you the beauty of such an amazing test. The white structure in the middle is the heart with its white echo, dense muscle filled with black echo lucent blood. The arrow is pointing both to the thickened white band around the heart, which is the thickened pericardium with inflammation, and the echo lucent white area around the heart (pericardial effusion) that can be water-like, pus-like, or blood. I want to emphasize here that a CT of the chest is not as good as actually visualizing the fluid with an echocardiogram. Even if a CT is done first, an echocardiogram is absolutely necessary; thus, a CT of the chest is redundant and mostly an excessive and expensive test.

The blood test in the ER can be confusing as the troponin levels that are increased in damaged heart muscles due to angina or a heart attack can also be elevated with pericarditis. Aside from the echocardiogram, the most useful test for pericarditis is the EKG. There are some very classical changes on the EKG, which can aid in the immediate diagnosis of pericarditis as the cause of the patient's chest pain. These are similar to that seen with a heart attack but have some subtle differences that make them extremely accurate positive findings (Fig.86).

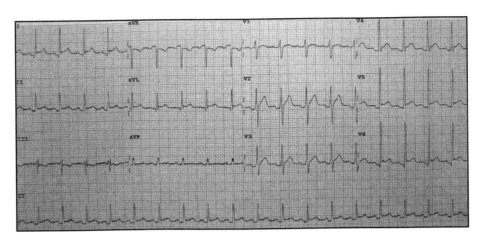

(Fig.86) (en.wikipedia.com) This is an EKG from a patient with a classical pericarditis. Note the elevation in the ST segment in all leads of the EKG except in lead aVR. This is a very accurate "pathognomonic" (definitive) finding for pericarditis and an absolute diagnosis. In lead II, the PR segment between the P wave and the QRS is actually depressed, which is another pathognomonic sign of pericarditis. Other signs that can be seen include a low voltage of the QRS if the heart becomes covered with a large pericardial effusion and the QRS voltage or size that can alternate beat to beat called appropriately "QRS alternans."

Lastly, the treatment of pericarditis can be a real challenge. Most of the time, the inflammation subsides by itself if it's viral and lasts only a few days. However, if the pain is persistent, the best treatment is the use of aspirin or a non-steroidal, anti-inflammatory agent like ibuprofen. If this is the second episode of pericarditis, then the treatment can include colchicine, which is usually a drug used to treat gout. In the persistent or severe cases, IV or oral corticosteroids can be used to treat the inflammation. If the fluid or effusion around the heart causes dysfunction of the heart called pericardial tamponade, the cardiologist may elect to place a needle guided by the echocardiogram into the pericardium to drain the fluid in a procedure called a pericardiocentesis.

In summation, pericarditis can be a very challenging diagnosis to make. The ER diagnosis of a simple viral pericarditis will often result in patient going home with aspirin for follow-up in his office as an outpatient. Unfortunately, the patient is often admitted for custodial care in a telemetry unit. In this scenario, it doesn't qualify as an inpatient admission but rather as observation services, and you should be discharged the next morning barring any complications such as the finding on a repeat echocardiogram that the pericardial effusion is markedly enlarging and becoming pericardial tamponade. If that's the case, the admission would convert to inpatient and meet the two-midnight rule of inpatient status.

SYNCOPE

This will be one of the last conditions to be covered in this book after a final review of the association of heart disease and the mind. I might've omitted something that would be of interest, but I've done my best to cover the salient cardiac conditions. After this review of syncope and mental disorders associated with premature heart disease, I'll go over some general medical situations that are plaguing the American medical system.

Syncope can lead to a very difficult and controversial discussion. Second to diastolic dysfunction, syncope is the most over or underdiagnosed condition that is used as a rationale for hospital admission and by far the least understood. There are estimates that the diagnosis of syncope accounts for 3% of Medicare ER admissions in the hospital, and more than 90% are not true syncope that require either no hospitalization or no more than observation status. A high proportion of workups could be done in an outpatient non-hospital setting. I will stress that a simple loss of consciousness can be present in up to 75% of the population while true syncope is present in 35% of patients over the age of 75 (Fig.87). In my estimate, 90% of these admissions are simply unwarranted and driven by financial incentive rather than the true practice of correct medicine.

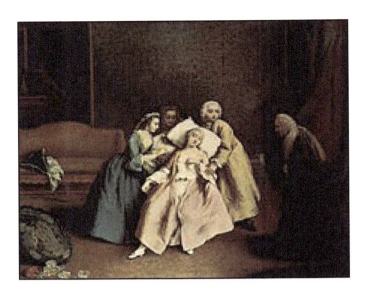

(Fig.87) (Wikipedia) This is an oil painting from 1744 called "Fainting." Fainting in women was a common occurrence in Victorian England and Europe, which was partially due to the over-tightened corsets that made it difficult to breathe. However, the overwhelmingly common cause was because it was fashionable for women to feign frailty by fainting at a particularly emotional moment and creating an attention-causing scene. This isn't too different from ending up with an inappropriate hospital admission based on the family's insistence, which is due to the ignorance of a perfectly benign phenomenon that doesn't require an acute hospitalization. Also, fainting can be due to kneeling and saying the emotional hallelujahs and amens in church, which is referred to "church syncope." However, most ER physicians just do a barrage of expensive, useless tests to justify a totally inept admission out of sheer convenience and to add to the bottom line for the doctor and the hospital's profit. (Wikipedia)

However, a true syncope is a major contributor to morbidity and mortality (disease and death) in the elderly population over 75. Prevalence and incidence (how common) figures for syncope in older adults are confounded by a very high incidence of overlap with simple falls and weakness. These patients almost always present with some physical injury such as a leg or pelvic fracture with a history of almost 100% functional dependency on outside care. The costs in the quality of life are very hard to quantify. 60% of geriatric patients in community (home) or in institutional care experience a fall or true syncope, and these events consume enormous psychological and economic expense. Within this population, one out of three will have an episode of true syncope or just falling out of sheer weakness and frailty.

True syncope as a diagnosis has three primary components: short loss of consciousness, fast onset with some brief symptoms before they pass out (prodrome), and spontaneous recovery. These three components are rarely met as most syncope diagnoses are improperly given to the patient who is found on the floor and possibly unconscious for a prolonged period of time. Under these circumstanced, the family almost universally reports that the patient is disoriented for minutes to hours. This type of presentation is not syncope but an episode of long periods of unresponsiveness or a fall with prolonged weakness and disorientation and often just a deep sleep in the elderly.

The prodrome in syncope before the true loss of consciousness can be dizziness, sweating (diaphoresis), blurred vision, nausea, and feeling flush or warm. Syncope is usually associated with some twitching of the muscles and the eyes rolling back. There are some estimates that this is attributed incorrectly to a seizure. 95% of the time, this leads to numerous, useless consults and EEGs (electroencephalograms) along with anti-seizure medicine, not to mention being branded with a diagnosis of seizures for the rest of their lives. The incorrect diagnosis of seizures can frequently lead to totally bogus disability payments. The use of electronic medical records follow the patient forever. If the government was checking the records with competent personnel, this could be appropriate. However, it's all done by computerized algorithms programmed by non-medical workers, who have no clue as to the permanent consequences of what they are doing and are directed by a government intent on having every citizen in a big medical databank for an ultimate single payer (government socialized) medical system.

Presyncope is considered same as syncope and is associated with the same prodrome but not complete loss of consciousness. In presyncope, the individual often falls to their knees but never completely loses consciousness. It's important to understand that presyncope can have the same causes as syncope and deserves to be evaluated.

The causes of syncope can range from the totally benign (no medical consequence and non-serious) to the potentially life threatening. Over 90% of syncope is benign, but the 10% that can be life threatening are of great concern. The most important is in the category of heart. These can be of the most concern and deserve the most intense investigation. However, even with the possibility of a life threatening cause of syncope, this workup in the hospital almost never meets the standard of complexity to warrant inpatient hospitalization.

The causes of this type of syncope is almost always an arrhythmia of the heart: bradycardia (too slow) such as heart block in the various levels of the conduction system, tachycardia (too fast) as in ventricular tachycardia, and irregularly such as with atrial fibrillation. One has to recognize that if the heart goes to fast or too slow, the blood supply to the brain can be decreased, leading to loss of consciousness. The reason this occurs in the heart going too fast is that the blood never has time to adequately fill and be ejected into the blood stream. At its most extreme is a full cardiac arrest; however, the precursor toward a future arrest may be a true syncopal spell predating the arrest and giving the electrophysiologist a chance to intervene before a fatal event with a possible ICD or ablation.

The primary tool in the hospital for detecting an arrhythmia is the EKG and placing the patient in a cardiac ward that has telemetry or the EKG patches one wears with an EKG machine by the bed or in a central bank of EKG machines transmitting the EKG over the airwaves. Syncope, which a transient (lasting for a short time) event, may not repeat itself in the hospital (the most common scenario), and the diagnosis will be made with outpatient follow-up at the doctor's office. The key test in this circumstance is a 24-hour EKG called a holter monitor. A longer term heart monitoring system called ambulatory arrhythmia monitoring entails wearing the transmitter that makes the EKG transmit to a satellite and a central station that monitors the heartbeat in real times, 24 hours a day, and 7 days a week. These newer technologies are remarkably effective in picking up a short-lived arrhythmia, particularly if there are symptoms like dizziness noted on the patient's log, which can then be correlated to correspond to a simultaneous arrhythmia identified on the monitor.

At the most extreme, the doctor may elect to place a loop monitor, which is machine the size of a stick of gum, under your skin in a very simple surgical procedure to store a computer chip that tracks all your heartbeats for up to two years. There are no electrodes involved as the machine simply records like electrodes hooked up to an EKG machine. The doctor is able to download the EKG beats, and if there are symptoms recorded by the patient in a diary, then the doctor has the ability to correlate the symptoms with a possible arrhythmia. Once the culprit arrhythmia is detected, such as a very slow heart rate or intermittent heart block in the conduction system, the doctor can take the appropriate steps such as a pacemaker, ablation, medicines, or ICD implant. At the same time, he can remove the loop monitor from under the skin.

If the patient has a syncopal spell and records it in his diary, the doctor will interrogate the loop monitor at the time of the event and see if there is a correlating culprit arrhythmia. If there's no heart rhythm abnormality at the time of the event, then the syncopal spells are not due to an arrhythmia but something else. If the patient has no more syncopal spells but the electrophysiologist is still concerned that the cause is an arrhythmia, then he can do an invasive electrophysiological study. Again, note that I place the electrophysiological (EP) study after the lack of success with a holter, event monitor, or an implanted loop monitor; it is the last resort, not the first line of diagnosis.

In the electrophysiological study, the electrophysiologist tests all aspects of the conduction system for impending heart block and for various arrhythmias that he can induce with the electrodes to correlate it to the syncopal spells. Thus, under most circumstances, the EP study is not the first test to be done. One exception is if the patient is found to have a low EF that is less than 35%. In this instance, the probability is high that a malignant type of arrhythmia such as ventricular tachycardia that has the potential of a cardiac arrest and death can be unmasked. The electrophysiologist would most likely place an ICD after an EP study. I must stress again, that the EP study, in no circumstance that I can envision, is to be done before the monitoring techniques in a patient with a normal EF.

Many electrophysiologists will elect to do an EP study on the first admission for syncope. This is absolutely contraindicated (should not be done), and Medicare may elect not to reimburse as they see it to be inappropriate as first line interventional procedure. The patient and the family, especially the patient over 80, must be very vigilant to this pattern of behavior and make sure that the electrophysiologist takes the time to outline his reasoning to do the test as a first line intervention rather than proceed to the appropriate outpatient monitoring. In a very common scenario, he may elect to place an implantable loop monitor, which may very well be an appropriate first step during the first hospitalization.

A very last ditch effort to unravel the cause of the syncopal spell may be a cardiac catheterization to determine whether or not there's an underlying coronary artery disease even if the patient has absolutely no chest pain. Many studies show that the incidence of coronary artery disease in the patient with a normal EF is less than 3%. Given this statistic, it seems irrational to initially do a cardiac catheterization especially before a stress test. Even in the face of a minimally positive stress test, it's an abuse of the system and should be strongly discouraged, especially in the patient with no chest pain. If the patient has a strong history of typical chest pains consistent with angina, it may be appropriate to do a cardiac catheterization in light of a positive stress test. Nevertheless, a treadmill and cardiac catheterization can all be done as an outpatient and not necessarily during the initial hospital stay for syncope. It could be denied by Medicare review as excessive and unrelated as it has no proven or documented relationship to the syncopal spell.

The second broad category of causes of syncope is blood vessel related reflexes known as neutrally medicated causes of loss of consciousness. This is a common cause of syncope and is based on the response of blood vessels and the blood pressure to various scenarios such a simple faint with a sudden drop in blood pressure and heart rate which is called vasovagal syncope. The most common type of faint in this situation is when the patient purposefully closes their throats and bears down. This causes an increase pressure in the lungs and activates a reflex called the Bezold reflex described in 1860 about animals that faint to mimic death as a defense mechanism under attack. In humans, this is frequently done by women to gain attention and is a harbinger of significant psychological diseases. There's an inordinate amount of psycho-neurological causes of syncope seen in the younger population versus the older population who have comorbities or risk factors associated with true pathological syncope.

In younger individuals, the treatment is to explain to the patient the mechanism of the faint, discuss causes of anxiety or fear, and optimize salt intake. Psychological counseling may be in order especially those who repeatedly come to the ER with a totally benign and psychologically related fainting spell. It's extremely important but regularly ignored fact that the general practitioner and the psychological team should work closely together for those patients. Many of these episodes are in response to needles, blood, dead bodies, simple perceived anxiety, or an expression of the Bezold normal reflex. With the added patient load now seen with Obamacare, these simple and time-consuming interventions will not be forthcoming and may lead to repeat of inappropriate and totally unnecessary hospital admissions.

Valvular diseases such as aortic and mitral stenosis are the most common cause of syncope with disease of the valves. Again, a simple complete history and physical exam for a pathological murmur are all that's needed but rarely done in the ER. The doctor frequently resorts to expensive technology and useless in-hospital admissions when the diagnosis and tests can be done as an outpatient basis without expensive hospitalizations. The importance of this diagnosis, especially in the elderly with a high incidence of aortic stenosis, is that syncope can be the first sign of a high-risk situation that can lead to death if untreated.

The formation of a clot in the pulmonary artery called a pulmonary embolism can cause a syncopal spell, and again, it can be sign of a significant pathology. This is a diagnosis that can be ascertained by a history and physical in 99% of the cases and substantiated by resorting to a CT of the lungs. The problem is that many times CTs of the lungs are done to rule out a pulmonary embolism in a patient with syncope when there is absolutely no clinical findings but is often done out of reflex by the ER or attending physician to avoid being accused of missing a diagnosis (WIGGS syndrome).

In general, faints triggered by true cardiac or pulmonary structural disease are very important to recognize as they can be a warning of potentially life-threatening conditions if the patients are prone to either reflex hypotension or bradycardia. Other important structural causes of syncope is hypertrophic cardiomyopathy (IHSS) and acute dissection of the aorta usually seen the elderly with a history of a known aneurysm picked up on a previous screening sonogram and accompanied by hypertension or profound hypotension at its acute stage.

An important but very rare structural situation causing syncope is vertebro-basilar arterial disease in the brain, which is arterial disease in the upper spinal cord or lower brain that causes recurrent dizziness and a true syncopal spell. This is a pure diagnosis that can be made in the majority of time by a medical student and a complete history. Nevertheless, it is remarkably uncommon and is the cause of syncope in less than 1/1000 cases of syncope. Yet, it's most under or over-diagnosed simply due to the lack of experience and knowledge. Often, the attending has not seen or been trained properly with appropriate years of experience, and this diagnosis is made incidentally (by accident) with further expensive testing such as an MRI of the brain. Probably, in 99% of cases that present with false or true syncope to the ER, the doctor or attending hospitalist will order a carotid echo and a CT of the head. The reality is that it that there is no mechanism for isolated carotid disease to cause syncope.

The use of CT scans can detect old or new strokes, but a stroke that doesn't cause brain stem or lower brain injury isn't a cause for true syncope but just weakness or prolonged lethargy and not quickly reversible loss of consciousness often by a seizure. So, the use of CT scanning and carotid ultrasound as initial tests as substitute for a good history and physical is not recommend by the guidelines of the American College of Neurology. Nevertheless, these tests are routinely done in nearly 100% of patients out of the fear of lawsuits and the desire of the doctor to "kill the ant with an atomic bomb" rather than take a knowledgeable and proper approach. Not to belabor a point, but this behavior is now the norm partially as a result of the lack of enough doctors with proper training and the time to see the patient accompanied by the WIIGS syndrome.

This apparent abuse of the system with syncope is primarily by these corporate physicians needing to add to their quota and metrics of ordered tests. The money made from these tests is justified for the corporation as paying for the initial expense of buying the CT scanner with the knowledge that they can simply get away with such egregious behavior.

Since 2014, 95% of these attending hospitalists ordering these tests have only one year of specialty training and are not board certified. They only have passed the American Boards, and in most cases, they're too culturally challenged to approach advanced American patients and medicine. Additionally, many of these doctors have a deep seeded-intolerance to American behavior and demands, and hospitals are now starting to operate on a third-world level. Furthermore, the doctor has become a low-paid technician rather than the highly trained and well-reimbursed individual, who is respected as part of the culture and community and who acts as a physician and counselor with the proper adherence to modern American standards of care. I sincerely hope this book has taught you to be a proactive patient who approaches and demands their proper cardiological care.

There are multiple benign syndromes associated with this vascular and neurally mediated forms of syncope that can be ascertained by a proper history and never requires in-hospital admissions and certainly not inpatient versus observation level of care. Most of these syndromes fall under the umbrella as vasovagal syncope or simple faints. One includes cough syncope associated with a chronic cough such as seen in a smoker or patient with the flu. It includes deglutination syncope seen when one gets food caught in their throats and bears down. Another category is micturition (urination) and defection syncope when the patient goes to the bathroom or is walking to the bathroom with a full bladder or rectal vault.

Another includes church syncope when the individual gets up from kneeling or is taken up in the emotions of the sermon. One other includes alcohol, which aside from making you drunk and pass out, the alcohol stimulus to the stomach may induce syncope lasting only seconds. Lastly, and most importantly, there are a variety of emotional triggers such as anxiety, family death, being at a funeral, and embarrassing or uneasy situations. The common thread of all these benign syndromes is that they all can be ascertained by a brief history and never warrant a CT of the head or a carotid ultrasound, and rarely warrant even a brief hospital admission.

Nevertheless, some estimates show 90% of these patients are not only admitted but never counseled as to the true nonthreatening nature of their episodes, which would go a long way to patient education and prevent useless repeat ER visits and expense. Again, the primary driving force behind this behavior is the WIIGS syndrome as well as the demands of the increasing culture of entitlement of the patient, which is fostered and perpetuated by our government at the highest levels.

Furthermore, most of these patients could benefit from at least some psychological treatment, but this is precluded by some low cost insurance policies and is not initiated by the doctor who often is culturally and professionally hindered. At least in America, there are some very progressive private insurance carriers such as United Healthcare and Blue Cross, which truly comprehend the importance of psychological care and are vigorously intent on preventing absolutely useless hospital admissions. I feel that if enforced, the new Medicare rules as of 2015, which will not pay the physician or consultant for inappropriate and unqualified care or admissions, but will go a long way to stop this fragrant abuse. Unfortunately, many regulations in the government go unenforced and are just window dressings to appear as if there is serious approach to the problem.

Thirdly, a basket of syncope can be classified as orthostatic syncope. This may be the most common form of syncope in the elderly and those with long standing diabetes. A combination of malnutrition with low salt intake, abnormal mechanisms to maintain vascular tone, and the ability to maintain sufficient blood pressure and blood flow to the brain lead to syncope upon sitting or standing. This is defined as greater than a 20 mm. of mercury in one's blood pressure when going from the lying or standing position to standing. Additionally, it's positive if the patient passes out or feels very dizzy when they stand. This is a very common mechanism in the frail or demented patient, who doesn't eat or drink enough food and with a low salt intake. Plus, orthostatic hypotension can become a reason that when an old person is found on the floor, they cannot get up or maintain an upright position.

The diagnosis of orthostatic hypotension is relatively easily made in the emergency room with a good history. Often, the paramedics, if called to the home for syncope, will make a special point due to their superb training to take postural blood pressure readings and report them to the ER. Nevertheless, it's simply remarkable that the orthostatic or postural blood pressure readings are either ignored or not repeated in the ER or by the attending. They're simply not done on a routine basis even though the history is that the patient is consistently passing out when they stand up!

It's far more common for the physician to proceed with a head CT, EKG, chest X-ray, carotid ultrasound, and even a head MRI before they finally decide to measure orthostatic blood pressure readings. I've been in medical practice for over 30 years, and it never ceases to amaze me in the stupidity of ordering over $20,000 dollars' worth of test when a simple BP check would've sufficed to make the diagnosis orthostatic hypotension. In this respect, it's not uncommon for the patient to be in the hospital 2 or 3 days before some highly trained board certified neurologists makes the suggestion that it may be appropriate to do orthostatic BP readings in a way not to offend the intelligence of the referring attending physician who failed to do simple vital signs on standing and is a source of many of his referral cases.

The bottom line is that the diagnosis of true syncope doesn't require inpatient hospitalization greater than two days in the overall majority of cases or even any hospital admission in the first place. It is especially important for the patient and the family of the elderly patient with advanced dementia to be diligent to misdiagnosis and the inappropriate use of advanced and expensive technology.

Lastly, before we leave syncope, I want to touch upon a very common clinical situation, which has become an occurrence of an ever-growing rate with epidemic proportions in the American medical system. An elderly, and often progressively demented patient, is brought to the ER for being found on the floor or altered mental status and weakness with prolonged episodes of passing out. I must emphasize that the majority of ER and attending physicians use the diagnosis of syncope to justify hospital admission in these patients. However, this isn't syncope as it isn't immediately reversible and is 99% of the time a result of severe weakness, dehydration, malnutrition, possible chronic urinary tract infection, and progressive dementia. In these patients, we see prolonged episodes of loss of consciousness or severe episodic disorientation and weakness. However, the real problem is that the family just can't care for their elderly parent. The family often is unaware of ancillary services such as home health care and would prefer that their loved one enter a nursing home or long-care facility.

The catch 22 is that if the doctor decides to admit the patient to the hospital, the only way Medicare will pay for a rehabilitation facility if there's a three-day inpatient hospital stay. As in syncope, these patients, at best, require a short-term infusion of fluids and physical therapy. They rarely, if ever, meet the level of inpatient services and don't require a three-day hospitalization. Yet, the families are often very insistent, and these patients usually become a pure social problem admitted for only custodial care. The families are simply unprepared and can no longer care for their spouse or parent and afford long term care.

There is some reasoning to this rule. It's to prevent the system from becoming overwhelmed by elderly patients, who need to be cared for by the families rather than in nursing homes. In other western societies, and certainly in eastern societies, there is a strong commitment in caring for the elderly as their cultures dictate. In America, there is no apparent forethought or resources to accommodate the elderly and the desire to make it someone else's problem. To be very honest, it may be discovered that there has been an acute stroke, and the patient may be a candidate for appropriate acute rehabilitation care. However, it's a rare exception, and if the patient is wrongly placed as an inpatient, and the patient subsequently placed in a rehabilitation facility, and the admission is subsequently denied by Medicare, the money for the rehabilitation services may need to be recouped from the family as of 2015. In this respect we are talking of thousand of dollars per day.

I frankly do not know the answer or solution to this recurring situation. The doctor is faced with a social problem who never should've been admitted in the first place but rather a patient that cannot care for themselves. Medicare does wisely pay for comprehensive home health services, but that requires a spouse or parent to be home but be able to perform basic supportive services for the patient such as simple feeding, drinking, and taking to the bathroom. In many of these cases, the families insist their loved one needs to be in the hospital and becomes indignant or hostile. The hospital has no choice but to give the patient a HINN letter, which states that Medicare will no longer pay for the hospitalization. So, the family may become responsible for the subsequent charges that can range in the thousands per day. This is the unfortunate reality of growing old in America where it seems the responsibility of one's care is passed on to someone else ion this destructive age of entitlement only perpetuated by the sheer ignorance and possibly greed of our leaders.

THE HEART AND THE MIND

This will be the last subject I'll cover in this book, but I saved it for last as it may be the most important but least understood aspect of cardiological care. There's no doubt that the majority of doctors, cardiologists, and electrophysiologists are ignorant of this strong association and don't offer the appropriate psychological support to their patients. At least, there is an attempt in this country to give the patients a letter at the end of their hospitalization explaining their procedures that were done and the long-term implications of their illness. However, these summaries fail to delve into the emotional or life-altering implications of their disease and fall short of giving the patients a comprehensive assessment of their illness. Additionally, most specialists and the busy hospitalists will not take the time to sit down and have a frank discussion with the patient about the life changing and emotional implications of their disease.

One reason for writing this book was to convey the knowledge to make you understand your treatment and allay some of the anxiety that invariably accompanies cardiological illness. Much of what I write in this section has been supplemented by ideas of a very good friend and physician, Dr. Claire Friend, who has kindly allowed me to share many of her ideas. She was a practicing physician and is now a psychiatrist, who has a keen understanding of the direct relationship of the patient's psychological state and the development of significant heart disease. Although this is the least understood aspect of cardiology by your treating cardiologist, the advent of remarkable new antidepressant drugs has given them and psychiatrists the tools to alter the relentless progression of heart disease associated with psychological dysfunction, specifically in the patients' invariable difficulty in altering their lifestyle to prolong their lives.

Before I introduce some history, it must be understood that 75% of chronic schizophrenics or patients with severe depression die before the age of 55 years of heart disease, diabetes, or cancer. This is a staggering number and suggests a very strong relationship of psychological disease with overt physical heart disease such as premature coronary disease with subsequent death from heart attacks and sudden cardiac death as well as severe congestive heart failure. Interestingly, these patients are totally ill-prepared to properly care for themselves and be compliant with medicines or the appropriate subsequent complex and intense medical care because of their severe psychological illnesses. Thus, they die prematurely without the aid of modern cardiological interventions and without lifestyle changes necessary to for simple control of their diabetes, high cholesterol, or blood pressure.

Also, an inordinate amount of these patients smoke cigarettes for relaxation and are unable or unwilling to stop. In many of these patients, smoking may offer their only avenue for some assemblance of a happy lifestyle. This problem is compounded by the fact that the doctor doesn't recognize these psychological problems in their patients. Without proper referral to a psychiatrist, the appropriate drug intervention is never initiated. With the knowledge of this book, a proactive patient or family will hopefully recognize such illness as severe depression after a heart attack and seek the proper psychological interventions.

Next, Schleifer (Archives of Internal Medicine, 1989) observed that minor depression occurred in 27% of patients after a myocardial infarction, and major depression occurs in 18%. What is truly remarkable is that in 2003, the ENRICH Heart Disease study revealed that SSRI treatment drugs for clinical depression and generalized anxiety (selective serotonin re-uptake inhibitors such as Paxil, Celexa, Zoloft, Lexapro, and Latuda) actually reduce the long-term death rate in post infarction patients with depression by a remarkable 44%. These numbers are extremely important as it has been shown by Ahern (Ahern, American Journal of Cardiology, 1999) that there's a 20 fold increase in overall death and cardiac arrest at one year post myocardial infarction in depressed patients. These are truly shocking numbers and simply attest to the physiological association of emotion and the heart.

This association is not really surprising as I've mentioned the remarkable observation by the ancient Chinese and Greeks that there was a strong emotional component to premature death by disease, which we now know to be coronary heart disease and cardiac arrhythmias. In Chinese philosophy, "xin" can refer to one's disposition or feelings, and it also has been translated to refer to the physical heart—thus the "heart-mind" association. In ancient Chinese medicine and the Suwen, or book of Plain Questions, the heart is associated with "fire and joy," and the physicians observed that these elements are related to heart palpitations and death. In the Suwen, it's said that "by striving to balance their the organ related to the person's emotional state the emotion can be balanced as well, and vice versa…this can relieve the symptoms." One must remember that these observations predate modern medicine by over 2,500 years, and one cannot help to be in awe at the remarkable wisdom, patience, and observational powers of these ancient physicians. I must stress again that these astute observations cannot be made in a cursory five-minute exam by a modern doctor, but it takes time and continual follow-up by a well-trained physician who has a familiarity with American culture to make these associations and the diagnosis of emotional disease and prevent the deterioration of the American medical system to that of a third world country.

Some modern Chinese writers feel that the practice of acupuncture was for physical and emotion health started more than 4,000 years ago (2000 B.C.E.). In actuality, the ancient philosophers, as recorded in ancient cave petroglyphs, felt that acupuncture started in the Stone Age when the Shaman used sharp stones to rupture abscesses and relieve pain! Nevertheless, the first recorded practice of acupuncture was 2,000 years ago in the Nei Ching Su Wen treatise where acupuncture is described as bringing health from disease. To this day, acupuncture has actually been shown to be effective in the treatment of cardiac arrhythmias. In this respect, some have demonstrated that acupuncture effects coronary artery disease due to specific concentration on the emotional state following a heart attack.

Now, back to modern times. William Harvey described the circulatory system but further proposed some revolutionary links between the mind and the heart. He notes that, "The mind, spirit, and emotion cause physical changes in the body sometimes causing death." He further writes, "I was acquainted with another strong man…who had suffered an injury and affront…and was so overcome by passion and spite…that at last he fell into a strange distemper, and suffering from extreme pain in the heart and the breast…in the course of a few years…became tabid and died." Modern medicine strongly makes the association of how stress can cause heart attacks, and how the heart attack itself can cause more stress and anxiety. In the man described by Harvey, he obviously developed angina pectoris and died of a heart attack. In De mutu cordis (1628), Harvey further wrote, "every affection of the mind… is the cause of agitation whose influence extends to the heart."

Later, Sir William Osler (Lancet 1910) made the observation that work and worry are major causes of heart disease. He reported the syndrome of irritable hearts often seen in soldiers returning from war, which was associated with a heightened emotional state that he felt caused heart arrhythmias. Perhaps, Osler's greatest contribution to medicine was the creation of the medical residency for further clinical training in the hospital after medical school and his insistence that "students learn from seeing and talking to patients." Again, back to the recurrent theme of the doctor taking time to examine and talk to the patient which is utterly lacking in American medicine. The hospitalist admitting 10 new patients in a day and rounding on 20 to 30 patients barely would have 5 minutes per patient for examination, analysis, and discussion.

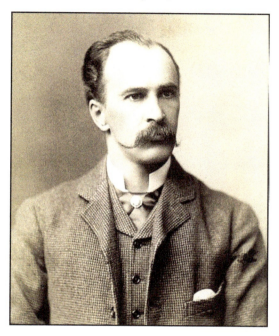

(Fig.) Sir William Osler circa 1880 (Wikipedia)

Next, and in my opinion, the most important point is that Dr. Bernard Lown (American Journal of Cardiology, 1977) made the monumental observation that sudden cardiac death is triggered by emotion. We now know that sudden intense emotion, specifically in women, can trigger a heart attack of a particular type called Takatsubo's Syndrome that can lead to sudden severe weakening of the LV, and in 12% of the patients, sudden death. In the prolonged QT syndrome, there are various genetic types that have specific emotional stimuli that can cause a cardiac arrest: emotional upheaval, an alarm clock ringing, jumping in cold water, door bells, and telephone ringing.

He made the remarkable observation that the threshold for ventricular fibrillation or sudden cardiac death (fibrillation threshold) was raised 50% in animals with increased levels of serotonin in their brain tissue. This 50% rise in the fibrillation threshold simply means it's 50% harder to have a cardiac arrest with increased brain levels of serotonin. Due to this observation, we now know that brain serotonin levels in humans are reduced in depression, and the SSRI medicines raises the amount of brain serotonin by blocking the metabolic breakdown of serotonin in the brain, raising the fibrillation threshold as observed by Lown. In this respect, in patients with ICDs, it's a very common occurrence that there are appropriate shocks to abort sudden cardiac death during high stress or emotion situations. The problem is that with more shocks increase in results in a cascade of arrhythmias causing what is called a "storm" of ICD shocks.

Interestingly, it has been repeatedly shown that patients with an ICD for prevention of sudden cardiac death often develop anxiety disorders and clinical depression. This can be easily explained by the simple fact that they're on a constant activation of their nervous system in the anticipation of a shock and sudden death. This has been found to be particularly frequent in the patient with an ICD, who has had repeated shocks in the past with their ICD and are constantly vigilant in the expectation of another shock. These patients suffer from extreme depression in a form of post-traumatic stress disorder (PTSD) and are unable to get a restful night's sleep due to their heightened vigilance, resulting in the lack of REM sleep and dreaming. Unfortunately, the doctor often simply puts the patient on medicines such as Xanax, Ativan, Valium, or Ambien to sedate the patient rather than a frank discussion and referral to a psychologist.

Interestingly, these sedative agents only compound the emotional problems because they mask them as well as increase the depression and blunt active dreaming. It leads to the development of lifelong physical drug dependency and concomitant dire implications. It's very important to realize that many of the private insurance companies such as United Heath and Blue Cross have comprehensive behavior therapy coverage. However, the cardiologist must be aware of the problem and must have the appropriate attitude to refer the patient for proper therapy. Unfortunately, this foresight on the part of the doctor is a rarity.

Additionally, it has been shown that very high levels of serotonin in the blood stream can cause valvular disease and fibrosis. Some patients taking weight-loss medications that markedly raised serotonin levels in the body and subsequently developed severe tricuspid and mitral valvular disease. At the same time, it was observed that lower levels of serotonin had the protective effect of reducing glucose in diabetics and cholesterol, which delayed development of coronary artery disease without the negative effects on valvular dysfunction. Also, etiological with the observation of prevalence (how common) studies demonstrated that there's a fourfold increase in CAD in otherwise healthy patients with depression. It was documented that with clinical depression, there is a 3-5 times increase of medium and long-term death due to progressive coronary artery disease with heart failure and sudden cardiac death.

Of equal importance was that treatment of depression had a direct lowering effect on the mortality in CAD. In post-acute myocardial infarction male patients with depression or socially isolated after their heart attack, the ENRICH study (Taylor, Archives of General Psychology, 2005) demonstrated that the group treated with antidepressants had a 43% lower risk of recurrent non-fatal heart attacks than those who were not treated. This is truly a staggering number and suggests very strongly that serotonin itself has a direct beneficial effect against the progression of coronary artery disease.

Similarly, the incidence of depressed patients going the ER for chest pain is significantly greater than the normal person. For this reason, there may be an overestimate of significant post MI recurrent heart attacks because with increased detection, these false chest pains may actually turn out to be a recurrent but often insignificant small heart attack. The sensitivity of blood test for even a minor heart attack has been shown to lead to inappropriate hospital admission for minor chest pain that is diagnosed as a clinical heart attack but is actually a reflection of stable angina. These chest pains are not a true heart attack in the sense of new heart damage but just a stunning of the myocardium. The bottom line is that depression leads to a component of paranoia regarding even minor chest pains, and the lifestyle of the patient is negatively affected and can cause a destruction of the family and social fabric. Thus, this further suggests the need for aggressive therapy of the depression with pharmacological and psychological intervention.

As I've said, the major insurance companies are keenly aware of the need in these patients for a psychiatric visit to reduce the costs of recurrent inappropriate hospitalizations and are very generous and liberal in their medical coverage for behavioral disease. However, this coverage is only afforded if the cardiologist orders and documents the appropriate need for psychiatric intervention. Unfortunately, in the majority of cases, this result can only be achieved by the proactive patient, who demands appropriate psychological diagnosis and referral. More often than not, the doctor is simply ill-informed and has no interest in the strong and well-proven relationship to heart attack with the mind. Although the doctor may seem offended by the patient taking proactive action, this behavior is a reflection of the physician not wanting to recognize or reveal his obvious lack of knowledge and his own limitations. Thus, it may take some persistence by the proactive family and patient to achieve the appropriate psychological referral without a fear of offending the doctor.

The bottom line is that the doctor must think about mood disorders in all chronic and acute cardiac illness. The cardiologist or electrophysiologist must think about depressive illness when their patient reports undue fatigue, poor appetite, failure to thrive, poor sleep habits, anger, a marriage in jeopardy, and non-specific aches and pains, 'I'm not my old self." Plus, the patient must seek help if they are unable to stop smoking and start to miss work for nonspecific illness. This lack of the ability to stop smoking, which is so common in these patients, should be a red flag for intervention and recognition of psychological illness and clinical depression. Furthermore, and especially in the case of patients with an ICD, the doctor must recognize the marked association of stress and depression with the increased risk of sudden death and initiate the appropriate interventions such as psychiatric consultation and SSRI treatment.

Lastly, I think the point to take home for the proactive patient with coronary artery disease and angina pectoris or a heart attack is that depression is very common with heart disease, and going untreated can lead to early death and progression of disease. The unfortunate reality is due to most cardiologists, and especially electrophysiologists, relying more upon coronary interventions and an ICD for treatment rather than the proper recognition of the underlying depression. If the patient complains of minor aches and pains, the cardiologist would initiate further testing for coronary artery disease progression and even another angiogram instead of properly recognizing depression as the cause of the non-specific and often unrelenting pains.

Thus, it's up to the patient and family to have the knowledge to direct their own therapy for depression. It's important to seek the help of a psychiatrist for pharmacological (medicines) treatment after your hospitalization, but if you feel very depressed in the hospital after a heart attack or CABG, ask your physician to see a psychiatrist before discharge. Then you will immediately be placed on the proper therapy as the dictum "silence is deadly" does more harm than good by perpetuating the depression. It's truly important if you're in the hospital having survived a cardiac arrest or having an appropriate shock with your ICD. The treatment for depression is absolutely critical for simple preservation of your sanity. If you're in the coronary care unit and don't have the opportunity to speak with the doctor, speak to the nurses as they generally have a much more open ear and will subsequently communicate concerns for your psychological dysfunction to the doctor.

CONCLUSION AND SUMMATION

I guess now is the time to take some literary license to add some important concepts and observations. Hopefully, by now, it's obvious that the medical system in America is totally dysfunctional and progressively becoming worse. It's my hope that I've taught the readers to be proactive patients who know how to deal with this broken system and obtain what was once considered the best and most advanced medical care in the world. In my opinion, the free enterprise system in this country resulted in the former excellence of our once top medical system. It's the misdirected interference of the government imposing their ill-advised attempts to control the system with artificial constraints and to keep a sham of universal coverage that is daily eroding the excellence of our medical care.

Before I proceed with offering some solutions to reverse the decline in our health system within the present established institutions, I must reiterate and point out the unfortunate reality of the Affordable Care Act (Obamacare). There's absolutely no ambiguity that there is unequivocal destructive intent of the law. There is no doubt that the changes brought on by Obamacare have jeopardized the life and well-being of the elderly and chronically ill at the expense of affording inexpensive coverage for the previously uninsured young population. It's my feeling that the private insurance companies have embraced the edicts of Obamacare simply because it's the only "game in town" even at the expense of inevitable loss of profit. It has to be remembered that medicine in America became the most advanced on the planet under free enterprise, not a socialistic universal system.

Medical care is rationed in almost all the socialistic universal health care systems in the world, and it has become a reality in America now. However, under the oppressive mandates and a result of Universal care, it's inevitable that rationing of medical care will become a necessity just to accommodate the increase physical demands and financial burden of this system of mandatory coverage. To simply compound the situation, this coverage is coerced by the punishment of a large financial penalty. Mind you, this is no different from how you force a two-year-old to obey your will with a threat of punishment for undesired behavior. This legislation is simply coercive to the most immature of levels and assumes that the public will just eventually acquiesce to such a system of their immature sense of entitlement.

For example, Obamacare offers inexpensive Bronze and Silver plans for medical coverage that are cheap and often government subsidized to attract the younger and poorer consumer. However, in order to be affordable, the prescription plan of all insurance companies, including those for the elderly under Medicare, have simply gone to a draconian switch involving increased cost-sharing. The healthcare overhaul bars insurers from denying coverage to people with prior illness. In the same breath, the Department of Health and Human Services said in a statement (Reuters Feb. 28, 2014) that the law does nothing to cap these patients' out-of-pocket expenses.

To make matters worse, there has not been one individual in this country who has not seen an exponential rise in their insurance deductible and prescription costs. The law caps the out-of-pocket expense for the young and elderly by capping these expenses at $12,700 for a family such as an elderly couple. As the young don't use many prescriptions, this is an onerous, if not feasible, expense for the elderly and chronically ill. To compound matters, in order for the insurance companies to simply remain viable, the costs of medicines have risen more than 300%, and the out-of-pocket deductibles for medicines has risen from "10% to 50%" according to Brian Rosen, senior vice president for public policy at the Leukemia and Lymphoma Society in a study commissioned to analyze Obamacare.

In the past, the patient could pay for his medicines over a year's time. Under these new plans, the patients will pay their $12,700, out-of-pocket expense in the first month that will force the majority of the elderly to give up their medicine or food. This bait and switch is often done by changing the tier classification of a drug. There are a multitude of Medicare HMO prescription plans in Las Vegas that changed insulin from a tier one to a tier-6 drug overnight. Since tier-6 drugs include specialized chemotherapeutic agents, the cost of insulin went up from $20 a month to $600 a month. In most cardiology patients, the cost of the new blood thinning agents for those with stents or atrial fibrillation went up more than 1,000%, and in many cases, they went up to thousands of dollars per month, which the patient is supposed to pay 50% of the cost-sharing proportion.

Although the chronically and elderly ill cannot be denied coverage, they simply cannot afford the medicines that can cost more than 100% of their incomes. Thus, the worthless promises of Obamacare are nothing less than hollow lies at the expense of the ever growing chronically-ill, elderly patients. As far as I'm concerned all those responsible for Obamacare are simply deceitful in their behavior and should be held accountable as Obamacare is the most destructive piece of medical legislation since the beginning of democracy, which is unfair to the poor, sick, and elderly. In reality because the elderly must often eat at the expense of not taking their medications, Obamacare is in one sense is simply killing the elderly and the poor. Not to seem overly dramatic, the elderly and poor go into Medicare and Obamacare with the expectation of medical care but are essentially exterminated as they must chose between eating and food and as a result die in droves off their medications in the hospital of stroke, heart attacks, and diabetic coma. You can bet the government does not keep statistics of this stark reality.

To make matters worse, the rising atmosphere of entitlement is simply overwhelming the system, and there's no doubt this will soon lead to rationing of medical care. As I have said, entitlement simply breaks the fabric of society. Rationing of medical care is already being seen in the VA system simply out of sheer patient neglect and is now leading to an almost arbitrary triaging of patients by the computer to see who is rendered the most immediate medical care. It's completely conceivable, which has occurred in almost all socialistic universal health care systems in most civilized countries, there will now be rationing of medical care based on age and need for pacemakers, CABG, PCI, stents, ICDs, transplants, LVADs, and ablations. This reality is a certainty, and the government will have no other options to cover the tide of new and rising health care demand with inadequate infrastructure, such as doctors, to handle the load. Thus, the universal coverage under a socialistic system will degenerate to denial of care to selected populations.

Before I proceed to some solutions, I'd like to mention those who argue that all this is the fault of the insurance companies. The reality is that private free enterprise health care has created our modern healthcare system. Many of these measures by insurance companies have been forced by the restrictions of Obamacare and threaten the viability of private health coverage. In my opinion, the most insidious aim of Obamacare is to actually place private insurance carriers out of business and switch to a totally one-payer government medical system. Thus, this would be the absolute in a socialist medical heath care system and would only open up the flood gates for "Big Brother Medicine" to completely control your medical care and lead to rationing of medical care by the bureaucracy rather than free choice. This country was founded on democracy, not on the oppression of an almost dictatorial socialistic system. We are a country of liberty, not of domination, which is the precise agenda of the present United States leaders when it comes to the freedom to choose appropriate and fair medical care.

However, rather than simply berate the system in this final chapter, I would like to suggest some very effective and rather logical ways to fix the system before it is irreversibly destroyed. Usually with any government, there are rules and regulations already on the books to alleviate and fix the situation, but they're simply not enforced or ignored in deference to new ideas that do nothing to fix the situation other than bring the writer of the new idea to public prominence and in the limelight as I feel the aim of Obamacare to create a legacy.

The most important endpoint is that the end game of delivery of medical care lies in the physician. All the bureaucracy, forms, computers, and support can never substitute for the physician but only act as secondary support for the end game and the actual delivery of medical care to the patient. The CEO of the hospital may run the business, but the doctors deliver and implement the proper care. The real problem develops in that as the amount of patient load has increased, and the threat of malpractice continues.

The doctor simply has become a technician with no time to converse with the patient and indiscriminately ordering a multitude of unnecessary tests to cover all contingencies and to assuage the uninformed patient, who feel they're entitled. This is irrespective of whether it has anything to do with the present diagnosis. Although one can argue that affording universal health coverage as proposed by legislatures is well intentioned. However this is resulting in complete destruction of our excellent medical system and a plague of inappropriate death to the elderly and poor, and which is now offering both substandard and remarkably expensive care.

Let us now examine four most remarkable statistics. The National Health Expenditure Accounts (NHEA) are the official estimates of total health care spending in the United States. (cms.gov). Dating back to 1960, the NHEA measures the total cost of health care in the United States including heath care goods and health care delivery, which are broken down to hospitalizations and procedures, insurance costs, government administration, and investments related to health care.

U.S. healthcare spending grew 3.6% in 2013, reaching 2.9 trillion dollars or $9,255 for every American. It's estimated that up to 40% of this money is spent on cardiological care! 2.9 trillion dollars and is equal to 17.4% of the nation's Gross Domestic Product. To put this in perspective, the United States, no different from a household, spent nearly 20% of all the money it made on healthcare in 2013. If your income is $100,000, then you would pay $20,000 on healthcare after taxes. Under the financial burdens of the Affordable Care Act, it's estimated that the cost of healthcare in America will rise 5-6% per year due to the subsidies to the uninsured in addition to the marked increase in their deductibles to those already insured.

This brings us to the second and what I feel to be another important two statistics that are the key to completely reversing not only the rise in medical costs but the dysfunction of the overall American medical system. This whole book has been aimed at giving the proactive patient the knowledge to receive the timely and proper care that avoids many of the pitfalls of the defensive medicine where doctors order inappropriate tests mainly out of the WIIGS syndrome. In an astounding study by Jackson Healthcare (jacksonhealthcare.com), an independent poll of doctors found that 92% of the physicians surveyed said they practiced some form of defensive medicine. As a cardiologist for 30 years, I can personally attest to that number as accurate. This is compounded by the fact that the physician is taught that they have to practice some form of defensive medicine to prevent frivolous lawsuits in every medical school and residency.

This form of medical practice is called "rule out medicine" rather than true "diagnostic medicine" in that they order many unnecessary and often dangerous procedures out of fear they will miss a diagnosis or be accused of delaying diagnosis and care with the perceived negative medical outcome for the patient. This is exactly the motivation for taking the patient with chest pain for an immediate heart catheterization before tying even a nuclear treadmill when medical therapy would suffice. To make matters worse, the majority of doctors surveyed responded that they also did the exact reverse often out of fear of adverse consequences of a test such as a cardiac catheterization when it's truly indicated. The doctor in fear of retribution would not order the test with increased risk of a complication.

Thus, this ill-health of the medical system works both ways, which are equally detrimental to proper "diagnostic medical care." One cardiology example could be the cardiologist who avoids a repeat and needed catheterization as he perceives the family or patient to be litigious (prone to sue). In this scenario, the doctor wants to avoid a complication or additional radiation so that if the patient develops a future cancer, where some unscrupulous lawyer can't blame the additional radiation exposure resulting from the indicated catheterization. The result is the patient not getting a diagnostic test that he actually needs, which exposes the patient to the added risk of a new heart attack.

The estimate in the costs of defensive medicine in 2014 is 850 billion dollars—25% to 30% of all medical expenditures for the year. This staggering cost is accounted primarily from improper ordering of tests and procedures in the private or corporate sector of medicine. Amazingly enough, doctors working for the federal government such as the VA system are protected from frivolous lawsuits by the Federal Tort Claims Act. However, this protection does not extend to the rest of medicine, and doctors can be held personally financially liable for patient afterward unlike in the other countries in the world. Furthermore, these lawsuit rewards are quantum steps greater compared to the other countries, and this is without any discernable effect on patient longevity and positive medical outcomes. Another evidence that fear of personal liability is motivating defensive medicine in the United States was found in the result of a 2011 survey of 700 physicians in New Zealand, the United Kingdom, Canada, and Sweden. None (0%) reported ordering tests, treatments, or consultations in an effort to avoid lawsuits (jacksonhealth.com).

One cannot help but be astonished by these results. Also, these countries enjoy protections under their medical malpractice systems that have not been implemented in the American system for over 50 years due from the pressure by American medical and legal Societies. The legal lobby groups and the fact that most legislatures themselves are lawyers are felt to be the primary impediment to the adoption of an effective reform. The savings of almost a quarter of all medical expense with a concomitant improvement in medical care and reversal of the relentless decline in the American medical system are simply ignored by these lobby groups. The lawyer group's defense in this posture is that tort reform would actually lead to a decline in our excellent medical system. Such thinking simply defies reality and the facts and only further supports that this defense is simply based on pure financial incentives rather than improvement in patient care.

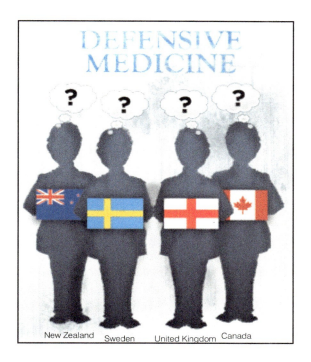

(Fig.81) Doctors in New Zealand, Sweden United Kingdom, and Canada report a 0% incidence of practicing defensive medicine in preference to diagnostic medicine (jacksonhealth.com).

As a parting point in this discussion of tort reform and the medical system, I would like to make a few suggestions about both tort reform and some solutions for reversal of the deteriorating medical system in America. Amazingly, most of these solutions are on the books but have been not been implemented for a multitude of reasons that are not within the bounds of this book. Nevertheless, I am hoping to provoke insightful thought and possibly appropriate legislative actions. Nevertheless, I can take some great satisfaction out of guiding the proactive patient to preserve the excellence of his own cardiological care armed with the knowledge of the ages.

Tort reform in this country must tackle two provisions that are an essential part of present legal provisions in all realms of American law. In a survey, 89% of doctors felt that in the case of true medical malpractice, the patient deserved a just settlement or monetary award. Nevertheless, almost all felt that there must be some form of binding arbitration in place regarding both the validity of the claim and reasonable compensation. The traditional attempts for tort reform in some states are by putting caps on the pain and suffering award. This has little to no effect on the sheer amount of frivolous and unjustified lawsuits that are filed each year in America. In reality, the only solution is for a no-fault, administrative compensation system out of arbitration similar to what is utilized often in no-fault car insurance. Without these changes, nearly 90% of doctors asked would not change their practice of defensive medicine irrespective of attempts at capping awards for pain and suffering.

Before I end this book, there's one last subject to cover in terms of medical care in America, and that is to analyze various options other that tort reform, which would return the doctor to a physician rather than technician and truly bring excellent medical care to all Americans—universal coverage. In actuality, the government always has had an excellent system of medical coverage for the needy, but that has been overshadowed by the desire of lawmakers to see their names on new legislation that is inferior to what was already in place for established routes of medical care delivery. This established system is simply neglected or underutilized with laws that are not enforced. The VA system has definite merits if there were enough well trained and adequately compensated physicians to cover the vast amount of veterans. It would also be of great benefit if informed doctors ran the program instead of incompetent political appointees.

The system of Medicaid, community mental health centers, and the excellent medical care afforded to the poor by Federally Qualified Heath Centers (FQHC) have been around for the past 10-15 years. They've been openly and freely available to the low income families and individuals to use for their mental and physical health concerns. These FQHCs are manned by federally contracted physicians, who are well compensated and protected by federal tort reform laws and are meant to offer medical care to the underserved population. These physicians are subject to regular utilization review for the delivery of proper medical care and are carefully scrutinized. The FQHCs can provide medical services, mental health care, and even dental services. The FQHCs serve

Medicaid and private insurance patients with a tiered payment system federally subsidized and based on the patient's income.

In that sense, these clinics can even serve the homeless if the homeless had the desire to seek medical treatment in the first place. The real problem is that the patients don't go the VA, don't apply for Medicaid, and don't avail themselves for their care to FQHC clinics that are present in most all low-income communities. All legislation such as Obamacare is doing is renaming universal coverage that was already available but now fines the individuals that don't avail themselves to the FQHSs or don't have the drive or the ability to go to a website to apply for coverage at the threat of a fine, which they can't pay or afford! In reality, any type of entitlement system that gives the pretense of universal coverage just acts as a replacement for the universal systems already in place and had been for 15 years; any pretense to the contrary is an all outright lie and meant to deceive the public in to the fantasy of better health coverage. Furthermore, this forced implementation of a mandatory medical entitlement system disrupts the whole fabric of a democratic society, forces more suffering on the poor, degrades the intellect, and irreversibly destroys the human spirit-it kills people and in an Orwellian way seeks to control the "stupid" populace.

In reality, Medicare and private insurance companies have already devised what may be the optimal model for health care delivery, the Accredited Care Organization (ACO). I've mentioned this briefly before, but it's my strong opinion that this model can offer the optimal universal medical care that is self-monitored and affords proper care and utilization of medical resources. The ACO will reverse over testing and afford far superior medical care. Basically, the ACO is an organization that is owned by a group of physicians in conjunction often with a hospital. The insurance company or Medicare pays the organization to care for an enrolled amount of patients—the more patients the more money. The ACO pays for any hospitalization or procedure out of this pool, and the rest of the money is profit for the ACO. In this regard, the ACO benefits to keep the patient healthy because it suffers if it doesn't do the appropriate timely procedures as the patient will ultimately get sicker and require more care and more expense.

The ACO has a monetary incentive and self-interest in educating and preventing the doctors from practicing defensive medicine and overutilization of test that they pay for, fostering a culture of appropriate diagnostic and therapeutic medicine. There's no doubt that many of the large private health insurers are working hand in hand with Medicare to foster the ACO model of medical care delivery. Importantly, in Pittsburgh Pennsylvania, the University of Pittsburgh medical system covers essentially all the residents of the city under their own health insurance. This is like a giant ACO where the insurance company has a financial incentive to afford well health care, appropriate medical delivery, and the proper utilization of resources. Most importantly, they have a vital self-interest to assure their physician members properly practice diagnostic and therapeutic medicine with appropriateness of care, which ultimately leads to delivery of excellent medical services.

If these models are adopted in addition to meaningful tort reform, I feel very strongly that the United States will again have a health system, which is the envy of the world and where the rich and poor all have equal access to the best medical care.

THE END

CPSIA information can be obtained at www.ICGtesting.com
Printed in the USA
BVOW11s0454141115

427088BV00007B/16/P